Induction and Modulation of Gastrointestinal Inflammation

FALK SYMPOSIUM 104

Induction and Modulation of Gastrointestinal Inflammation

EDITED BY

A. Stallmach
Innere Medizin II
Medizinische Klinik und Poliklinik
Universität des Saarlandes
Homburg/Saar
Germany

M. Zeitz
Innere Medizin II
Medizinische Klinik und Poliklinik
Universität des Saarlandes
Homburg/Saar
Germany

T. T. MacDonald
Department of Paediatric
Gastroenterology
St Bartholomew's and The Royal
London School of Medicine
and Dentistry, London, UK

W. Strober
National Institute of Allergy and
Infectious Diseases
National Institutes of Health
Bethesda, MD
USA

H. Lochs
IV. Medizinische Klinik
Schwerpunkt Gastroenterologie
Humboldt-Universität zu Berlin
Berlin
Germany

Proceedings of the Falk Symposium 104 held in Saarbrücken, Germany,
March 5–7, 1998

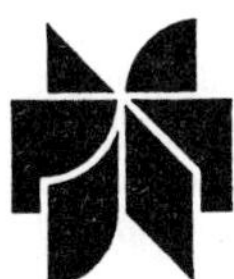

KLUWER ACADEMIC PUBLISHERS
DORDRECHT / BOSTON / LONDON

Library of Congress Cataloging-in-Publication Data is available.

ISBN 0–7923–8747–3

Published by Kluwer Academic Publishers,
P.O. Box 17, 3300 AA Dordrecht, The Netherlands

Sold and distributed in North, Central and South America
by Kluwer Academic Publishers
101 Philip Drive, Norwell, MA 02061, U.S.A.

In all other countries, sold and distributed
by Kluwer Academic Publishers,
P.O. Box 322, 3300 AH Dordrecht, The Netherlands

Printed on acid-free paper

Printed and bound in Great Britain by MPG Books, Bodmin, Cornwall.

Contents

CONTENTS

Section VI: IMMUNOMODULATORY STRATEGIES IN IBD

List of Principal Authors

T. Andus
Klinik und Poliklinik für Innere Medizin I
Klinikum der Universität Regensburg
D-93042 Regensburg
Germany

S. P. Balk
Cancer Biology Program
Beth Israel Deaconess Medical Center
Harvard Medical School
330 Brookline Avenue
HIM 1047
Boston, MA 02215
USA

R. S. Blumberg
Gastroenterology Division
Brigham & Women's Hospital
Harvard Medical School
75 Francis Street
Boston MA 02115-6195
USA

M. Boirivant
Immunology Department
Istituto Superiore di Sanita
Viale Regina Elena, 299
I-00161 Roma
Italy

R. Duchmann
Internal Medicine II
Saarland University
D-66421 Homburg/Saar
Germany

J. Emmrich
Abteilung für Gastroenterologie
Medizinische Klinik
Klinikum der Universität Rostock
Ernst-Heydemann-Str. 6
D-18057 Rostock
Germany

P. B. Ernst
Child Health Research Center
Department of Pediatrics
UTMB
301 University Blvd.
Galveston, TX 77555-0366
USA

I. Fuss
National Institute of Health
Bldg. 10, Rm. 11N238
NIAID
10 Center Drive
MSC 1890
Bethesda MD 20892-1890
USA

M. F. Kagnoff
Laboratory of Mucosal Immunology
University of California, San Diego
Department of Medicine 0623D
9500 Gilman Drive
La Jolla, CA 92093-0623
USA

B. L. Kelsall
Immune Cell Interaction Unit
Mucosal Immunity Section
Laboratory of Clinical Investigation
National Institute of Health
Bldg. 10 Rm. 11N238
10 Center Drive
Bethesda MD 20892-1890
USA

M. Kronenberg
La Jolla Institute for Allergy and
  Immunology
10355 Science Center Drive
San Diego, CA 92121
USA

T. Kühbacher
1 Medizinische Klinik der
  Christian-Albrechts-Universität zu
  Kiel
Labor für Mucosaimmunologie
Schittenhelmstr. 12
24105 Kiel
Germany

O. Liesenfeld
Institute of Infection Medicine
Department of Medical Microbiology
  and Immunology of Infection
Free University of Berlin
Hindenburgdamm 27
12203 Berlin
Germany

N Lügering
Department of Medicine B
University of Münster
Domagkstr. 3
D-48149 Münster
Germany

T. T. MacDonald
Dept of Paediatric Gastroenterology
St Bartholomew's and the Royal
  London School of Medicine and
  Dentistry
Suite 31, 3rd Floor, Dominion
  House
59 Bartholomew Close
London EC1A 7BE
UK

T. Marth
Internal Medicine II
Saarland University
D-66421 Homburg/Saar
Germany

J. R. McGhee
The Immunobiology Vaccine
  Center
The University of Alabama at
  Birmingham
761 BBRB 845 19th Street South
Birmingham, AL 35294-2170
USA

S. C. Meuer
Institute for Immunology
Ruprecht-Karls-University
Im Neuenheimer Feld 305
D-69120 Heidelberg
Germany

M. F. Neurath
Laboratory of Immunology
University of Mainz
Langenbeckstrasse
D-55101 Mainz
Germany

P. Parronchi
Istituto di Medicina Interna ed
  Immunoallergologia
University of Florence
Viale Morgagni 85
I-50134 Florence
Italy

E. Pringault
Laboratoire des Interactions
  Lympho-épitheliales
Department of Bacteriology and
  Mycology
Pasteur Institute
28 Rue du Dr Roux
F-75015 Paris
France

J. Reimann
Institut für Medizinische Mikrobiologie
Universitätsklinikum Ulm
Albert-Einstein-Allee 11
D-89069 Ulm
Germany

Y. Samstag
Institute for Immunology
Ruprecht-Karls-University
Im Neuenheimer Feld 305
D-69210 Heidelberg
Germany

R. B. Sartor
Division of Digestive Diseases &
  Nutrition
UNC School of Medicine
Room 030 Glaxo Bldg., CB# 7080
Chapel Hill, NC 27599-7080
USA

M. A. Schmidt
Institut für Infektiologie
Zentrum für Molekularbiologie der
  Entzündung
Universität Münster
Von-Esmarch-Str. 56
D-48149 Münster
Germany

LIST OF PRINCIPAL AUTHORS

T. Schneider
Internal Medicine II
Saarland University
D-66421 Homburg/Saar
Germany

A. J. G. Schottelius
Lineberger Comprehensive Cancer
  Center
University of North Carolina at Chapel
  Hill
Chapel Hill, NC 27599-7295
USA

F. Seibold
Medizinische Poliklinik
Universität Würzburg
Klinikstrasse 6
97070 Würzburg
Germany

A. Stallmach
Internal Medicine II
Saarland University
D-66421 Homburg/Saar
Germany

W. Strober
National Institutes of Health
Mucosal Immunity Section
Laboratory of Clinical Investigation
National Institute of Allergy and
  Infectious Diseases
Bldg. 10, Rm 11N 234-244
Bethesda, MD 20892-1890
USA

E. Stüber
I. Medizinische Uni.-Klinik
Abteilung für Allgemeine Innere
  Medizin
Schittenhelmstr. 12
24105 Kiel
Germany

I. Takahashi
Department of Mucosal Immunology
Research Institute for Microbiol
  Diseases
Osaka University
3-1 Yamadaoka
Suita-Osaka 565
Japan

C. Terhorst
Division of Immunology
Beth Israel Deaconess Medical
  Center
330 Brookline Avenue, RE-204
Boston, MA 02215
USA

J. Westermann
Zentrum Anatomie (4120)
Medizinische Hochschule Hannover
D-30623 Hannover
Germany

M. Zeitz
Internal Medicine II
Saarland University
D-66421 Homburg/Saar
Germany

Preface

It has been increasingly recognized that the immune system at the intestinal mucosal surface has distinct structural and functional features specifically adapted to its function at this important interface between the environment and the organism. These features include tolerance induction to orally administered antigens, local protective immune responses at the T and B cell level, and systemic and mucosal dissemination of stimulated T and B cells. In addition, it has become evident from gene knock-out animal models that disturbances in immune regulation lead to mucosal inflammation. Since this is a rapidly expanding field of knowledge in basic immunology and cell biology as well as clinical research, the aim of the Falk Symposium No. 104 in Saarbrücken was to provide the opportunity for an interchange between both basic scientists and clinicians.

The symposium focussed on immunological mechanisms of mucosal protection and their disturbances leading to inflammation and destruction in the gastro-intestinal tract. Extensive exchange of information and opinions on these topics yielded broad consensus on some issues and spirited controversy on others. There was general agreement that mucosal immune responses are highly regulated in the sense that responses to antigens associated with non-pathogenic organisms and food lead to immunological tolerance and that failure to achieve such tolerance is likely to be of importance in mucosal inflammation. Another area of consensus and controversy concerned the pathogenesis of various forms of chronic inflammatory bowel disease (IBD), i.e. ulcerative colitis and Crohn's disease, especially in its relation to the dominating cytokine profile. Analysis of the immunological mechanisms that underlie tolerance induction may have major impact on new therapeutic strategies of autoimmune diseases, gastrointestinal infections and IBD. Antigen presentation in the mucosal immune system is still incompletely understood and remains a subject of ongoing research. This book collects the presentations of the speakers and represents an impressive spectrum of the scientific work done by international experts in the field of mucosal immunology.

The topics discussed at this symposium reflect the many years of joint activities of the organizers. They are very grateful to the speakers and discussants for their willingness to participate and present their most recent data and particularly to the Falk Foundation for their generous support. Both have made this symposium possible.

The Editors

Section I
Antigen uptake, presentation and epithelial cell biology

1
Molecular and functional characterization of M cells: targeting restriction, molecular markers, and effects of an intestinal inflammation model on rat M cells

C. CICHON, A. FREY, K. RAUTENBERG, T. KUCHARZIK,
W. DOMSCHKE and M. A. SCHMIDT

INTRODUCTION

In higher organisms the approximately 300–400 m² of mucosal surfaces of the gastrointestinal, respiratory and urogenital tract are covered by a layer of epithelial cells representing a three-dimensional 'frontier' to the outside world. These surfaces are in permanent contact with masses of largely foreign and often harmful antigens and, furthermore, represent a barrier against a continuous onslaught of microbial pathogens (bacteria[1–3], viruses[4,5], and parasites[6]). For the immunological surveillance of this vast surface area a special branch of the immune system has evolved, the 'common mucosal immune system', again subdivided in different compartments which nevertheless remain in continuous contact. Thus, besides exhibiting a physical barrier function, the mucosa also serves as the inductive site for mucosal as well as systemic immune responses[7–9] via the mucosa-associated lymphoid tissue (MALT). In the gastrointestinal tract these responses are mediated by the gut-associated lymphoid tissue (GALT). Corresponding tissues have been identified in the respiratory tract as the bronchio-associated lymphoid tissue (BALT) and in the nasal mucosa (NALT: nasal-associated lymphoid tissue). These tissues form the connected and cooperative common mucosal immune system. Lymphocytes in the gastrointestinal tract are either diffusely distributed in the lamina propria as intraepithelial lymphocytes (IEL), or are found in organized form as in the Peyer's patches and mesenteric lymph nodes. Due to the antigen contacts on the mucosa it is not surprising that the total number of immunocompetent cells in the gastrointestinal tract alone by far exceeds the number of immune cells in the bone marrow, the spleen, lymph nodes and the thymus combined.

As, in general, food antigens present no threat to an individual the GALT must be able to differentiate locally between potentially harmful and nutritional antigens, desirably before mucosal and systemic immune responses are induced. A mucosal immune response against food antigens in the gut would not only interfere with or even prevent their uptake but would also lead to inflammatory reactions (e.g. as in coeliac disease) resulting in pathological changes in the gut and in the development of disease. Thus, luminal antigens have to be under constant immunological surveillance by the mucosal immune system. For this, antigens have to be transported across the epithelial layer, to be subsequently processed and presented to immunocompetent cells. The criteria on which the mucosal immune system discriminates between hostile (pathogenic) and friendly (food-borne) antigens are largely unknown. The current concepts favour discrimination on the basis of different transport routes. Transport via the epithelial lining cells may lead to immunological tolerance[10], while uptake via the M cell route is believed to induce a mucosal and systemic immune response.

This seems to be the major function of M cells ('microfold, manyfold, or membranous'), as these cells are specialized in antigen uptake and transport[11,12] and are interspersed in the follicle-associated epithelium (FAE) of the Peyer's patches. Due to its deficiency of goblet cells the FAE of the domes lacks most of the protective mucin layer covering the neighbouring regular epithelia. This is thought to facilitate the access of luminal antigens, and especially of particulate antigens, to the FAE. After uptake, M cells pass on antigens by transcytosis to macrophages and lymphocytes which initiate local and/or systemic immune responses[10,13]. Therefore, M cells play a crucial role in the monitoring and surveillance of antigens which come into closer contact with mucosal surfaces. However, a growing number of microbial pathogens, such as reoviruses, polioviruses, HIV-1, *Salmonella*, *Yersinia* and mycobacteria, have learned to take advantage of M cells as a port of entry[5,14–17]. Thus, M cells represent the true 'gateway' for mucosal infections and immunizations[18].

The presence and number of Peyer's patches and M cells varies with age and development stages and also among species[19,20]. To our knowledge M cells were first discovered in 1965 by J. Smidtje based on histochemical studies and further described by R. Owen and A. Jones[12]. Compared to normal enterocytes in the intestine M cells do not possess microvilli but small membrane folds (microfold – M cell). A striking feature of M cells is the presence of a basolateral invagination or pocket which, in most M cells, seems to be occupied by lymphocytes and macrophages (Figure 1). Antigens taken up by endocytosis are transcytosed through a very thin cellular bridge and again released towards antigen-presenting cells (APC) usually residing in the M cell pocket. There, the transcytosed antigens are further processed for induction of the immune response.

At present it is not quite understood what exactly targets an antigen to be transcytosed by M cells. Although it is tempting to speculate that there might be a mechanism to discriminate between wanted and unwanted antigens already at the level of transcytosis there has been no experimental evidence to support this notion.

Most of what we know about M cells still results from studies by electron microscopy, where M cells in the FAE can be identified due to their charac-

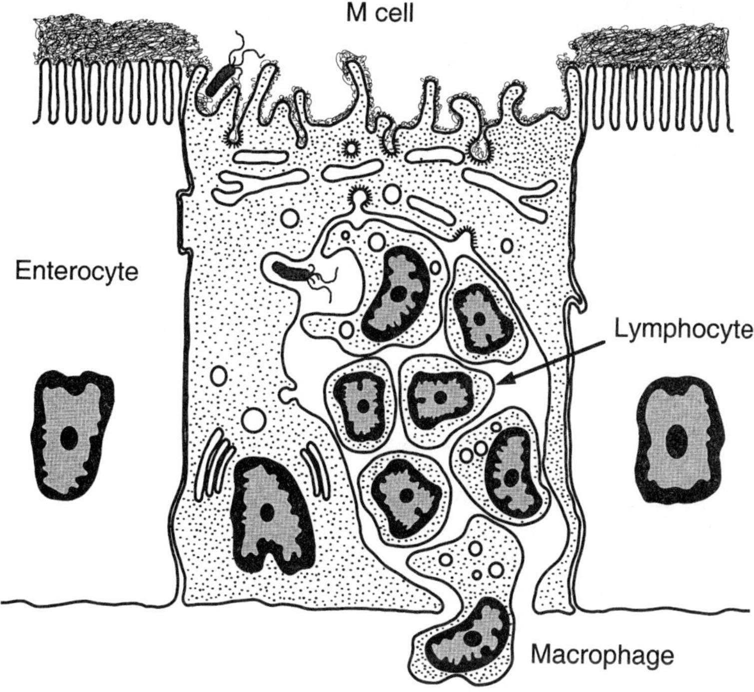

Figure 1 Schematic representation of a Peyer's patch M cell. The basal membrane of the M cell forms an intraepithelial pocket that is populated with lymphocytes and macrophages. The apical surface of the M cell displays an irregular array of membrane extensions and lacks a dense, thick glycocalyx

teristic morphology. Further progress in the understanding of the cell and molecular biology of antigen recognition and uptake has been restrained by the so far unsuccessful attempts to isolate and culture M cells and, as a result, by the lack of M cell-derived *in vitro* model systems. The availability of a specific or at least selective immunological marker would greatly facilitate the isolation and also the further characterization of M cells. Thus, several attempts have been made to establish histochemical markers for their identification (with e.g. monoclonal antibodies or lectins). The markers identified (Table 1) for rat (this study), rabbit,

Table 1 M cell reactivities with molecular markers in different species

Species	Reactivity with marker	Reference
Mouse	UEA-1 lectin (Fucose) (Balb/c mice)	34
Pig	cytokeratin 18	32
Rabbit	Mab	31
Rat	cytokeratin 8 annexin I	36, 37 This study

porcine and mouse M cells in Peyer's patches have been shown to be highly restricted to the respective species[21–24]. Moreover, despite intense efforts no histochemical markers have so far been established in man.

As a third aspect, M cells might not only represent the interface between exterior and interior but might also be involved during the pathogenesis of inflammatory bowel diseases (IBD). It is tempting to hypothesize that under certain conditions normally harmless luminal antigens might be recognized as potential threats to the organism, the mounted immune response leading to pathological changes in the gut. On the other hand remote, not M cell-related inflammatory reactions in the gut might well have a deleterious effect on the integrity of M cells in the intestine. Subsequently, destruction of M cells would breach the gastrointestinal barrier further and would open the floodgates for all kinds of luminal antigens – which under normal circumstances are meant to be excluded from the mucosa and the immune system – resulting in a self-fuelling inflammatory reaction.

In this report we will therefore discuss some experimental approaches to the following questions related to M cell function; first, is the access of particulate antigens to M cells and the FAE also affected by particle size due to a physical sieving effect? Second, can one define molecular markers for M cells in the rat animal model? Finally, what is the effect of an experimental drug-induced inflammatory condition in the small intestine on the integrity of M cells?

RESULTS

Size restriction of M cell-bound antigens – role of the glycocalyx

For efficient transcytosis of infectious agents or particulate mucosal vaccines, antigens have to reach the apical surface of M cells in the FAE on the dome of the Peyer's patches. As very little is known about surface components serving as potential receptors of M cells, the B subunit of cholera toxin (CTB) has been used quite successfully as a targeting device to deliver antigens via ganglioside G_{M1} as receptor which is present in the membrane of every nucleated cell type. Though CTB-mediated binding is not M cell-specific, mucosal immune responses against soluble antigens can be dramatically enhanced when the antigen is conjugated to CTB. Along that line, it has been suggested that conjugation of CTB to microparticles might enhance endocytosis by M cells and, in addition, prevent endocytosis by enterocytes. In this way these microparticles would efficiently be targeted to M cells provided the CTB moieties retain their G_{M1}-binding capacity. In contrast to the rigid, highly organized and dense microvilli structures of enterocytes[25], which express mucin-like glycoproteins forming a 400–500 nm layer covering the tips of the microvilli, the apical surface of M cells generally lacks densely packed microvilli-like structures and is usually devoid of a thick glycoprotein coat. Though M cells are usually devoid of mucin-like structures, (particulate) antigens (CTB-conjugates) will still have to pass the glycocalyx coat to access potential glycolipid receptors. Access of glycolipid receptors on the apical surface of M cells might decide on success or failure of a particular CTB conjugate. Thus, it might well be that by exerting a sieving effect based mainly on the overall size of the particle the very nature of

the carbohydrate and glycoprotein coat covering the apical surfaces of enterocytes and/or M cells might decisively influence the fate of a mucosal vaccine or,
potentially, a mucosal pathogen.

To address the influence of particle size on the ability of CTB to target particulate antigens to enterocyte or M cell apical surfaces different sized CTB
probes and control antigen probes were prepared[26]. The probes included soluble
CTB–FITC (Ø ~ 6.4 nm), CTB–gold (14 nm gold; final diameter ~ 28.8 nm)
nanoparticles and CTB conjugated to fluorescent microspheres (Ø ~ 1.1 μm).
When rabbit Peyer's patches were exposed either as explants for 30–45 min at
15°C or for 1 h *in vivo* to soluble CTB–FITC (1 μg/ml) access of soluble
CTB–FITC to apical surfaces of all intestinal epithelial cells could be demonstrated[26]. In contrast, when CTB conjugates with colloidal gold (Ø 28.8 nm)
were incubated with Peyer's patch explants the particles selectively bound to the
apical surface of M cells. Incubation of the larger 1.1 μm CTB conjugates with
ligated jejunal/ileal segments of rabbit Peyer's patch mucosa for 1 h *in vivo*
revealed that these particles were still able to selectively access the dome of the
Peyer's patches. However, as shown in Figure 2, microparticles used as controls

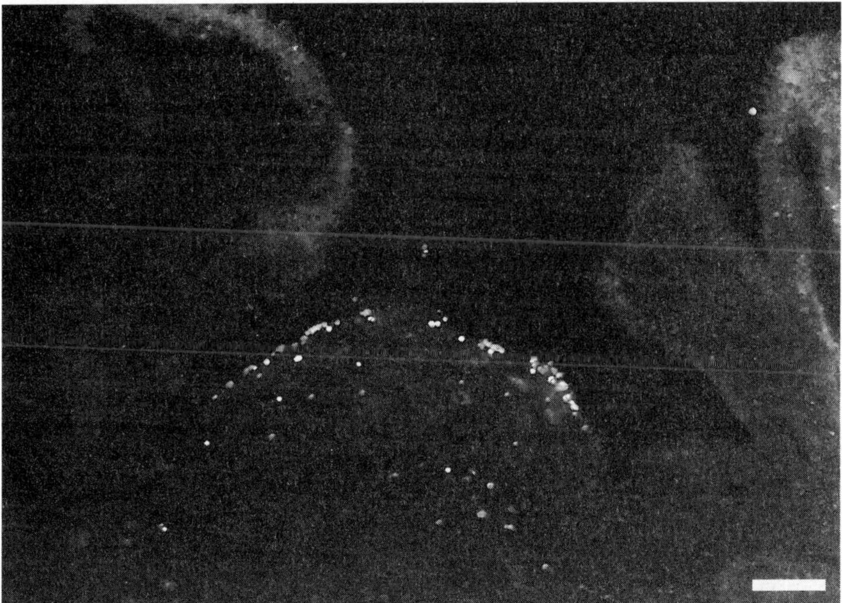

Figure 2 Restricted accessibility of intestinal epithelial cell membranes. Ligated jejunal/ileal
segments of rabbit Peyer's patch mucosa were exposed to equal numbers (2.5 × 10⁸ particles) of red
fluorescent cholera toxin B subunit-coated and green fluorescent biocytin-quenched avidin-coated
1 μm particles for 1 h *in vivo*. Fluorescence microscopy of a representative cryostat cross-section
shows that both types of particles are taken up into the dome but not into adjacent villi. Control
microparticles (green) were taken up in greater numbers than cholera toxin B subunit-coated
microparticles (red), suggesting that the cholera toxin receptor GM_1 was not accessible for
the microparticle probes and that uptake was due to nonspecific interaction. (For details see ref. 26).
The original colour image was reproduced as a monochrome figure. Red fluorescence appears white,
green fluorescence grey. Scale bar = 100 μm

(avidin-coated; green) were taken up in even greater numbers, than the CTB-coated microparticles (red). This indicates that the specific targeting property of CTB for M cell apical surfaces demonstrated with the colloidal gold microspheres is apparently lost in the larger microparticles[26] and that the residual uptake by the FAE is due to nonspecific binding. The property of CTB to specifically target antigens to the apical surface of M cells is, therefore size-restricted to antigens in the nanometre range. Experimental data obtained thus far suggest that the size restriction is imposed by the glycocalyx[26,27]. Thus, for the specific delivery of particulate antigens to M cells to be transcytosed the size of the antigen is a decisive factor. This finding has important implications for the development of oral delivery systems, such as mucosal vaccines or therapeutic drugs. Experiments to further define the permissive size range for specific M cell targeting by CTB of antigens between about 30 nm and 1000 nm diameter are currently under way in our laboratory.

Molecular markers for rat M cells

In an alternative approach, the FAE of Peyer's patches of the small intestine of rats, which represent a valuable animal model, has been investigated by immuno-cytochemistry to identify and characterize M cell markers. M cell markers would not only be useful as novel receptors for vaccine targeting without size restrictions, but would potentially also open new possibilities for M cell isolation.

M cells in the follicle-associated epithelium (FAE) of the dome of rat Peyer's patches cannot be distinguished from normal enterocytes by cell staining techniques for light microscopy. The identification of M cells by electron microscopy (Figure 3) allows only *post mortem* identification of M cells and, moreover, previous studies have indicated morphological criteria alone are not always sufficient[22,28]. Thus, numerous efforts have been made to develop histo-chemical markers. Histochemical markers for the recognition of M cells have been established in rabbits by generating monoclonal antibodies and by the reactivity of certain lectins[21,22,28–31], or by the investigation of the expression of particular intermediate filaments in pigs[32,33], certain strains of mice[34] and rats[35] (Table 1). These studies emphasized that in the FAE M cells are commonly present as single dispersed cells in very low numbers.

The FAE of Peyer's patches of rats was therefore investigated for the detection of relatively rare single dispersed cells which should, additionally, comply with other known criteria for M cells.

A large panel of monoclonal antibodies directed against different antigens was assessed on cryosections for the specific or at least selective detection of single dispersed cells in the FAE of Peyer's patches in the small intestine of Wistar rats[36,37]. The reactivity of these cells was compared with the reaction of epithelial cells in the neighbouring villus epithelium. The selection of the mono-clonal antibodies employed was biased towards recognizing those antigens which might be involved in functional aspects of M cells, such as MHC antigens (immune functions), certain CD antigens (receptor functions) or antigens po-tentially associated with intracellular traffic (transport functions). A selection of the monoclonal and polyclonal antibodies involved in this study is given in Table 2.

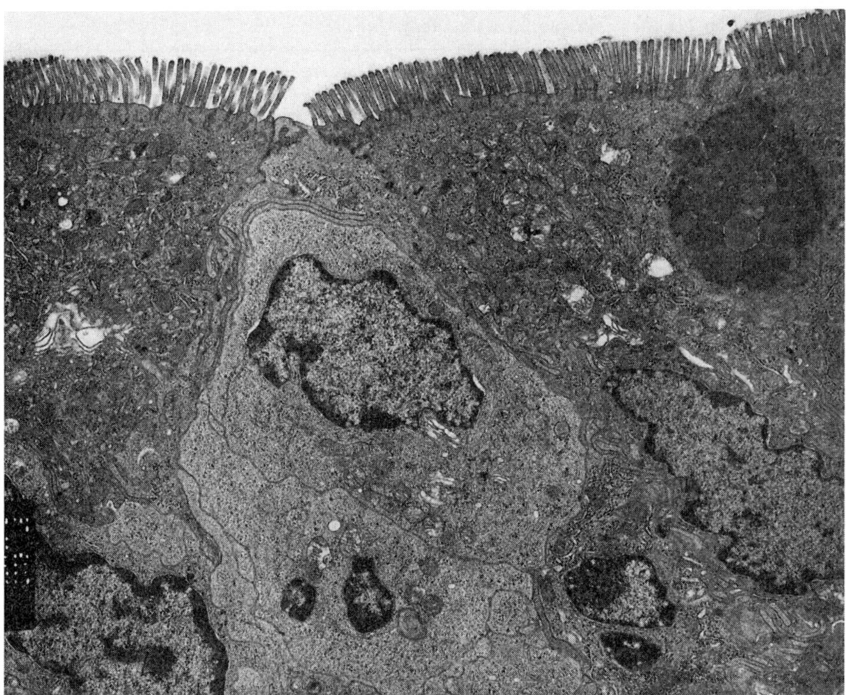

Figure 3 Electron micrograph of a typical M cell of a Peyer's patch in the rat intestine. The M cell is flanked by two enterocytes and a goblet cell with granula. The basolateral pocket harbours lymphoid cells. Briefly, the excised PPs were prepared as follows: the tissue was washed with cold PBS, cut in small pieces and fixed for at least 1 h in ice-cold Karnovsky's fixative[46] composed of 1.6% paraformaldehyde and 1.75% glutaraldehyde in 80 mM cacodylate buffer, pH 7.4. After washing overnight in PBS at 4°C, the tissue was postfixed in 1.0% osmium tetroxide in 0.1 M cacodylate buffer, pH 7.4 for 2 h at 4°C, rinsed again, dehydrated through a graded series of ethanol which was in the last step replaced with propylene oxide. After embedding in epoxy resin the block was hardened overnight at 65°C. Sections were cut on an ultramicrotome (0.05 μm) and mounted. Thin sections were stained with 5% uranyl acetate and 0.1% lead citrate. Magnification = × 5250

Monoclonal antibodies directed against clathrin (clone $C_{HC}5.9$), desmoplakin I and II (DPmix), ICAM-1 (clone 1A29), LFA-1 (clone WT.1), MHC class I (clone R4-8B1), macrophages (clone HIS-36) and FDC (clone ED5) did not exhibit a distinct staining pattern, such as the recognition of single dispersed cells in the FAE of the dome. The monoclonal pan B cell antibody (HIS-14) also detected intraepithelial B cells in the FAE. The staining for B cells was congruent with the reaction with a MHC class-II specific antibody (HIS-19), indicating that most of the MHC class-II cells in the FAE are probably B cells.

The distribution and composition of cytokeratins, which are normally expressed in the simple epithelium of the small and large intestine of several species[38–40], may serve as a 'fingerprint' for the presence of a distinctly different cell type. Moreover, as the property of transcytosis is a special function of M cells in the FAE this function might well be reflected in an unusual quality of cytoskeletal proteins. Therefore, in addition to monoclonal antibodies directed at

Table 2   Selected antibodies employed in this study

Antibodies specificity	Antibody specificity
Anti-Cytokeratins	
Anti-Cytokeratin Nr. 8 clone 4.1.18	Monoclonal mouse Ab
Anti-Cytokeratin Nr. 8 clone 4.1.17	Culture supernatant, IgG enriched via protein G FPLC
Anti-Cytokeratin Nr. 13 clone Ks 13.1	Monoclonal mouse Ab
Anti-Cytokeratin 8 u. 13 clone CAM 5.2	Monoclonal mouse Ab
Anti-Cytokeratin Nr. 18 clone CK2	Monoclonal mouse Ab
Anti-Cytokeratin Nr. 19 clone 170.2.14	Monoclonal mouse Ab
Anti-Cytokeratin 18 clone Ks 18.04	Culture supernatant
Anti-Cytokeratin 20 clone IT-K_S 20.15	Culture supernatant
Anti-Cytokeratin 20 clone IT-K_S 20.15	Monoclonal mouse Ab
Anti-Annexins	
Anti-Annexin I	Polyclonal rabbit serum 656
Anti-Annexin II	Polyclonal rabbit serum 419
Anti-Annexin III	Polyclonal rabbit serum
Anti-Annexin VI	Affinity-purified IgG from sheep
Miscellaneous Antibodies	
RT1D anti-rat-RT1D (MHC II) clone MRC OX-17 FITC-conjugated	Monoclonal mouse Ab
LECAM anti-rat-LECAM-1(L-selectin) clone GRL 3	Monoclonal mouse Ab
ED1 anti-monocyte, macrophages and dendritic cells	Monoclonal mouse Ab
OX2 anti-rat follicular dendritic cells Monoclonal mouse Ab marker III	
5D9 anti-New Zealand rabbit M cells	Culture supernatant
5B11 anti-New Zealand rabbit M cells	Culture supernatant
Anti-CD14 anti-receptor for LPS and LPS-binding protein	Monoclonal mouse Ab

surface exposed antigens, several monoclonal antibodies against cytokeratins were tested to detect dispersed cells in the FAE of Peyer's patches (Table 2). Detection of antigens in the FAE by anti-cytokeratin antibodies was very much dependent on the particular clone used in immunohistochemistry. While the monoclonal antibody against cytokeratin 18 (clone CK2) stained the whole dome of Peyer's patches but not the FAE, interestingly, anti-CK 18 clone Ks18.04 stained villi epithelia and the FAE of the dome with equal intensity. In the area of the crypts, however, distinct single epithelial cells apparently expressed CK 18 in substantially higher amounts and were thus more intensely stained. On the basis of our previous results[35] three different monoclonal antibodies were employed for the detection of cytokeratin 8 expression in the epithelium of the small intestine. Clone 17.2 (courtesy of W. W. Franke, Heidelberg) reacted on cryosections with all epithelial cells as did the cytokeratin 19 mAb (clone 170.2.14, Boehringer Mannheim). Reactions at the apical membrane were somewhat stronger than the reaction in the middle and basolateral parts of the cells. A mAb directed at cytokeratin 8 (clone 4.1.17) which was obtained from

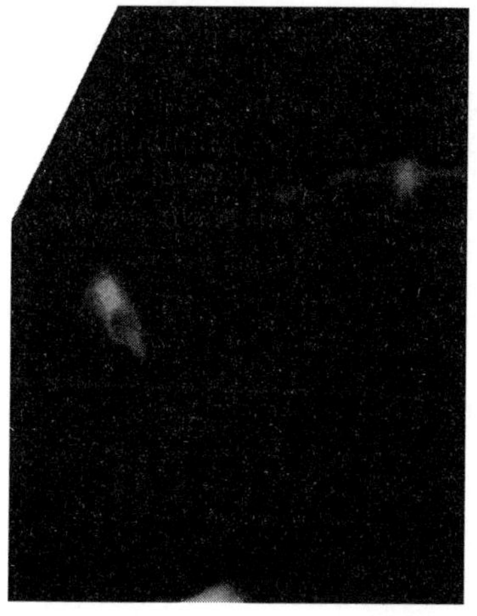

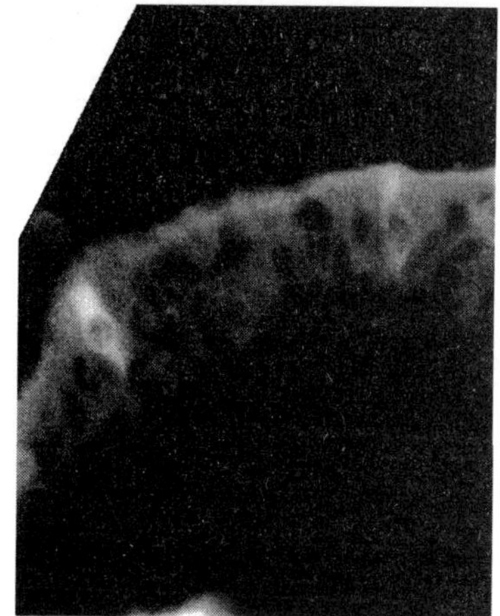

Figure 4 Cytokeratin 8 and annexin 1 reactivity as molecular markers for rat M cells. Cryosections of follicle-associated epithelium (FAE) of rat appendix were reacted with an anti-cytokeratin 8 mouse monoclonal antibody (clone 4.1.18) and a polyclonal rabbit antiserum directed against annexin 1. Double staining was performed with DTAF-labelled (green) anti-mouse secondary antibodies and AMCA-labelled (blue) anti-rabbit antibodies. Clearly, anti-CK 8 and anti-annexin 1 antibodies stain the same cell. The original colour image was reproduced as a monochrome figure. DTAF: dichloro triazinyl aminofluorescein; AMCA: 7-amino-4-methyl coumarin-3-acetic acid

M. Osborn (Göttingen) uniformly stained the FAE as well as the neighbouring epithelia. In contrast, staining for cytokeratin 8 with mAb clone 4.1.18[39,41] exhibited a completely different pattern: only single and distinct cells in the FAE were recognized (Figure 4), whereas the staining of the villus epithelial cells was almost indescernible from non-specific background reactions. In villus epithelia located between neighbouring domes of the Peyer's patches a few single cells also reacted occasionally. As shown by double staining experiments the anti-CK 8, clone 4.1.18-positive cells did not stain for alkaline phosphatase in their apical membranes. This is regarded as a criterion for the identification of M cells[42]. Furthermore, staining for mucin with Alcian Blue (data not shown) was also negative, indicating that these cells are not goblet cells. Thus, clone 4.1.18 against cytokeratin 8 selectively recognized M cells in the FAE of rat Peyer's patches.

In line with the observed species specificity of the few molecular M cell markers identified so far, the detection of M cells with the anti-cytokeratin 8 mAb (clone 4.1.18) also turned out to be specific for rats. Studies on the expression of intermediate filaments in human intestinal M cells demonstrated that in humans these components of the cellular architecture seem to be expressed in enterocytes and M cells alike[43].

Annexins are a family of proteins which often play a role in endo- and exocytotic processes[44]. As M cells are characterized by their endocytotic and transcytotic function we were interested to see whether annexins might be involved in these functions. Cryosections of rat Peyer's patches were incubated with anti-bodies against annexins I, II, III, and VI (courtesy of V. Gerke, ZMBE). While anti-annexin III and VI did not stain any cells in the rat intestine, anti-annexin II stained the whole FAE. Interestingly, only monodisperse cells were stained by anti-annexin I antibodies which, by double staining, were shown to be the same cells as those recognized by the anti-CK 8 mAb clone 4.1.18 (Figure 4). Thus, in the rat intestine, annexin I seems to be solely expressed in M cells of the FAE of Peyer's patches. This is especially remarkable as annexin I and II are only rarely expressed together and, moreover, annexin I expression has so far not been reported for intestinal epithelia.

The anti-CK 8 mAb (clone 4.1.18) and the anti-annexin I antibodies represent two molecular markers for the detection of M cells in the FAE of Peyer's patches of the rat small intestine. Though these antibodies recognize intracellular antigens it is expected that they will greatly facilitate further attempts to isolate the elusive M cells from rat Peyer's patches.

M cells in the indomethacin-induced inflammation model of chronic ileitis in the rat

As proposed above, in inflammatory bowel diseases (IBD) intestinal M cells might either be directly involved in the pathogenesis of localized inflammatory reactions in the intestine, e.g. as a gateway for harmful antigens, or might fall victim to acute distantly localized or chronic inflammatory conditions of the gastrointestinal tract.

An experimental model to test the latter hypothesis would be the chronic ileitis which can be induced in the rat animal model by two intracutaneous injections of the drug indomethacin ([1-(p-chlorobenzoyl)-5-methoxy-2-methyl indol-3-yl] acetic acid)[45]. A subcutaneous injection of only one dose of indomethacin induces an acute self-limiting inflammation of the intestine. In humans, indomethacin is used orally for its analgetic effect in rheumatic inflammatory diseases. However, due to incompatibilities some 30–50% of the patients have to abandon this treatment. If the drug is used for longer (e.g. 6 months), or even chronically, frequent side-effects affecting the gastrointestinal tract are observed (e.g. increased mucosal permeability, ulcerations, allergic reactions) and, especially in children, latent infections have been found to be reactivated.

We were interested to see whether the chronic inflammatory reaction induced by indomethacin in the rat model would have any effect on M cells in the FAE of the Peyer's patches. To induce chronic intestinal inflammation (ileitis) rats were injected intracutaneously with two doses of indomethacin (7.5 mg/kg body weight for each daily injection) 24 h apart. After 14 days the animals were sacrificed and the small intestine was removed for analysis. To follow the fate of M cells by immunohistochemistry the two molecular markers described above were very useful and the morphology of the M cells was also investigated by electron microscopy. Indomethacin induced a transient increase in the number of M cells detectable in the FAE of Peyer's patches. After about 14 days analysis of the FAE of intestinal Peyer's patches by electron microscopy revealed a progressive destruction; this seemed to be M cell-specific as neighbouring enterocytes

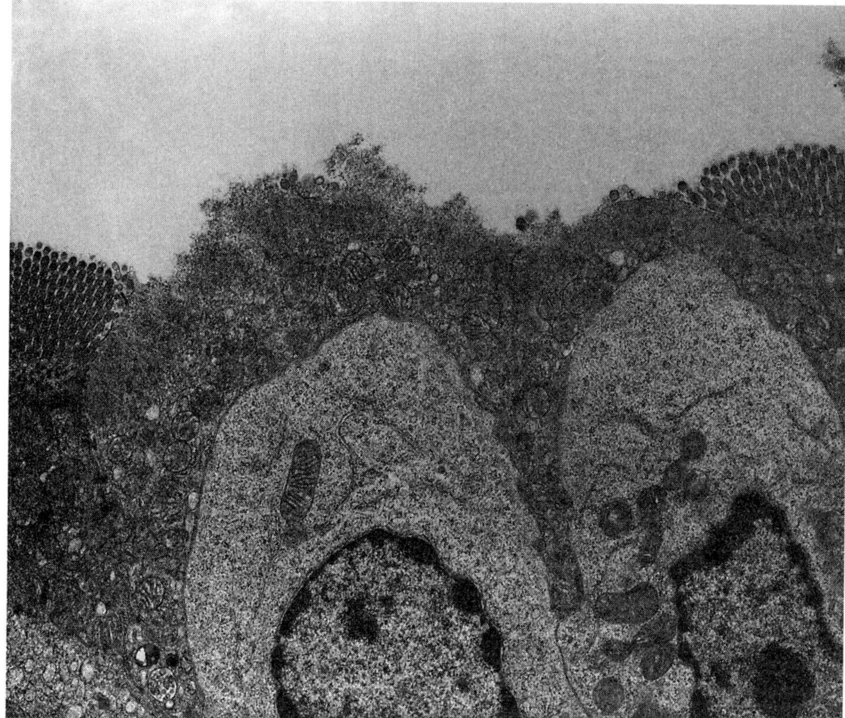

Figure 5 Electron micrograph of an M cell in the chronic ileitis model in the rat as a model for experimental inflammatory bowel disease induced by intracutaneous injection of indomethacin. Two doses of indomethacin (7.5 mg/kg body weight) given intracutaneously 24 h apart induce a chronic ileitis in the rat. Magnification: × 25 190

appeared perfectly normal and were apparently not affected (Figure 5). The morphology of the cells and the disintegration of the apical membrane of the M cells indicates a necrotic mechanism of cellular destruction. The specific destruction of M cells resulting from the indomethacin-induced inflammatory reaction would open the gateway for massive bacterial translocation, as has indeed also been observed in the rat model[45]. This finding might have important implications for the situation in humans, where at least some of the side-effects of indomethacin treatment could be attributed to a similar effect. Studies to investigate this hypothesis are currently being performed in our laboratories.

DISCUSSION

One of the key processes for the induction of mucosal immune responses is the recognition and transcytosis of antigens through the mucosa to the underlying mucosal lymphoid tissues. Uptake and transcytosis of antigens, and especially of particulate antigens, is accomplished by a specialized epithelial cell type, the

M cells, which are interspersed nearly exclusively in the follicle-associated epithelia (FAE) of the Peyer's patches in the mucosa[8,9].

For the induction of mucosal and also systemic immune responses luminal antigens have to be able to reach the apical membrane of M cells. Studies of orally applied antigens, such as candidate mucosal vaccines, have used the B-subunit of cholera toxin (CTB) to target antigens for delivery via its G_{M1} glycolipid receptor. This has been shown to dramatically increase mucosal as well as systemic immune responses against soluble antigens. As M cells are proposed to preferably transcytose particulate antigens it has been suggested that conjugating CTB to microparticles might also enhance endocytosis, though the G_{M1} receptor for CTB is also present on enterocytes. However, as it is generally accepted that the mucin layer covering enterocytes is markedly reduced on M cells, it could be envisaged that access to the apical membrane of M cells is facilitated for particulate antigens. To address this question in the study discussed here CTB was conjugated to soluble antigens and nano- and microparticles. Targeting of CTB-conjugated nano- and microparticles apparently reveals a size restriction brought about by the glycocalyx. Thus, CTB is able to specifically target soluble antigens and nanometre size particles to M cells. In contrast, with micrometre sized particles the targeting effect was found to be lost. This has implications not only for the development of mucosal (oral) vaccines but also for other applications where the intention is delivery by the M cell route. Studies are currently under way in our laboratory to further investigate and define the permissive particle size for M cell targeting.

To identify molecular markers for rat M cells a panel of monoclonal antibodies was assessed for specific or selective recognition of M cells in the FAE of rat Peyer's patches. Anti-cytokeratin 8 (clone 4.1.18) monoclonal antibodies, as well as anti-annexin I antibodies, specifically recognized single dispersed cells in the FAE of Peyer's patches; these cells did not show alkaline phosphatase activity in their apical membrane, an accepted criterion for M cells. The identification of two M cell markers associated with the cytoskeleton and endocytotic processes is in line with markers identified in other species. Interestingly, antibodies directed at cytokeratins were found to exhibit a clone-specific staining pattern in the FAE of rat Peyer's patches.

It is somewhat puzzling that, at present, all molecular markers for M cells identified are highly species specific, as vimentin is only over-expressed in rabbit M cells[29,30], cytokeratin 18 reactivity is found only in pigs[32], and the reactivity with the UEA-1 lectin has been found only in a certain strain of mice[34]. Also, to our knowledge, cross-reactivity of the monoclonal antibodies generated against rabbit M cells has not been observed[31]. The reasons for these findings are not known.

A third part of this study investigated a possible effect on M cells caused by the intestinal inflammation during indomethacin-induced chronic ileitis in the rat. At the present stage of the studies the results from electron microscopy strongly indicate that M cells are primarily affected by inflammation and destroyed by a process showing signs of necrosis. Destruction of M cells would result in massive translocation of luminal contents, including endogenous microorganisms. This would probably further enhance the inflammatory reactions leading to an even more severe pathology of the intestine. Since a large proportion of human patients treated with indomethacin develop side effects comparable to the conditions observed in the rat model, it is possible that M cells also have a central role in the development of this gastrointestinal pathology. This possibility is currently under investigation in our laboratories.

ACKNOWLEDGEMENTS

The authors are grateful to M. Osborn (Göttingen), W. W. Franke (Heidelberg), and V. Gerke (Münster) for their generous donation of antibodies. This project was supported in part by the Deutsche Forschungsgemeinschaft (SFB 310, C6 and FR958/2-1), by the Interdisziplinäres Klinisches Forschungszentrum (IKF) of the University of Münster and by a personal grant from the Bundesministerium für Bildung, Wissenschaft, Forschung und Technologie (BMBF) to AF.

References

1. Owen RL, Pierce NF, Apple RT, Cray Jr WC. M cell transport of *Vibrio cholerae* from the intestinal lumen into Peyer's patches: a mechanism for antigen sampling and for microbial transepithelial migration. J Infect Dis. 1986;168:1108–1118.
2. Walker RI, Schmauder-Chock EA, Parker JL, Burr D. Selective associations and transport of *Campylobacter jejuni* through M cells of rabbit Peyer's patches. Can J Microbiol. 1988;34:1142–1147.
3. Wassef JS, Keren DF, Mailloux JL. Role of M cells in initial antigen uptake and in ulcer formation in the rabbit intestinal loop model of shigellosis. Infect Immun. 1989;57:858–863.
4. Sicinsky P, Rowinski J, Warchol JB et al. Poliovirus type 1 enters the human host through intestinal M cells. Gastroenterology. 1990;98:56–58.
5. Wolf JL, Rubin DH, Finberg R et al. Intestinal M cells: a pathway for entry of reovirus into the host. Science. 1981;212:471–472.
6. Marcial MM, Madara JL. *Cryptosporidium*: cellular localization, structural analysis of absorptive cell-parasite membrane-membrane interactions in guinea pigs, and suggestion of protozoan transport by M cells. Gastroenterology. 1986;90:583–594.
7. Dougan G, Hormaeche CE, Maskell DJ. Live oral *Salmonella* vaccines; potential use of attenuated strains as carriers of heterologous antigens to the immune system. Parasite Immunol. 1987;9:151–160.
8. Neutra MR, Kraehenbuhl JP. Cellular and molecular basis for antigen transport in the intestinal epithelium. In: Ogra PL, Mestecky J, Lamm ME, Strober W, McGhee JR, Bienenstock J (eds.): Handbook of Mucosal Immunology. San Diego: Academic Press, 1994:27–39.
9. Trier JS. Structure and function of intestinal M cells. Gastroenterol Clin N Am. 1991;20:531–547.
10. Bland PW, Warren LG. Antigen presentation by epithelial cells of the rat small intestine. II. Selective induction of suppressor T cells. Immunology. 1986;58:9–14.
11. Kato T, Owen RL. Structure and function of intestinal mucosal epithelium. In: Ogra PL, Mestecky J, Lamm ME, Strober, W, McGhee JR, Bienenstock J (eds.): Handbook of Mucosal Immunology. San Diego: Academic Press, 1994:11–26.
12. Owen RL, Jones AL. Epithelial cell specialization within human Peyer's patches: an ultrastructural study of the intestinal lymphoid follicles. Gastroenterology. 1974;66:189–203.
13. Weiner DB, Girard L, Williams WV, McPhillips T, Rubin DH. Reovirus type 1 and type 3 differ in their binding to isolated intestinal epithelial cells. Microb Pathogenesis 1988;5:29.
14. Amergongen HM, Weltzin R, Farnet CM, Michetti P, Haseltine WA, Neutra MR. Transepithelial transport of HIV-1 by intestinal M cells: a mechanism for transmission of AIDS. J Acquired Immune Def Syndr. 1991;4:760–765.
15. Grutzkau A, Hanski C, Hahn H, Riecken EO. Involvement of M cells in the bacterial invasion of Peyer's patches: a common mechanism shared by *Yersinia enterocolitica* and other enteroinvasive bacteria. Gut 1990;31:1011–1015.

16. Jones BD, Ghori N, Falkow S. *Salmonella typhimurium* initiates murine infection by penetrating and destroying the specialized epithelial M cell of the Peyer's patches. J Exp Med. 1994;180:15–23.

17. Neutra MR, Kraehenbuhl JP. Transepithelial transport and mucosal defence I: the role of M cells. Trends Cell Biol. 1992;2:134–138.

18. Neutra MR, Frey A, Kraehenbuhl JP. Epithelial M cells: gateway for mucosal infection and immunization. Cell. 1996;86:345–348.

19. Orlic D, Lev R. An electron microscopic study of intraepithelial lymphocytes in human fetal small intestine. Lab Invest. 1977;37:554–561.

20. Liebler E. Gut-associated lymphoid tissue in the large intestine of calves. Vet Pathol. 1988;25:503–508.

21. Clark MA, Jepson MA, Simmons NL, Booth TA, Hirst BH. Differential expression of lectin-binding sites defines mouse intestinal M cells. J Histochem Cytochem. 1993;41:1679–1687.

22. Gebert A, Hach G. Differential binding of lectins to M cells and enterocytes in the rabbit cecum. Gastroenterology. 1993;105:1350–1361.

23. Giannasca PJ, Neutra MR. Interactions of microorganisms with intestinal M cells: mucosal invasion and induction of secretory immunity. Infect Agents Dis. 1994;2:242–248.

24. Owen RL. M cells – entryways of opportunity for enteropathogens. J Exp Med. 1994;180:7–9.

26. Frey A, Giannasca KT, Weltzin R et al. Role of the glycoclayx in regulating access of microparticles to apical plasma membranes of intestinal epithelial cells: implications for microbial attachment and oral vaccine targeting. J Exp Med. 1996;184:1045–1059.

27. Frey A, Neutra MR. Targeting of mucosal vaccines to Peyer's patch M cells. Behring Inst Mitt. 1997;98:376–389.

28. Inman LR, Cantey JR. Specific adherence of *Escherichia coli* (strain RDEC-1) to membraneous (M) cells of the Peyer's patch in *Escherichia coli* diarrhea in the rabbit. J Clin Invest. 1983;71:1–8.

29. Gebert A, Hach G, Bartels H. Co-localization of vimentin and cytokeratins in M cells of rabbit gut-associated lymphoid tissue (GALT). Cell Tissue Res. 1992;269:331–340.

30. Jepson MA, Mason CM, Bennett ML, Simmons NL, Hirst BH. Co-expression of vimentin and cytokeratin in M cells of rabbit intestinal lymphoid follicle-associated epithelium. Histochem J. 1992;24:33–39.

31. Pappo J. Generation and characterization of monoclonal antibodies recognizing follicle epithelial M cells in rabbit gut-associated lymphoid tissues. Cell Immunol. 1989;120:31–41.

32. Gebert A, Rothkötter HJ, Pabst R. Cytokeratin 18 is an M cell marker in porcine Peyer's patches. Cell Tissue Res. 1994;276:213–221.

33. Pabst R. The anatomical basis for the immune function of the gut. Anat Embryol (Berl.) 1987;176:135–144.

34. Giannasca PJ, Giannasca KT, Falk P, Gordon JI, Neutra MR. Regional differences in glycoconjugates of intestinal M cells in mice: potential targets for mucosal vaccines. Am J Physiol. 1994;267:G1108–G1121.

35. Demel M, Heyer G, Knochenhauer S, Schmidt MA. Cytokeratin 8 as possible intracellular marker for M cells of rat Peyer's patches (Abstract). 7th International Congress of Mucosal Immunology Prague. p. 54 (1992).

36. Rautenberg K, Cichon C, Heyer G, Demel M, Schmidt MA. Immunocytochemical characterization of the follicle-associated epithelium of Peyer's patches: anti-cytokeratin 8 antibody (clone 4.1.18) as a molecular marker for rat M cells. Eur J Cell Biol. 1996;71:363–370.

37. Rautenberg K, Cichon C, Schmidt MA. Towards targeting strategies for oral immunization – identification of marker antigens in rat M cells. Behring Inst Mitt. 1997;98:361–375.

38. Franke WW, Winter S, Overbeck J, Gudat F, Heitz P, Stahli C. Identification of the conserved, conformation-dependent cytokeratin epitope recognized by monoclonal antibody (lu-5). Virchows Arch A Pathol Histopathol. 1987;411:137–147.

39. Moll R, Franke WW, Schiller DL, Geiger B, Krepler R. The catalog of human cytokeratins: patterns of expression in normal epithelia, tumors and cultured cells. Cell. 1982;31:11–24.

40. Osborn M, Weber K. Tumor diagnosis by intermediate filament typing: a novel tool for surgical pathology. Lab Invest. 1983;48:372–394.

41. Osborn M, van Lessen G, Weber K, Kloppel G, Altmannsberger M. Differential diagnosis of gastrointestinal carcinomas by using monoclonal antibodies specific for individual keratin polypeptides. Lab Invest. 1986;55:497–504.

42. Owen RL, Bhalla DK. Cytochemical analysis of alkaline phosphatase and esterase activities and of lectin binding and anionic sites in rat and mouse Peyer's patch M cells. Am J Anat. 1983;168:199–212.

43. Kucharzik T, Lügering N, Schmid KW, Schmidt MA, Stoll R, Domschke W. Human intestinal M cells exhibit enterocyte-like intermediate filaments. Gut. 1998;42:54–62.

44. Gerke V. Annexins and membrane traffic. In: Seaton BA (ed.) Annexins: Molecular Structure to Cellular Function. Austin, TX: R. G. Landes Co; 1996: 67–79.

45. Yamada T, Deitch E, Specian RD, Perry MA, Sartor RB, Grisham MB. Mechanism of acute and chronic intestinal inflammation induced by indomethacin. Inflammation. 1993;17:641–662.

46. Kohbata S, Yokoyama H, Yabuuchi E. Cytopathogenic effect of *Salmonella typhi* GIFU 10007 on M cells of murine ileal Peyer's patches ligated ileal loops: an ultrastructural study. Microbiol Immunol. 1986;30:1225–1237.

2
Lymphoepithelial interactions trigger M cell formation and permeability to microorganisms

E. PRINGAULT and S. KERNÉIS

FOLLICLE-ASSOCIATED EPITHELIUM, M CELLS AND EPITHELIAL PERMEABILITY TO ANTIGENS AND MICROORGANISMS

Simple or stratified epithelia that constitute mucosal surfaces are usually impermeable to macromolecules and microorganisms. This is not the case for the lymphoid follicle-associated epithelium, which provides entry sites for macromolecules and microorganisms due to its vectorial transcytosis activity. This normal, physiological function allows the triggering of local immune responses that protect mucosal surfaces: indeed, antigens have to cross the epithelial barrier in order to interact with the immune cells of the mucosa-associated lymphoid tissues (MALT)[1]. These lymphoid follicles are the primary sites of antigen sampling and processing in the small intestine and are separated from the lumen by the follicle-associated epithelium (FAE) that contains specialized antigen transporting cells, the so-called M cells. These epithelial cells take up foreign material and microorganisms and deliver them by transepithelial transport from the external environment to MALT[2]. Thus, M cells play a key role in mucosal immune responses by addressing antigens to lymphoid follicle[1]. They are also involved in pathogenesis of many bacteria and viruses, since they represent a port of entry for these microorganisms[3].

M cells are scattered in the FAE and represent 10–50% of epithelial cells of this epithelium, depending on species. They are characterized by large intraepithelial pockets formed by the invagination of the basal plasma membrane. These pockets are filled with B and $CD4^+$ T lymphocytes, macrophages and dendritic cells which shuttle between the underlying follicles and the epithelium[4,5].

DIFFERENTIATION OF THE FOLLICLE-ASSOCIATED EPITHELIUM

The cells of the FAE, like all intestinal epithelial cells, are derived from stem cells in the crypts which form clonal units. A ring of anchored stem cells near the base of each crypt gives rise to multiple cell types that migrate upward in columns onto several adjacent villi[6,7]. The follicle-associated crypts are unusual in that they contain two distinct axes of migration from the same ring of stem cells. The cells on one wall of the crypt differentiate into absorptive enterocytes, goblet and enteroendocrine cells that migrate onto the villi, while cells on the opposite wall acquire features of M cells and distinct follicle-associated entero-cytes[8,9]. That the follicle-facing side of follicle-associated crypts shows distinct features, including a lack of goblet cells, M cell-like glycosylation patterns[10] and a lack of polymeric immunoglobulin receptor expression[11] suggests that factors or cells produced by MALT may regulate the differentiation programme. These factors may act very early in the differentiation pathway, inducing crypt cells to commit to FAE phenotypes. Whether they can also act later, to convert some of the FAE enterocyte-like cells to antigen-transporting M cells, is presently not known.

M cell formation: conversion of differentiated enterocytes or induction of a specific differentiation genetic programme in crypt cells?

A rapid and probably reversible conversion of enterocytes from the FAE into M cells has been proposed[12]. Different results described previously support this hypothesis. Indeed, the number of M cells in the FAE of mice dramatically increased following bacterial challenge with kinetics much faster than the gener-ation time of M cells[13,14]. An opposing view is that M cells originate from crypt stem cells and constitute a distinct cell lineage resulting from a distinct differ-entiation programme. This hypothesis lacks definitive experimental support because no M-cell specific markers are known.

Induction of follicle-associated epithelium by immune cells

Since cells from the FAE display strong functional differences when compared with the epithelium lining the villi, one can postulate that cross-talk with the underlying follicle cells could trigger a distinct differentiation programme, trans-criptionally and/or post-translationally regulated, into the whole FAE. These 'committed' enterocytes would undergo further conversion to give typical M cells. The interaction of lymphoid cells with the follicle-associated epithelium of Peyer's patch induces two types of changes *in vivo*: a general transcriptional down-regulation of digestive functions in all FAE cells (digestive enzymes and membrane transporters, in particular lactase, α-glucosidase, intestinal alkaline-phosphatase and H^+/di-tripeptide transporter[15–18]), and dramatic local morpho-logical changes restricted to M cells.

The importance of lymphoid cells in the induction of the FAE is shown by experiments in which injection of Peyer's patches lymphocytes into the submu-cosa of syngeneic mice resulted in local assembly of new lymphoid follicles and the *de novo* appearance of FAE with typical M cells[19]. Immunodeficient SCID mice[20] and B cell-deficient mice[21] lack mucosal follicles and identifiable M cells. In contrast, T cell-deficient nude mice still have small Peyer's patches with FAE with M cells[22]. Taken together, these observations suggest that B lymphocytes may play a critical role in FAE formation. The fact that Peyer's patches do not form in lymphotoxin (LT) knock out mice[23,24] suggests that LT is involved in the ontogeny of MALT. This is further supported by recent experiments in which soluble LTβ–receptor fusion protein expressed in transgenic mice altered the development of Peyer's patches but not peripheral lymph nodes[25]. The disruption of a B cell-specific chemokine receptor gene (BRL1) impaired the formation of Peyer's patches and inguinal lymph nodes[26], suggesting that a distinct set of chemokines mediate B cell recruitment and MALT formation.

IN VITRO RECONSTITUTION OF FOLLICLE-ASSOCIATED EPITHELIUM AND M CELLS

Study of M cell biology has been hampered by the lack of M cell-specific molecular markers and systems that reproduce the M cell phenotype *in vitro*. The few monoclonal antibodies that label M cells[27] have been found to recognize other cell types. Currently, M cells are identified by morphological criteria and by their capacity to sample and transport macromolecules[28,29], microorganisms[30–32] and inert particles[33,34]. They have not been biochemically characterized, because they are a minor population in the FAE and are difficult to purify to homogeneity. No M cell lines have been established so far.

We have recently demonstrated that murine Peyer's patch lymphocytes co-cultured with human differentiated Caco-2 cell monolayers are able to induce a phenotypic conversion of enterocytes into cells sharing structural and functional properties with M cells. In particular, this co-cultured system shows efficient transport of bacteria and the disorganization of the brush border and the loss of cell-surface expressed sucrase-isomaltase. The loss of digestive functions is concomitant with a gain of transcytotic activity characterized by the temperature-dependent translocation of inert particles and *Vibrio cholerae* from the apical to the basolateral compartment. An important conclusion drawn from this model *in vitro* is that differentiation of cultured intestinal epithelial cell is plastic and can be modulated by lymphoepithelial interactions[19].

In this study, we confirmed by an *in vitro* approach the role of immune cells of mucosa-associated lymphoid tissue (MALT) in M cell formation. We showed that FAE-like properties could be reconstituted in culture, by providing experimental evidence that immortalized, differentiated enterocytes can be converted by Peyer's patch lymphocytes into cells that share major features of M cells. Whether this conversion results from modulation of intestinal cell transcriptional activities or post-translational events has not yet been established, but this can now be tested using this co-culture system.

In the co-culture system, cell polarity and tightness of the epithelial monolayers were not altered by contact with lymphocytes, indicating that cytotoxic effects cannot account for the observed changes in all characteristics. The interaction of lymphocytes with epithelial cells triggers at least two distinct but related processes. The first of these is the reorganization of the actin network and the second is the vectorial transepithelial translocation of inert particles. The loss of the brush border requires the destabilization of a specialized cytoskeletal complex that controls brush border morphogenesis, in which villin has been shown to play a crucial role[35–37]. In Peyer's patches, the modification of the apical actin network affects a subset of enterocytes, including M cells[9,15]. In the Caco-2 monolayers cultured with Peyer's patch lymphocytes most enterocytes display a redistribution of villin to the cytosol, probably as a result of a more efficient lymphoepithelial interaction than *in vivo*.

The reorganization of the cytoskeleton in the co-culture system occurs in parallel with the downregulation of sucrase-isomaltase cell surface expression. A similar result was reported for Caco-2 cells transfected with a cDNA encoding antisense villin. In these cells the lack of villin production is associated with the inability to assemble a brush border[36]. The disruption of the specialized microfilament network leads to a lack of apical insertion of intestinal enzymes such as sucrase-isomaltase and alkaline phosphatase. These modified Caco-2 cells are unable to transport latex beads even though the beads efficiently adhere to their apical cell surface. Considering these results, we can conclude that the inability of normal Caco-2 cells to translocate inert particles when cultured alone cannot be explained by restricted accessibility of the plasma membrane linked to the brush border structure and its thin glycocalyx. Thus, lymphocytes activate at least two distinct cellular effectors mediating brush border disassembly and transcytosis of inert particles. It is possible that molecules that critically control phagocytosis[38] are up-regulated in Caco-2 cells following their contact with lymphocytes. The analysis of temperature-dependent transport of latex beads across the Caco-2 cell monolayers in presence of lymphocytes reveals a 10 min lag period followed by a high number of particles transported 30 min later. This time course is similar to the time course of the transport of fluorescein-labelled beads across mouse M cells *in vivo*[34], and similar to the receptor-mediated transcytosis of immunoglobulins through neonatal enterocytes[39].

V. cholerae, a non-invasive microorganism transported exclusively by M cells[31,40], can pass through converted cells after co-culture with PP lymphocytes. This interaction is characterized by tight interactions with the apical membrane. *V. cholerae* is present in intracytoplasmic vacuoles and released into the intraepithelial pocket in close contact with immune cells.

CONCLUSION

Results from different laboratories suggest that differentiation of the epithelium of Peyer's patches is controlled by the lymphoid follicle. Based upon these data we were able to develop a co-culture system of cells that share *in vitro* several characteristics with M cells. The ability to culture these cells will allow the study of different topics in M cell biology. Indeed several important questions can now be pursued, such as the nature of the inductor/s of this conversion and the mechanisms mediating cytoskeletal reorganization and transcytosis. With an *in vitro* model of M cells, we will also be able to analyse the cellular machinery allowing the translocation of microorganisms and antigens. It is also possible that in the future the understanding of the translocation of antigens and microorganisms will facilitate the design of oral vaccines and efficient mucosal drug delivery systems.

ACKNOWLEDGEMENTS

We thank R. M. Golsteyn for suggestions and criticisms. This work was supported by grants from the ANRS (French national Agency for AIDS Research) and the Fondation pour la Recherche Médicale (Paris, France).

References

1. Neutra MR, Pringault E, Kraehenbuhl JP. Antigen sampling across epithelial barriers and induction of mucosal immune responses. Annu Rev Immunol. 1996;14:275–300.
2. Neutra MR, Giannasca PJ, Troidle K, Kraehenbuhl JP. M cells and microbial pathogens. In: Blaser MJ, Smith PD, Ravdin JI, Greenberg HB, Guerrant L (eds). Infections of the Gastrointestinal Tract. New York: Raven Press, 1994:163–178.
3. Siebers A, Finlay BB. M cells and the pathogenesis of mucosal and systemic infections. Trends Microbiol. 1996;4:22–29.
4. Ermak TH, Steger HJ, Pappo J. Phenotypically distinct subpopulations of T cells in domes and M-cell pockets of rabbit gut-associated lymphoid tissues. Immunology. 1990;71:530–537.
5. Farstad IN, Halstensen TS, Fausa O, Brandtzaeg P. Heterogeneity of M-cell-associated B and T cells in human Peyer's patches. Immunology. 1994;83:457–464.
6. Schmidt GH, Wilkinson MM, Ponder BAJ. Cell migration pathway in the intestinal epithelium: an *in situ* marker system using mouse aggregation chimeras. Cell. 1985;40:425–429.
7. Gordon JI, Hermiston ML. Differentiation and self-renewal in the mouse gastrointestinal epithelium. Curr Opin Cell Biol. 1994;6:795–803.
8. Bye WA, Allan CH, Trier JS. Structure, distribution and origin of M cells in Peyer's patches of mouse ileum. Gastroenterology. 1984;86:789–801.
9. Kernéis S, Bogdanova A, Colucci-Guyon E, Kraehenbuhl JP, Pringault E. Cytosolic distribution of villin in M cells from mouse Peyer's patches correlates with the absence of a brush border. Gastroenterology. 1996;110:515–521.
10. Giannasca PJ, Giannasca KT, Falk P, Gordon JI, Neutra MR. Regional differences in glyco-conjugates of intestinal M cells in mice: potential targets for mucosal vaccines. Am J Physiol. 1994;267:1108–1121.
11. Pappo J, Owen RL. Absence of secretory component expression by epithelial cells overlying rabbit gut-associated lymphoid tissue. Gastroenterology. 1988;95:1173–1177.
12. Brown D, Smith MW, James PS, Savidge TC. Possible models describing enterocyte replacement in mouse Peyer's patch follicle-associated epithelial tissue. Epith Cell Biol. 1993;2:135–142.
13. Savidge TC, Smith MW, James PS, Aldred P. *Salmonella*-induced M-cell formation in germ-free mouse Peyer's patch tissue. Am J Pathol. 1991;139:177–184.
14. Regoli M, Borghesi C, Bertelli E, Nicoletti C. Uptake of a gram-positive bacterium (*Streptococcus pneumoniae* r36a) by the M cells of rabbit Peyer's patches Ann Anat. 1995;177:119–124.
15. Owen RL, Bhalla DK. Cytochemical analysis of alkaline phosphatase and esterase activities and of lectin-binding and anionic sites in rat and mouse Peyer's patch M cells. Am J Anat. 1983;168:199–212.
16. Savidge TC, Smith MW. Evidence that membranous (M) cell genesis is immunoregulated. In: Mestecky J (ed.) Advances in Mucosal Immunology. New York: Plenum, 1995:239–241.
17. Smith MW. Selective expression of brush border hydrolases by mouse Peyer's patch and jejunal villus enterocytes. J Cell Physiol. 1995;124:219–225.
18. Freeman TC, Bentsen BS, Thwaites DT, Simmons NL. H$^+$/ditripeptide transporter (PepT1) expression in the rabbit intestine. Pflügers Arch. 1995;430:394–400.
19. Kernéis S, Bogdanova A, Kraehenbuhl JP, Pringault E. Conversion by Peyer's patch lymphocytes of human enterocytes into M cells that transport bacteria. Science. 1997;277:948–951.
20. Savidge TC, Smith MW, Mayel-Afshar S, Collins AJ, Freeman TC. Selective regulation of epithelial gene expression in rabbit Pfeyer's patch tissue. Pfluger Arch Eur J Physiol. 1994;428:391–399.
21. Loffert D, Schaal S, Ehlich A et al. Early B-cell development in the mouse: insights from mutations introduced by gene targeting. Immunol Rev. 1994;137:135–153.

22. Ermak TH, Owen RL. Phenotype and distribution of T lymphocytes in Peyer's patches of athymic mice. Histochemistry. 1987;87:321–325.

23. De Togni P, Goellner J, Ruddle NH et al. Abnormal development of peripheral lymphoid organs in mice deficient in lymphotoxin. Science. 1994;264:703–706.

24. Eugster, HP, Müller M, Karrer U et al. Multiple immune abnormalities in tumor necrosis factor and lymphotoxin a double-deficient mutant. Int Immunol. 1995;8:23–36.

25. Ettinger R, Browning JL, Michie SA, van Ewijk W, McDevitt HO. Disrupted splenic architecture, but normal lymph node development in mice expressing a soluble lymphotoxin-beta receptor-IgG1 fusion protein. Proc Natl Acad Sci USA. 1996;93:13102–13107.

26. Förster R, Mattis AE, Kremmer E, Wolf E, Brem G, Lipp M. A putative chemokine receptor, BLR1, directs B cell migration to defined lymphoid organs and specific anatomic compartments of the spleen. Cell. 1996;87:1037–1047.

27. Pappo J. Generation and characterization of monoclonal antibodies recognizing follicle epithelial M cells in rabbit gut-associated lymphoid tissues. Cell Immunol. 1989;120:31–41.

28. Owen RL. Sequential uptake of horseradish peroxidase by lymphoid follicle epithelium of Peyer's patches in the normal unobstructed mouse intestine: an ultrastructural study. Gastroenterology. 1977;72:440–451.

29. Neutra MR, Phillips TL, Mayer EL, Fishkind DJ. Transport of membrane-bound macromolecules by M cells in follicle-associated epithelium of rabbit Peyer's patch. Cell Struct Funct. 1987;247:537–546.

30. Wolf JL, Rubin DH, Finberg R et al. Intestinal M cells: a pathway for entry of reovirus into the host. Science. 1981;212:471–472.

31. Owen RL, Pierce NF, Apple RT, Cray WC Jr. M cell transport of *Vibrio cholerae* from the intestinal lumen into Peyer's patches: a mechanism for antigen sampling and for microbial transepithelial migration. J Infect Dis. 1986;153:1108–1118.

32. Kohbata S, Yokobata H, Yabuchi E. Cytopathogenic effect of *Salmonella typhi* GIFU 10007 on M cells of murine ileal Peyer's patches in ligated ileal loops: An ultrastructural study. Microbiol Immunol. 1986;30:1225–1237.

33. Lefevre ME, Olivo R, Joel DD. Accumulation of latex particles in Peyer's patches and their subsequent appearance in villi and mesenteric lymph nodes. Proc Soc Exp Biol Med. 1978;159:298–302.

34. Pappo J, Ermak TH. Uptake and translocation of fluorescent latex particles by rabbit Peyer's patch follicle epithelium: a quantitative model for M cell uptake. Clin Exp Immunol. 1989;76:144–148.

35. Friederich E, Vancompernolle K, Huet C et al. An actin-binding site containing a conserved motif of charged amino acid residues is essential for the morphogenic effect of villin. Cell. 1992;70:81–92.

36. Costa de Beauregard MA, Pringault E, Robine S, Louvard D. Suppression of villin expression by antisense RNA impairs brush border assembly in polarized epithelial intestinal cells. EMBO J. 1995;14:409–421.

37. Gumbiner BM. Cell adhesion: the molecular basis of tissue architecture and morphogenesis. Cell. 1996;84:345–357.

38. Maniak M, Rauchenberger R, Albrecht R, Murphy J, Gerish G. Coronin involved in phagocytosis – dynamics of particle-induced relocalization visualized by a green fluorescent protein tag. Cell. 1995;83:915–924.

39. Rodewald RD, Kraehenbuhl JP. Receptor-mediated transport of IgG. J Cell Biol. 1984;99:159–164.

40. Apter FM, Michetti P, Winner LSI, Mack JA, Mekalanos JJ, Neutra MR. Analysis of the roles of antilipopolysaccharide and anti-cholera toxin immunoglobulin A (IgA) antibodies in protection against *Vibrio cholerae* and cholera toxin by use of monoclonal IgA antibodies in vivo. Infect Immun. 1993;61:5279–5285.

3
Subsets of dendritic cells in the Peyer's patch

B. L. KELSALL

INTRODUCTION

The Peyer's patch is thought to be the primary site for antigen processing in the intestine. However, little is known regarding the cellular basis for antigen handing in the Peyer's patch. This chapter will discuss recent studies defining different subpopulations of dendritic cells in the Peyer's patch and their ability to present orally administered antigens to T cells. IL-12 production by Peyer's patch dendritic cells and its regulation by factors present in the mucosal environment is postulated to play an important role in the induction of mucosal immune responses.

DENDRITIC CELLS AND MACROPHAGES OF THE PEYER'S PATCH

Luminal antigens gain access to the Peyer's patch via transfer across specialized epithelial cells, known as M cells (microfold cells), that are scattered amongst the columnar epithelial cells above the Peyer's patch dome (follicle-associated epithelium, reviewed in reference 1). Once antigens are transported into the Peyer's patch, the cell that is likely to play a key role in the processing of oral antigens is the dendritic cell. To examine this possibility, using immuno-peroxidase techniques, we stained frozen sections of murine Peyer's patches with a variety of monoclonal antibodies identifying various murine cell types. In initial studies we found that the murine Peyer's patch contains a striking concentration of cells in the subepithelial dome and the interfollicular region that express an antigen recognized by a mAB against murine CD11c (N418)[2], an antibody that in the mouse stains non-follicular dendritic cells[3]. In additional studies we showed that cells in the subepithelial dome in the same position as the CD11c$^+$ cells express an intracellular antigen of murine dendritic cells and B cells recognized by mAb 2A1[4,5]. Finally, we found that the vast majority of the same subepithelial dome cells express MHC class II, and that a subpopulation express low levels of the β_2 integrin CD11b/Mac-1, similar to dendritic cells from other organs. In contrast to these findings, only scattered cells in the sub-epithelial dome stained positively for the T cell markers (CD3 and CD4, not CD8), and the pattern of staining did not suggest that the N418[+] cells expressed these T cell markers, as has been demonstrated for populations of spleen[6], blood[7], or skin-derived dendritic cells[8].

A second population of N418[+], 2A1[+] cells were also present in the inter-follicular region of the Peyer's patch. This population, in contrast to the cells in the subepithelial dome, also express antigens recognized by the mAbs NLDC-145[9], an antibody that stains a novel protein (named DEC-205)[10] on the surface of interdigitating dendritic cells, veiled cells, and Langerhans' cells, as well as the thymic epithelium; in addition, these cells stain with mAb M342, which reacts with an intracellular antigen of dendritic cells and some B cells[11]. These dendritic cells present in the interfollicular regions of the Peyer's patch are more typical of the interdigitating dendritic cells described by others.

Based on these studies, one can conclude that there are at least two different populations of dendritic cells in the Peyer's patch. One is present in the subepithelial dome and poised for the direct uptake of antigens transported in to the Peyer's patch by overlying M cells. This cell population is similar to an N418[+], NLDC-145[-], M342[-] population of spleen dendritic cells that form a dense network in the periphery of the white pulp, where they are in the direct path of migrating T cells[2,11]. A separate population of dendritic cells is present in the interfollicular region that stained with the mAbs NLDC-145 and M342, in addition to N418, and these dendritic cells are typical of interdigitating cells of the lymph node or periarteriolar lymphoid sheaths of the spleen. It can be argued that the M342[-] cells of the Peyer's patch subepithelial dome are in a less differentiated state than the M342[+] dendritic cells of the Peyer's patch interfollicular region, since freshly isolated M342[-] spleen dendritic cells acquire this antigen[11], along with high levels of MHC antigens, co-stimulatory molecules, and antigen-presenting functions upon overnight culture[2,12]. In further studies, we went on to isolate Peyer's patch and spleen dendritic cells by transient plastic adherence, and analyse their surface phenotype by flow cytometry[3]. We found that CD11c[+] Peyer's patch dendritic cells expressed 5–10-fold higher levels of MHC class II molecules than similar cells isolated from the spleen. Levels, and percentages of cells expressing dendritic cell markers, such as N418, 33D1, and NLDC-145, as well as surface co-stimulatory molecules such as B7-1, B7-2, and CD40 (B. Kelsall, unpublished observation) were similar between spleen and Peyer's patch dendritic cells. These studies suggest that Peyer's patch dendritic cells in the subepithelial dome are immature, or resting, and that the dendritic cells of the interfollicular region are more mature, or more activated. Whether the dendritic cells of the interfollicular region arise directly from the cells in the subepithelial dome, e.g., after antigen processing or stimulation with endotoxin or cytokines, such as TNF-α (see discussion below), or whether they originate from circulating dendritic cells entering the Peyer's patch via the high endothelial venules present in the interfollicular region, is presently unclear.

To determine if dendritic cells are, in fact, the main antigen presenting cells in the Peyer's patch, we cultured Peyer's patch dendritic cells, macrophages, or B cells, with T cells from cytochrome c(CyC)-T cell receptor (TCR) transgenic mice in the presence of CyC, and the capacity of each cell population to induce

T cell proliferation and cytokine production was determined. We found that Peyer's patch dendritic cells were potent antigen presenting cells, and were, in this respect, far better than macrophages or B cells also derived from the Peyer's patches (Kelsall, unpublished observations). In addition, we demonstrated using T cells from TCR-transgenic mice with TCRs specific for either CyC or ovalbumin (OVA), that Peyer's patch dendritic cells are as effective as spleen dendritic cells in processing CyC or OVA for presentation to antigen-specific naive T cells. Finally, to extend these findings to the role of dendritic cells in antigen processing *in vivo*, we fed OVA to mice 12–18 hours prior to Peyer's patch dendritic cell isolation, and then determined the capacity of these *in vivo* loaded cells to present antigen to antigen-specific naive T cells. We found that the *in vivo*-loaded cells presented antigen to the T cells resulting in T cell proliferation. Thus, Peyer's patch dendritic cells do indeed manifest antigen-presenting function *in vivo*[3].

THE ROLE OF IL-12 IN T CELL RESPONSES IN THE PEYER'S PATCH

T cell responses in the Peyer's patch are variable, in that under certain conditions, the predominant response in the Peyer's patch is dominated by Th2 cytokines, such as IL-4 and IL-5, as when antigens are repeatedly administered with cholera toxin. Under other conditions, however, the response is dominated by the production of IFN-γ, as follows infection with pathogenic microorganisms, such as *Toxoplasma gondii*[13] or *Salmonella typhimurium*[14–18], which directly stimulate antigen-presenting cells, like macrophages and dendritic cells to produce IL-12. In addition, studies of TCR-transgenic mice have provided evidence that under certain conditions, soluble protein antigens elicit an initial T cell response in the Peyer's patch that is dominated by the production of IFN-γ[19,20]. Thus, it was shown that when either intact TCR-transgenic mice[20] or normal mice into which TCR-transgenic T cells have been transferred[19] are fed a high dose of the antigen recognized by the transgenic TCR, T cells develop in the Peyer's patch which produce IFN-γ out of proportion to IL-4 following restimulation *in vitro*. Consistent with this possibility, we found that Peyer's patch dendritic cells, when compared to spleen dendritic cells (both isolated by transient plastic adherence and FACs sorting for N418+ cells) manifest a greatly increased capacity to induce IFN-γ production by T cells from TCR transgenic mice following primary and secondary stimulation[21]. Interestingly, *in vivo* blockade of Th1 induction in the TCR-transgenic mice by systemic administration of antibodies to interleukin-12 during the feeding protocol results in Peyer's patch T cells that now produce lower levels of IFN-γ and higher levels of TGFβ, but which do not change their production of IL-4[20]. Finally, with low dose or repeated high dose oral antigen administration to these TCR-transgenic mice, the development of IFN-γ-producing cells is either prevented, or eliminated, respectively, and this is accompanied by the emergence of T cells producing TGFβ and IL-4[22].

These studies demonstrate that under a variety of fairly common circumstances of mucosal stimulation, such as high dose antigen administration, and infection with intracellular organisms, IFN-γ producing (Th1) T cells are induced to differentiate in the Peyer's patch. Under other conditions, such as when cholera toxin is used as a mucosal adjuvant, a predominant Th2 response occurs. Finally, with low dose or repetitive antigen administration[19], the induction of IFN-γ producing T cells is prevented, or in the case of repetitive high dose administration[20,22], eventually eliminated by apoptosis of Th1 cells, and the result is induction of T cells that produce TGFβ, with or without the concomitant production of IL-4.

The precise mechanism underlying these various response pathways is not completely clear. One possibility is that IL-12 may be a key regulatory cytokine for mucosal immune responses. In this way, factors that suppress IL-12 production by antigen presenting cells, such as dendritic cells, result in T cells producing TGFβ and possibly, but not necessarily, IL-4, while factors that induce IL-12 production result in T cells producing IFN-γ. One such factor could be IL-10, a cytokine produced by a number of cells and which has been shown to be a potent inhibitor of IL-12 production by dendritic cells[23]. While the conditions leading to the production of such IL-10 have not been defined, naive T cells stimulated in such conditions, i.e., the presence of IL-10 (and the absence of IL-12) have recently been shown to differentiate into cells capable of producing not only TGFβ, but also IL-10[24]. This would not only establish conditions in the Peyer's patch important for IgA production, but also result in suppressor T cells that, following migration out of the patch, could actively suppress peripheral responses. In addition, IL-10 production would provide for autocrine growth of IL-10-producing T cells. Other factors that could play a primary role in the suppression of IL-12 production by antigen presenting cells of the Peyer's patches include TGFβ, prostaglandin E_2[25], adrenergic agonists[26], complement components, such as iC3b (via complement receptor 3)[27,28], or C3b (via CD46)[29], or IgG-immune complexes (via Fc-receptors)[28,30].

CONCLUSION

In conclusion, we speculate that the dendritic cell network in the subepithelial dome of Peyer's patches provides an important mechanism for the uptake and processing of luminal antigens. Such uptake may occur by endocytosis, or even by phagocytosis, as has been demonstrated for Langerhans' cells[31] and dendritic cell precursors grown from bone marrow[32]. The dendritic cells then present the processed antigen to CD4[+] T cells in the subepithelial dome or, after maturation and migration to the interfollicular region, to CD4[+] or CD8[+] T cells in the latter area. Such presentation may be qualitatively different from similar processes occurring in other organs, since there is a special propensity for T cells developing in Peyer's patches to mediate oral tolerance and IgA B cell development. The regulation of IL-12 production from dendritic cells may be of primary importance in the regulation of such responses.

References

1. Owen R. Sequential uptake of horseradish peroxidase by lymphoid follicle epithelium of Peyer's patches in the normal unobstructed mouse intestine: An ultrastructural study. Gastroenterology. 1977;72:440–451.

2. Metlay JP, Witmer-Pack MD, Aggar R, Crowley MT, Steinman RM. The distinct leukocyte integrins of mouse spleen dendritic cells as identified with new hamster monoclonal antibodies. J Exp Med. 1990;171:1753.

3. Kelsall BL, Strober W. Distinct populations of dendritic cells are present in the subepithelial dome and T cell regions of the murine Peyer's patch. J Exp Med. 1996;183:237–247.

4. Witmer-Pack MD, Hughes DA, Schuler G et al. Identification of macrophages and dendritic cells in the osteopetrotic (op/op) mouse. J Cell Sci. 1993;104:1021–1029.

5. Inaba K, Steinman RM, Witmer-Pack M et al. Identification of proliferating dendritic cell precursors in mouse blood. J Exp Med. 1992;175:1157.

6. Crowley MT, Witmer-Pack MD, Gezelter S, Steinman RM. Use of the fluorescence cell sorter to enrich dendritic cells from mouse spleen. J Immunol Methods. 1990;133:55.

7. O'Doherty U, Steinman RM, Peng M et al. Dendritic cells freshly isolated from human blood express CD4 and mature into typical immunostimulatory dendritic cells after culture in monocyte-conditioned medium. J Exp Med. 1993;1067.

8. Wood GS, Warner NL, Warnke RA. Anti-Leu3/T4 antibodies react with cells of monocyte/macrophage and Langerhans lineage. J Immunol. 1983;131:212.

9. Kraal GM, Breel M, Janse M, Bruin G. Langerhans' cells, veiled cells and interdigitating cells in the mouse recognized by a monoclonal antibody. J Exp Med. 1986;163:981.

10. Swiggard WJ, Mirza A, Nussenzweig MC, Steinman RM. DEC-205, a 205-kDa protein abundant on mouse dendritic cells and thymic epithelium that is detected by the monoclonal antibody NLDC-145: purification, characterization, and N-terminal amino acid sequence. Cell Immunol. 1995;165:302–11.

11. Aggar R, Witmer-Pack N, Romani N et al. Two populations of spleen dendritic cells detected with a new monoclonal antibody to an intracellular antigen of interdigitating dendritic cells and some B cells. J Leuk Biol. 1992;52:34.

12. Larsen CP, Ritchie SC, Pearson, TC, Linsley PS, Lowry RP. Functional expression of the costimulatory molecule, B7/BB1, on murine dendritic cell populations, J Exp Med. 1992;176:1215.

13. Liesenfeld O, Kosek J, Remington JS, Suzuki Y. Association of CD4[+] T cell-dependent, interferon-gamma-mediated necrosis of the small intestine with genetic susceptibility of mice to peroral infection with *Toxoplasma gondii*. J Exp Med. 1996;184:597–607.

14. Everest P, Allen J, Papakonstantinopoulou A, Mastroeni P, Roberts M, Dougan G. Salmonella typhimurium infections in mice deficient in interleukin-4 production: role of IL-4 in infection-associated pathology. J Immunol. 1997;159:1820–7.

15. George A. Generation of gamma interferon responses in murine Peyer's patches following oral immunization. Infect Immun. 1996;64:4606–11.

16. Hess J, Ladel C, Miko D, Kaufmann SH. Salmonella typhimurium aroA-infection in gene-targeted immunodeficient mice: major role of CD4[+] TCR-alpha beta cells and IFN-gamma in bacterial clearance independent of intracellular location. J Immunol. 1996;156:3321–6.

17. Karem KL, Kanangat S, Rouse BT. Cytokine expression in the gut associated lymphoid tissue after oral administration of attenuated Salmonella vaccine strains. Vaccine. 1996;14:1495–502.

18. Yamanoto M, Vancott JL, Okahashi N et al. The role of Th1 and Th2 cells for mucosal IgA responses, Ann N Y Acad Sci. 1996;778:64–71.

19. Chen Y, Inobe J, Weiner HL. Inductive events in oral tolerance in the TCR transgenic adoptive transfer model, Cell Immunol. 1997;178:62–8.

20. Marth T, Strober W, Kelsall BL. High dose oral tolerance in ovalbumin TCR-transgenic mice: Systemic neutralization of IL-12 augments TGF-β secretion and cell apoptosis. J Immunol. 1996;157:2348–57.

21. Kelsall BL, Ehrhardt RO, Strober W. Peyer's patch dendritic cells: Phenotypic characterization by FACS analysis and *in vitro* primary and secondary T cell responses using a TCR-transgenic mouse model. J Cell Biochem. 1994; Suppl.18D:310.

22. Chen Y, Inobe J, Marks R, Gonella P, Kuchroo VK, Weiner HL. Peripheral deletion of antigen-reactive T cells in oral tolerance [published erratum appears in Nature 1995 Sep 21;377(6546): 257], Nature. 1995;376:177–80.

23. Kelsall BL, Stuber E, Neurath M, Strober W. Interleukin-12 production by dendritic cells. The role of CD40-CD40L interactions in Th1 T-cell responses. Ann N Y Acad Sci. 1996;795:116–26.

24. Groux H, O'Garra A, Bigler M, Rouleau M, Antonenko S, de VJ, Roncarolo MG. A CD4[+] T-cell subset inhibits antigen-specific T-cell responses and prevents colitis. Nature. 1997;389:737–42.

25. van der Pouw Kraan TC, Boeije LC, Smeenk RJ, Wijdenes J, Aarden LA. Prostaglandin-E$_2$ is a potent inhibitor of human interleukin 12 production. J Exp Med. 1995;181:775–9.
26. Panina BP, Mazzeo PD, Lucia PD et al. Beta$_2$-agonists prevent Th1 development by selective inhibition of interleukin 12. J Clin Invest. 1997;100:1513–19.
27. Marth T, Kelsall BL. Regulation of interleukin-12 by complement receptor 3 signalling. J Exp Med. 1997;185:1987–95.
28. Sutterwala FS, Noel GJ, Clynes R, Mosser DM. Selective suppression of interleukin-12 induction after macrophage receptor ligation, J Exp Med. 1997;185:1977–85.
29. Karp CL, Wysocka M, Wahl LM et al. Mechanism of suppression of cell-mediated immunity by measles virus [published erratum appears in Science 1997 Feb 21;275(5303):1053], Science. 1996;273:228–31.
30. Sutterwala FS, Noel GJ, Salgame P, Mosser DM. Reversal of proinflammatory responses by ligating the macrophage fcgamma receptor type I. J Exp Med. 1998;188:217–22.
31. Reis e Sousa C, Stahl PD, Austyn JM. Phagocytosis of antigens by Langerhans' cells *in vitro*. J Exp Med. 1993;178:509.
32. Inaba K, Inaba M, Naito M, Steinman RM. Dendritic cell progenitors phagocytose particulates, including bacillus Calmette–Guerin organisms, and sensitive mice to myocobacterial antigens *in vivo*. J Exp Med. 1993;178:479.

4
Antigen presentation by epithelial cells

S. P. BALK, M. EXLEY and R. S. BLUMBERG

INTRODUCTION

Intestinal epithelial cells (IECs) are in direct contact with intraepithelial lymphocytes (IELs), and these lymphocytes are a major cell type in the intestinal epithelium. This is particularly true in the small intestine, where there is approximately one IEL for every 6–10 IECs[1]. The intestinal epithelium clearly represents an important line of defence against ingested pathogens and it makes intuitive sense that a major function of these IELs would be to respond to antigens derived from these pathogens and presented by IECs. However, phenotypic and functional analyses of IELs in humans and mice indicate that responding to such diverse IEC presented antigens may not be their major function in normal intestine.

PHENOTYPIC AND FUNCTIONAL STUDIES IN HUMANS

One piece of evidence against significant antigen presentation by IEC through the MHC class II pathway is that CD4, the MHC class II co-receptor, is expressed by only a small fraction of normal IELs in human intestine. The majority ($> 90\%$) of small intestinal IELs express CD8 and the $\alpha\beta$ T cell antigen receptor (TCR$\alpha\beta$)[2–5]. CD8$^+$ TCR$\alpha\beta$ T cells are also the major population in human colon, but the number of IELs in the colon is much smaller than in the small intestine and other T cell subsets are more represented[6,7]. It should be noted that CD4$^+$ T cells are prevalent in the lamina propria and IEC antigen presentation to these cells by projections through the basement membrane remains possible. Nonetheless, at least with respect to the majority of IELs, IEC antigen presentation through a class II pathway would not appear to be of major importance in normal intestine.

The prevalence of CD8$^+$ T cells in the intestinal epithelium suggests that antigen presentation by IEC may be predominantly through MHC class I proteins. The immunological function of MHC class I proteins expressed by most non-professional antigen-presenting cells is to display on the cell surface peptide antigens derived from intracellular pathogens and hence target infected cells for destruction by MHC class I-restricted CD8$^+$ cytolytic T cells. Therefore, an alternative reasonable hypothesis is that the display of pathogen-derived peptides by infected IEC is the major antigen presentation function of IECs.

Evidence in favour of this latter hypothesis would be cytolytic activity by IELs. Functional studies have shown that IELs from human intestine proliferate in response to stimulation by anti-CD2 antibodies[8–10] or IL-7[11], indicating that the majority of intestinal IELs are activated *in situ*. Murine intestinal IELs appear to be activated cytolytic T cells, based upon their large granular lymphocyte morphology and cytolytic activity in redirected lysis assays[12–16]. However, most human intestinal IELs do not have large cytotoxic granules and appear to have only weak cytolytic activity when freshly isolated[17,18]. Moreover, recent data indicate that these cells *in situ* in normal intestine do not express any of the proteins associated with cytolytic function[19,20]. Specifically, we have shown that IELs in normal human intestine do not express perforin, granzyme B, Fas ligand or tumour necrosis factor[20]. Therefore, to the extent that IELs are activated *in vivo*, cytolysis of infected or otherwise abnormal IEC does not appear to be their major function in human intestine.

Further evidence against IEC presentation to IELs of antigens from diverse pathogens is the observation that IEL are oligoclonal in normal intestine[21–24]. In order to assess whether there might be restricted TCR variable region usage by human IELs, we initially sequenced TCRs used by freshly isolated human small intestinal IELs and a short term IEL line[21]. In both cases the analysis yielded a small number of unique TCRs, indicating that the majority of these IELs were derived from a small number of clones. This analysis was subsequently extended to a larger number of normal donors and to IELs isolated from multiple segments of the intestine and confirmed that a large fraction of TCR$\alpha\beta$ IELs in the small or large intestine were derived from a small number of clones[22–24]. More recently, the presence of dominant clones amongst human intestinal IELs has been confirmed by flow cytometry with a panel of TCR Vβ specific antibodies (M. Exley and S. Balk, unpublished data).

This massive expansion of relatively few T cell clones indicates that IELs are normally responding to a very limited number of antigens. Unfortunately, it has not yet been possible to obtain adequate samples of intestine for IEL purification from the same donor over a period of years to determine whether these clones persist. Such an analysis has been possible for human TCR$\gamma\delta$ IELs, which are enriched in human intestinal epithelium compared with lamina propria and peripheral blood, although not to the same extent as in mouse intestine. Sequence analyses in several normal donors have shown one or a small number of dominant clones expressed by IELs throughout the small intestine, with a distinct sequence identified in the colon[25]. In one donor, persistence of a clone for one year was shown. These results have been interpreted similarly to indicate that TCR$\gamma\delta$ IELs are responding to one or a very limited number of antigens, which recent data suggests are the MICA and B protein[26] (see below). Finally, we have recently been able to demonstrate persistence of a dominant clone in biliary tract epithelium[27].

PHENOTYPIC AND FUNCTIONAL STUDIES IN MICE

There are a number of important differences between human and murine intestinal IELs. The TCR$\gamma\delta$ is used at much higher frequency by murine IELs[28–30].

The CD8 protein expressed by approximately half of murine TCR$\alpha\beta$ and TCR$\gamma\delta$ IELs is a CD8$\alpha\alpha$ homodimer[31], rather than the CD8$\alpha\beta$ heterodimer expressed by peripheral blood T cells. In contrast, the CD8$\alpha\alpha$ homodimer is expressed by only a very small fraction of human IELs[32]. The significance of these two forms of CD8 is unclear, although use of the CD8$\alpha\alpha$ homodimer may reflect recognition of a nonclassical MHC class I-like protein or extrathymic T cell maturation. There are potentially significant strain differences between IELs in the small and large intestine which could reflect allelic differences in antigen presentation[33,34]. Finally, as noted above, a large fraction of murine IELs may be cytolytic. These and other differences between human and murine intestinal IELs indicate that there may be similarly important differences between antigen presentation by human and murine IECs.

Nonetheless, it is likely that the biology of the TCR$\alpha\beta$, CD8$\alpha\beta$ IEL population in humans and mice is similar, and studies in mice suggest that there are dominant TCR$\alpha\beta$ IEL clones in murine intestine[35]. Murine IELs can mount allogeneic immune responses and, in particular, MHC-restricted responses to viral infections[36]. This clearly indicates that some IELs use the classical MHC proteins for antigen recognition. However, the precursor frequency of these cells for a particular virus appears to be low ($< 0.1\%$)[36], making it unlikely that they correspond to the markedly expanded populations of TCR$\alpha\beta$ CD8$\alpha\beta$ IELs found in normal human and murine intestine.

A number of observations in mice support the idea that IELs recognize nonclassical antigen presenting molecules[37]. Initial evidence that some IELs do not recognize the classical MHC proteins was based upon their failure to undergo negative selection in response to endogenous superantigens. Mice which express the M1s-1^a and IE^d antigens delete T cells expressing certain Vβ genes from their peripheral blood pool. In contrast, T cells using these TCRs are present in normal numbers amongst the IEL subpopulation which expresses the CD8$\alpha\alpha$ homodimer[38]. This observation has been taken as evidence of extrathymic maturation of these IELs, but may also be evidence for peripheral expansion of IELs by nonclassical antigen-presenting molecules in the intestine. Either interpretation is consistent with the finding that transgenic TCRs which recognize autoantigens expressed on the cell surface of intestinal epithelial cells (TL or HY) are present at high frequency on IELs[39,40]. Further experiments are needed to determine precisely how IELs expressing these autoreactive TCRs develop in the intestine and why they are not autoreactive *in vivo*.

IELs expressing the $\gamma\delta$ TCR are found at normal or increased numbers in mice that are MHC class I or class II deficient, which suggests that a large fraction of these IELs use other proteins for positive selection and antigen presentation[41,42]. In contrast, IELs using the $\alpha\beta$ TCR are diminished in class I-deficient mice. However, the class I-deficient mice are generated by inactivation of the β2-microglobulin (β2m) gene, which would also be expected to prevent expression of some MHC class I-like proteins. Therefore, the possible role of class I-like proteins in antigen presentation to TCR$\alpha\beta$ IELs cannot be clearly assessed from these experiments.

Mice deficient in MHC class I expression have also been generated by knocking out the transporter associated with antigen processing (TAP). Cells from TAP-deficient mice do not efficiently generate peptide antigens for MHC class I proteins and have markedly diminished MHC class I expression. These mice have a corresponding deficiency of CD8[+] MHC class I restricted T cells in the periphery. In contrast, large numbers of CD8[+], TCR$\alpha\beta$ IELs remain in these animals[43]. These results suggest IEC antigen presentation by a TAP-independent MHC class I-like protein such as CD1d or TL.

STRUCTURE AND FUNCTION OF CD1d EXPRESSED BY IEC

The human CD1 locus encodes five homologous MHC class I-like proteins, CD1a–e. Sequence comparisons among the CD1 genes demonstrate that CD1d is divergent from CD1a, b and c[44]. Limited data from other species and the tissue distribution of the CD1 genes indicate that there are two classes of CD1 genes, those that are CD1a, b, c-like (which are deleted in rodents) and those that are CD1d-like[45]. CD1a–c are expressed by immature thymocytes and professional antigen-presenting cells[46], but have not been detected on IECs. In contrast, CD1d is expressed by human IECs (and at low levels by a variety of other cell types) and is, therefore, a potential ligand or antigen-presenting molecule for IELs[47,48].

Similarly to other MHC class I and class I-like proteins, CD1d is in most cases expressed as a glycosylated and β2m-associated protein (S. P. Balk, unpublished data). However, biochemical analyses of freshly isolated human IECs demonstrated that CD1d was expressed on the IEC surface in a non-glycosylated form which was not detectably associated with β2m[49]. These conclusions have been confirmed through the use of additional antibodies generated against human CD1d (S. P. Balk, manuscript in preparation). These more recent studies also suggest that this cell surface form of CD1d may be derived from a fully glycosylated and β2m-associated form (S. P. Balk, manuscript in preparation).

The immunological function of CD1d expressed on the cell surface of IEC remains to be clarified. CD1d has been clearly shown to be the antigen-presenting molecule or ligand for a novel regulatory population of NKR-P1 T cells found in human and murine peripheral blood, thymus, liver and bone marrow (ref. 50, and references therein), but not seen at high frequency in the intestine (S. P. Balk, unpublished data). We reported previously that a short-term IEL line and clone could recognize CD1d, but this was not specific as other CD1 proteins were also recognized[21]. Recent success in establishing long-term IEL lines and clones derived from dominant *in vivo* clones will allow for this recognition to be further addressed. In other studies, CD1d expressed by human IECs was shown to stimulate a fraction of peripheral blood CD8[+] T cells[51]. Further work to determine the molecular basis of this latter interaction is underway (L. Mayer, personal communication).

Recent reports indicate that CD1 proteins present hydrophobic, probably glycolipid antigens[52–54], consistent with the crystal structure of murine CD1d which shows a deep hydrophobic antigen-binding cleft[55]. Cell trafficking studies indicate that these hydrophobic antigens may be acquired in an endosomal compartment similar or identical to the compartment where MHC class II proteins acquire antigens[56]. The CD1d protein (as well as CD1b and c) has in its cytoplasmic tail an endosomal targeting signal which appears to mediate cycling of the protein between the plasma membrane and endosomes (D. Rodionov *et al.*, submitted for publication). The CD1d protein may acquire antigen as a result of this cycling and display it on the plasma membrane. Alternatively, CD1d may play a role in sampling luminal antigens and bringing them into the endosomal compartment. This latter function would be consistent with the apical and lateral expression of CD1d on human IECs (R. S. Blumberg, manuscript in preparation). Further studies are clearly needed to define the immunological functions of CD1d expressed by human IEC.

STRUCTURE AND FUNCTION OF CD1D EXPRESSED BY MURINE IEC

In contrast to the human CD1 locus, mice have only a recently duplicated CD1d gene. The first derived anti-mouse CD1d antibodies, 1H1 and 3C11, indicated that murine CD1d was expressed by hepatocytes, IEC and at low levels by thymocytes and spleen cells[57]. The lymphoid and hepatocyte expression of murine CD1d has been confirmed with other antibodies, but CD1d was not detected on IEC with the 1B1 anti-CD1d mAb[58]. There are also reports suggesting a more widespread CD1d tissue distribution[59,60], but definitive conclusions regarding murine IEC expression await biochemical studies similar to those carried out on human IEC. We have noted in the intestines of CD1d knockout mice decreased reactivity with the 3C11 anti-CD1d mAb, but no change in 1B1 reactivity (S. P. Balk, unpublished data). Finally, no marked intestinal abnormalities have yet been noted in CD1d knockout mice.

STRUCTURE AND FUNCTION OF MICA AND B EXPRESSED BY HUMAN IEC

The MIC genes are MHC encoded and distantly related to MHC class I molecules[61]. However, their expression is not dependent upon β2m or class I peptide ligands. The promoter regions of MICA and B contain heat shock elements, indicating that their expression is at least in part stress regulated[62]. MICA is expressed largely or exclusively by IEC[62,63] and a recent report indicates that MICA and MICB are recognized by diverse TCR$\gamma\delta$ IELs using Vδ1[26]. These observations indicate TCR$\gamma\delta$ lEL recognition of stressed (damaged, infected or transformed) IEC may be mediated by IEC expression of MICA and B. The effector function mediated by these TCR$\gamma\delta$ IELs could be immune destruction. However, these cells have also been shown to make keratinocyte growth factor in response to activation[64], suggesting that the biological function of this system may be to aid in the healing of damaged intestinal epithelium. A similar yet to be defined system presumably functions in murine intestine.

CONCLUSIONS

IEC are capable of antigen presentation through classical MHC class I and class II pathways, but several lines of evidence suggest that the presentation of diverse luminal antigens to IEL is not the primary antigen-presenting function of IEC. It now appears that one function of IEC is to present MICA or B to TCR$\gamma\delta$ IEL, which are oligoclonal in normal intestine. The oligoclonal expansion of TCR$\alpha\beta$ IEL in normal intestine suggests that IEC may similarly present novel antigens to these cells. However, MHC class I-restricted presentation by IEC of a small number of conventional antigens, presumably derived from a persistent or very frequent pathogen, remains possible. Further *in vitro* analyses of IEL clones expanded *in vivo* should clarify the function of these cells and the nature of the IEC-presented antigens.

References

1. Ferguson A, Murray D. Quantitation of intraepithelial lymphocytes in human jejunum. Gut. 1971;12:988–994.
2. Cerf-Bensussan N, Schneeberger EE, Bhan AK. Immunohistologic and immunoelectron microscopic characterization of the mucosal lymphocytes of human small intestine by the use of monoclonal antibodies. J Immunol. 1983;130:2615–2622.
3. Brandtzaeg P, Bosnes V, Halstensen TS, Scott H, Sollid LM, Valnes KN. T lymphocytes in human gut epithelium preferentially express the alpha/beta antigen receptor and are often CD45/UCHL 1-positive [published erratum appears in Scand J Immunol. 1989;30:653]. Scand J Immunol. 1989;30:123–128.
4. Trejdosiewicz LK, Smart CJ, Oakes DJ et al. Expression of T-cell receptors TcR1 (gamma/delta) and TcR2 (alpha/beta) in the human intestinal mucosa. Immunology. 989;68:7–12.
5. Jarry A, Cerf-Bensussan N, Brousse N, Selz F, Guy-Grand D. Subsets of CD3$^+$ (T cell receptor alpha/beta or gamma/delta) and CD3$^-$ lymphocytes isolated from normal human gut epithelium display phenotypical features different from their counterparts in peripheral blood. Eur J Immunol. 1990;20:1097–1103.
6. Deusch K, Luling F, Reich K, Classen M, Wagner H, Pfeffer K. A major fraction of human intraepithelial lymphocytes simultaneously expresses the gamma/delta T cell receptor, the CD8 accessory molecule and preferentially uses the V delta 1 gene segment. Eur J Immunol. 1991;21:1053–1059.
7. Lundqvist C, Baranov V, Hammarstrom S, Athlin L, Hammarstrom ML. Intra-epithelial lymphocytes. Evidence for regional specialization and extrathymic T cell maturation in the human gut epithelium. Int Immunol. 1995;7:1473–1487.
8. Ebert EC, Roberts Al, Brolin RE, Raska K. Examination of the low proliferative capacity of human jejunal intraepithelial lymphocytes. Clin Exp Immunol. 1986,65:148–157.
9. Ebert EC. Proliferative responses of human intraepithelial lymphocytes to various T-cell stimuli. Gastroenterology. 1989;97:1372–1381.
10. Pirzer UC, Schurmann G, Post S, Betzler M, Meuer SC. Differential responsiveness to CD3-Ti vs. CD2-dependent activation of human intestinal T lymphocytes. Eur J Immunol. 1990;20:2339–2342.
11. Watanabe M, Ueno Y, Yajima T et al. Interleukin 7 is produced by human intestinal epithelial cells and regulates the proliferation of intestinal mucosal lymphocytes. J Clin Invest. 95:2945–2953.
12. Lefrancois L, Goodman T. In vivo modulation of cytolytic activity and Thy-1 expression in TCR$^-$ $^-$ gamma delta$^+$ intraepithelial lymphocytes. Science. 1989;243:1716–1718.
13. Guy-Grand D, Malassis-Seris M, Briottet C, Vassalli P. Cytotoxic differentiation of mouse gut thymodependent and independent intraepithelial T lymphocytes is induced locally. Correlation between functional assays, presence of perforin and granzyme transcripts, and cytoplasmic granules. J Exp Med. 1991;173:1549–1552.
14. Gramzinski RA, Adams E, Gross JA, Goodman TG, Allison JP, Lefrancois L. T cell receptor-triggered activation of intraepithelial lymphocytes in vitro. Int Immunol. 1993;5:145–153.
15. Viney JL, Kilshaw PJ, MacDonald TT. Cytotoxic alpha/beta$^+$ and gamma/delta$^+$ T cells in murine intestinal epithelium. Eur J Immunol. 1990;20:1623–1626.
16. Sydora BC, Mixter PF, Holcombe HR et al. Intestinal intraepithelial lymphocytes are activated and cytolytic but do not proliferate as well as other T cells in response to mitogenic signals. J Immunol. 1993;150:2179–2191.

17. Taunk J, Roberts Al, Ebert EC. Spontaneous cytotoxicity of human intraepithelial lymphocytes against epithelial cell tumors. Gastroenterology. 1992;102:69–75.
18. Russell GJ, Nagler-Anderson C, Anderson P, Bhan AK. Cytotoxic potential of intraepithelial lymphocytes (IELs). Presence of TIA-1, the cytolytic granule-associated protein, in human IELs in normal and diseased intestine. Am J Pathol. 1993;143:350–354.
19. Oberhuber G, Vogelsang H, Stolte M, Muthenthaler S, Kummer AJ, Radaszkiewicz T. Evidence that intestinal intraepithelial lymphocytes are activated cytotoxic T cells in celiac disease but not in giardiasis. Am J Pathol. 1996;148:1351–1357.
20. Chott A, Gerdes D, Spooner A et al. Intraepithelial lymphocytes in normal human intestine do not express proteins associated with cytolytic function. Am J Pathol. 1997;151:435–442.
21. Balk SP, Ebert EC, Blumenthal RL et al. Oligoclonal expansion and CD1 recognition by human intestinal intraepithelial lymphocytes. Science. 1991;253:1411–1415.
22. Van Kerckhove C, Russell GJ, Deusch K et al. Oligoclonality of human intestinal intraepithelial T cells. J Exp Med. 1992;175:57–63.
23. Blumberg RS, Yockey CE, Gross GG, Ebert EC, Balk SP. Human intestinal intraepithelial lymphocytes are derived from a limited number of T cell clones that utilize multiple V beta T cell receptor genes. J Immunol. 1993;150:5144–5153.
24. Gross GG, Schwartz VL, Stevens C, Ebert EC, Blumberg RS, Balk SP. Distribution of dominant T cell receptor beta chains in human intestinal mucosa. J Exp Med. 1994;180:1337–1344.
25. Chowers Y, Holtmeier W, Harwood J, Morzycka-Wroblewska E, Kagnoff MF. The V delta 1 T cell receptor repertoire in human small intestine and colon. J Exp Med. 1994;180:183–190.
26. Groh V, Steinle A, Bauer S, Spies T. Recognition of stress-induced MHC molecules by intestinal epithelial gammadelta T cells. Science. 1998;279:1737–1740.
27. Probert CS, Christ AD, Saubermann LJ et al. Analysis of human common bile duct-associated T cells: evidence for oligoclonality, T cell clonal persistence, and epithelial cell recognition. J Immunol. 1997;158:1941–1948.
28. Itohara S, Farr AG, Lafaille JJ et al. Homing of a gamma delta thymocyte subset with homogeneous T-cell receptors to mucosal epithelia. Nature. 1990;343:754–757.
29. Bonneville M, Janeway CA, Jr, Ito K et al. Intestinal intraepithelial lymphocytes are a distinct set of gamma delta T cells. Nature. 1988;336:479–481.
30. Asarnow DM, Goodman T, Lefrancois L, Allison JP. Distinct antigen receptor repertoires of two classes of murine epithelium-associated T cells. Nature. 1989;341:60–62.
31. Guy-Grand D, Cerf-Bensussan N, Malissen B, Malassis-Seris M, Briottet C, Vassalli P. Two gut intraepithelial CD8+ lymphocyte populations with different T cell receptors: a role for the gut epithelium in T cell differentiation. J Exp Med. 1991;173:471–481.
32. Taplin ME, Frantz ME, Canning C, Ritz J, Blumberg RS, Balk SP. Evidence against T-cell development in the adult human intestinal mucosa based upon lack of terminal deoxynucleotidyltransferase expression. Immunology. 1996;87:402–407.
33. Camerini V, Panwala C, Kronenberg M. Regional specialization of the mucosal immune system. Intraepithelial lymphocytes of the large intestine have a different phenotype and function than those of the small intestine. J Immunol. 1993;151:1765–1776.
34. Beagley KW, Fujihashi K, Lagoo AS et al. Differences in intraepithelial lymphocyte T cell subsets isolated from murine small versus large intestine. J Immunol. 1995;154:5611–5619.
35. Regnault A, Cumano A, Vassalli P, Guy-Grand D, Kourilsky P. Oligoclonal repertoire of the CD8 alpha alpha and the CD8 alpha beta TCR-alpha/beta murine intestinal intraepithelial T lymphocytes: evidence for the random emergence of T cells. J Exp Med. 1994;180: 1345–1358.
36. Cuff CF, Cebra CK, Rubin DH, Cebra JJ. Developmental relationship between cytotoxic alpha/beta T cell receptor-positive intraepithelial lymphocytes and Peyer's patch lymphocytes. Eur J Immunol. 1993;23:1333–1339.
37. Blumberg RS, Balk SP. Intraepithelial lymphocytes and their recognition of non-classical MHC molecules. Int Rev Immunol. 1994;11:15–30.
38. von Boehmer H, Kirberg J, Rocha B. An unusual lineage of alpha/beta T cells that contains autoreactive cells. J Exp Med. 1991;174:1001–1008.
39. Rocha B, Vassalli P, Guy-Grand D. The V beta repertoire of mouse gut homodimeric alpha CD8+ intraepithelial T cell receptor alpha/beta+ lymphocytes reveals a major extrathymic pathway of T cell differentiation. J Exp Med. 1991;173:483–486.
40. Barrett TA, Tatsumi Y, Bluestone JA. Tolerance of T cell receptor gamma/delta cells in the intestine. J Exp Med. 1993;177:1755–1762.

41. Correa l, Bix M, Liao NS, Zijlstra M, Jaenisch R, Raulet D. Most gamma delta T cells develop normally in beta 2-microglobulin-deficient mice. Proc Natl Acad Sci USA. 1992;89:653–657.

42. Schleussner C, Ceredig R. Analysis of intraepithelial lymphocytes from major histocompatibility complex (MHC)-deficient mice: no evidence for a role of MHC class II antigens in the positive selection of V delta 4+ gamma delta T cells. Eur J Immunol. 1993;23:1615–1622.

43. Sydora BC, Brossay L, Hagenbaugh A, Kronenberg M, Cheroutre H. TAP-independent selection of CD8+ intestinal intraepithelial lymphocytes. J Immunol. 1996;156:4209–4216.

44. Balk SP, Bleicher PA, Terhorst C. Isolation and characterization of a cDNA and gene coding for a fourth CDI molecule. Proc Natl Acad Sci USA. 1989;86:252–256.

45. Calabi F, Jarvis JM, Martin L, Milstein C. Two classes of CD1 genes. Eur J Immunol. 1989;19:285–292.

46. Blumberg RS, Gerdes D, Chott A, Porcelli SA, Balk SP. Structure and function of the CD1 family of MHC-like cell surface proteins. Immunol Rev. 1995;147:5–29.

47. Blumberg RS, Terhorst C, Bleicher P et al. Expression of a nonpolymorphic MHC class I-like molecule, CD1D, by human intestinal epithelial cells. J Immunol. 1991;147:2518–2524.

48. Canchis PW, Bhan AK, Landau SB, Yang L, Balk SP, Blumberg RS. Tissue distribution of the non-polymorphic major histocompatibility complex class I-like molecule, CD1d. Immunology. 1993;80:561–565.

49. Balk SP, Burke S, Polischuk JE et al. Beta 2-microglobulin-independent MHC class Ib molecule expressed by human intestinal epithelium. Science. 1994;265:259–262.

50. Exley M, Garcia J, Balk SP, Porcelli S. Requirements for CD1d recognition by human invariant Valpha24+ CD4– CD8– T cells. J Exp Med. 1997;186:109–120.

51. Panja A, Blumberg RS, Balk SP, Mayer L. CD1d is involved in T cell-intestinal epithelial cell interactions. J Exp Med. 1993;178:1115–1119.

52. Beckman EM, Porcelli SA, Morita CT, Behar SM, Furlong ST, Brenner MB. Recognition of a lipid antigen by CD1-restricted alpha beta+ T cells (see comments). Nature. 1994;372:691–694.

53. Sieling PA, Chatterjee D, Porcelli SA et al. CD1-restricted T cell recognition of microbial lipoglycan antigens (see comments). Science. 1995;269:227–230.

54. Joyce S, Woods AS, Yewdell JW et al. Natural ligand of mouse CD1d1:cellular glycosyl-phosphatidylinositol. Science. 1998;279:1541–1544.

55. Zeng Z, Castano AR, Segelke BW, Stura EA, Peterson PA, Wilson IA. Crystal structure of mouse CD1: An MHC-like fold with a large hydrophobic binding groove (see comments). Science. 1997;277:339–345.

56. Sugita M, Jackman RM, van Donselaar E et al. Cytoplasmic tail-dependent localization of CD1b antigen-presenting molecules to MICs. Science. 1996;273:349–352.

57. Bleicher PA, Balk SP, Hagen SJ, Blumberg RS, Flotte TJ, Terhorst C. Expression of murine CD1 on gastrointestinal epithelium. Science. 1990;250:679–682.

58. Brossay L, Jullien D, Cardell S et al. Mouse CD1 is mainly expressed on hemopoietic-derived cells. J Immunol. 1997;159:1216–1224.

59. Mosser DD, Duchaine J, Martin LH. Biochemical and developmental characterization of the murine cluster of differentiation 1 antigen. Immunology. 1991;73:298–303.

60. Ichimiya S, Kikuchi K, Matsuura A. Structural analysis of the rat homologue of CD1. Evidence for evolutionary conservation of the CD1D class and widespread transcription by rat cells. J Immunol. 1994;153:1112–1123.

61. Bahram S, Bresnahan M, Geraghty DE, Spies T. A second lineage of mammalian major histo-compatibility complex class I genes (see comments). Proc Natl Acad Sci USA. 1994;91: 6259–6263.

62. Groh V, Bahram S, Bauer S, Herman A, Beauchamp M, Spies T. Cell stress-regulated human major histocompatibility complex class 1 gene expressed in gastrointestinal epithelium. Proc Natl Acad Sci USA. 1996;93:12445–12450.

63. Zwirner NW, Fernandez-Vina MA, Stastny P. MICA, a new polymorphic HLA-related antigen, is expressed mainly by keratinocytes, endothelial cells, and monocytes. Immunogenetics. 1998;47:139–148.

64. Boismenu R, Havran WL. Modulation of epithelial cell growth by intraepithelial gamma delta T cells. Science. 1994;266:1253–1255.

5
Functional role of FcRn on intestinal epithelial cells

R. S. BLUMBERG, N. SIMISTER and W. LENCER

MUCOSAL IMMUNITY AND EPITHELIAL CELL BIOLOGY

The passage of antigens into or across the epithelial barrier is the first step in the complex sequence of events that lead to mucosal, and potentially systemic, immunity. As such, a major function of the epithelial cells lining the mucosal surfaces is the management of immune responses to luminal antigens. Luminal antigens are either totally excluded from transport across the epithelial barrier or are taken up for processing and presentation to subjacent lymphoid tissue within the epithelium and lamina propria. Antigen uptake is selective, the selectivity probably being determined by interactions between the physicochemical characteristics of the antigen, luminal factors (including mucus, enzymes, bacteria, etc.) and the attributes of the epithelium. Many specific details governing the uptake of luminal antigens, however, remain unknown. In addition, very few data are available on the influence of such antigen uptake on host biological responses, notably on the factors which control immune versus tolerance induction.

The microfold villous cell (M cell) and absorptive enterocyte (AEC) represent two discrete types of epithelial cells that are being increasingly recognized as playing a role in regulation of antigen uptake and consequent biological responses[1-3]. These cell types probably differentiate from a common crypt stem cell, possibly under the influence of intestinal lymphoid elements[4]. Although morphologically distinct, recent data suggest that both cell types may transmit antigen either in a nominal form through the ability of the M cell[5] and AEC[3] to function directly as an antigen-presenting cell or as an intact antigen via paracellular and transcellular pathways. These two cell types may differ, however, in the types of antigens that are targeted for selective uptake; the specific details of their function as an antigen presenting cell; the specific features of their potential paracellular and transcellular pathways; the types of lymphoid tissue with which they associate[2,6,7]; and the types of host biological responses that are elicited in response to antigen (e.g. immune induction versus tolerance, T_H1 versus T_H2 responses)[1].

Intact proteins may be able to breech the epithelial barrier by entering the transcellular pathway of absorptive intestinal epithelia[8–12]. This pathway is a part of a large vesicular compartment whose components are just being elucidated[13–15]. Useful in characterizing this pathway are the bacterial toxins (e.g., cholera toxin; CT) which co-opt the transcellular pathway defined in AEC model systems similar to the manner in which certain pathogens co-opt the M cell pathway for the purposes of tissue invasion[8–12]. Importantly, if this exists *in vivo*, the transcellular pathway across absorptive enterocytes is likely to be quantifiably large due to the vast surface area of the intestinal epithelial cell surface[16].

Evidence that transcytosis of intact macromolecules may affect the mucosal immune system is provided by studies on CT, which is arguably the most effective intestinal immunogen known and, in addition, is a powerful mucosal adjuvant for other proteins[17]. Unlike most other protein antigens, small (microgram) quantities of CT delivered orally elicit a specific secretory IgA and plasma IgG response in rodents[18] and humans[19]. In addition, and in contrast to the oral administration of other protein antigens, feeding of CT to mice does not lead to systemic tolerance, and can abrogate oral tolerance to a second unrelated protein antigen[18,19]. The mechanism by which oral CT acts as a strong immunogen and adjuvant for unrelated protein antigens remains incompletely defined. Available data indicate, however, that the B-subunit may act as a 'carrier' for unrelated antigens[20], and that small quantities of the holotoxin may have an essential 'enzymatic' effect on components of the intestinal epithelia or mucosal immune system, or both[20]. These effects depend on the ability of CT to enter or breech the epithelial barrier.

For a number of years, we have used the human intestinal T84 cell line to examine the cell biology of CT action on polarized cells. In nature, CT makes initial contact with ganglioside G_{M1} in the intestinal apical membrane and subsequently activates adenylate cyclase on the cytoplasmic surface of the basolateral membrane. This process takes 30–40 min, which corresponds to the time required for CT to enter the cell via apical endosomes and move to its site of action on the basolateral membrane by transcytosis[21]. We have obtained evidence that the toxin actually breeches the epithelial barrier by entering this pathway. Movement to the basolateral membrane, however, may not be direct. Both CT and LT appear to transit through Golgi cisternae and possibly ER en route to the basolateral cell surface[9]. We have introduced the term 'indirect transcytosis' to describe this process[9,12,21]. These data may explain the paradoxical observations that in nature, these large toxins, while restricted from transepithelial diffusion[6,11,22], are able to transmit signals to subepithelial cells of the mucosal immune system[23,24]. We have now turned our attention to whether IgG antigen complexes may also breech the epithelial barrier by binding the major histocompatibility complex (MHC) class I-related molecule, FcRn.

MHC CLASS I-RELATED MOLECULES

The basic structure of the MHC class I-related molecules reflects that encoded by the classical MHC class I or class Ia genes[25,26]. These genes are encoded within the MHC class I locus on human chromosome 6 and consist of the human leukocyte antigens (HLA)-A, B and C. The open reading frame of these genes consists of structural domains encoded by discrete exons that translate into an approximately 43–45 kDa glycoprotein containing three membrane distal domains (α1, α2 and α3), a transmembrane domain and a cytoplasmic tail. The most membrane-proximal ectodomain (α3) provides the major contact sites for the noncovalently associated, 12 kDa, β2-microglobulin (β_2m) molecule which is encoded outside the MHC class I locus[27]. β_2m association with the MHC class I heavy chain is a prerequisite for functional expression of the protein complex on the cell surface. The most membrane distal (α1 and α2) domains contribute to the formation of a series of β-pleated sheets bounded on the sides by two α-helices forming a groove consisting of a series of pockets capable of binding nine amino acid peptides for presentation to the T-cell receptor (TCR) of CD8-bearing T cells[26,28]. In making contact with the α-helices and peptide of the α1 and α2 domains, stabilized by interactions between CD8 on the T cell and clusters of amino acids within the α3 domain of the MHC class Ia molecule[29], the T cell is activated to fulfil its effector function, whether it be proliferation, cytolysis and/or cytokine secretion. Since the peptides contained within the groove of the MHC class Ia molecules are predominantly derived from the degradation of intracellular molecules by proteasomes, CD8$^+$ T cells are concerned with monitoring the intracellular health of MHC class Ia-bearing cells such as epithelial cells. Delivery of peptides to the MHC class Ia molecule/β_2m complex is assisted by ER-associated proteins, the transporter associated with antigen presentation (TAP) 1 and 2[30]. The vast majority of intraepithelial lymphocytes which reside above the basal lamina adjacent to the basolateral surface of the epithelial cells of the intestine are CD8$^+$, indicating the potential importance of this pathway in dealing with deleterious intracellular events as might occur during viral infection, cellular stress and neoplastic transformation – common events for epithelial cells[31]. The MHC class Ia genes display significant allelic polymorphism, due to variations in the amino acid composition of the α1 and α2 domains, each capable of binding a slightly different large array of nonameric peptides[25]. In addition, each individual is endowed with six different alleles predicting that the peptide binding capacity of an individual is enormous and well suited to dealing with unforeseen antigenic assaults. This pathway of antigen presentation is so efficient that microorganisms, especially viruses, have spent a great deal of evolutionary energy devising strategies to subvert this pathway, such as the expression of molecules which interfere with cell surface display of MHC class Ia molecules[32,33] and the generation of decoy molecules encoded by the genome of the pathogen which structurally resemble the MHC class I molecule[34]. The common gastrointestinal pathogens adenovirus[33] and cytomegalovirus[34] can accommodate each of these mechanisms of immune evasion, respectively.

The classical MHC class I molecules not only serve as ligands for the TCR of CD8-bearing lymphocytes capable of eliciting cytolysis but also for killer inhibitory receptors (KIR) on the cell surface of natural killer (NK) cells[35]. When ligated by MHC class Ia, KIRs transmit inhibitory signals to the NK cell bearing the KIR. As a consequence, MHC class Ia-bearing cells are not lysed. However, in the absence of MHC class I, as commonly occurs during neoplasia, including tumours of the epithelium[36], NK-mediated lysis can be induced by ligation of killer activating receptors (KAR) on the NK cell[30]. KIRs exhibit allelic specificity for MHC class Ia molecules and their binding can be affected by the nonameric peptides which specific MHC class Ia alleles present. Although NK cells are not a prominent component of the epithelial compartment, the increasing recognition that subsets of T cells, such as so-called natural T cells[37], are capable of expressing KIRs indicates the potential importance of this mechanism of cytolysis induction for T cells and the utility of these regulatory mechanisms at epithelial surfaces.

Human evolution has been so enamoured with the general utility of this MHC structure in performing discrete tasks of immunological recognition, that a plethora of human genes have developed from the ancestral MHC class I gene. These MHC class I-related genes, other than the classical class I genes, are called non-classical MHC class I molecules or MHC class Ib molecules[29]. The MHC class Ib molecules are either encoded by genes linked to the classical HLA-A, B and C genes on chromosome 6 (HLA-E, F, G, H and MHC class I chain-related gene A [MICA]) or by genes outside the MHC class I locus. These latter genes include the CD1 family and a gene of unknown function, MR1[38], on chromosome 1, the human homologue of the rodent neonatal Fc receptor for IgG [FcRn] on chromosome 19 and the zinc-α2-glycoprotein [ZAG], a soluble serum protein of unknown function[39] encoded on chromosome 7. In mouse species, an even larger number of MHC-linked genes is encoded within three genetic loci (Q, T and M) on chromosome 17[29].

These genes are considered MHC class I-like on the basis of similarities of exon–intron structure with MHC class Ia molecules (α1–α3 ectodomains, transmembrane domain, and cytoplasmic tail encoded by discrete exons) and dependence on β_2m for cell surface display and function, with some exceptions. CD1d (see below), MICA[40,41], and ZAG[39] can be expressed without β_2m, suggesting an element of independence from β_2m in function. However, the MHC class Ib molecule molecules differ in their general lack of polymorphism in the amino acid composition of their respective α1 and α2 domains such that they are considered to be nonpolymorphic[25,29]. This lack of polymorphism, with some exceptions (as described below) suggests that the α1 and α2 domains of the MHC class Ib molecules bind very distinct structures. This further suggests that they have evolved to specialize in binding distinct ligands. In conjunction with other structural information encoded in their primary amino acid sequences, their specific ligand recognition also correlates with specific types of functions as a consequence of ligand binding. Finally, the MHC class I molecules, in contrast to MHC class Ia molecules which are ubiquitously expressed, exhibit a restriction in their expression to specific cell types and tissues[29]. This is especially relevant to human epithelial cells, which appear to be a particularly prominent cell type that exhibits expression of several MHC class Ib molecules, including CD1, FcRn, HLA-G, MICA, and HLA-H.

CLASS I-RELATED MOLECULES EXPRESSED BY AECs

The human CD1 gene family consists of five genes, CD1A–E[42]. A gene product for CD1E has not yet been defined. (By convention, CD1 genes are represented by capital letters and CD1 proteins by lower case letters.) Nucleotide and deduced amino acid homologies predict that these gene products segregate into two groups: CD1a–c and CD1d. CD1A–C homologues are not present in mice and rats, which do, however, have CD1D homologues highly related to human CD1D. Whereas CD1a–c are expressed by thymocytes and certain professional antigen-presenting cells such as B lymphocytes, Langerhans cells of the skin and activated monocytes, CD1d is expressed by thymocytes, B cells, hepatocytes and, importantly, epithelial cells in a wide variety of organs. CD1b and c appear to function in the presentation of exogenous and, possibly, endogenous lipid antigens to T cells[43]. In general, these CD1 restricted, lipid responsive T cells, are either CD8+ or lack CD4 and CD8 (double negative). The response of double negative cells suggests either no need for co-receptor function in TCR binding or the use of another novel, not yet described, co-receptor molecule. The antigen presenting pathway by which CD1b and c acquire lipid-related antigens is TAP independent and overlaps with that utilized by MHC class II molecules[44]. The MHC class II homologies include similarities in the nucleotide sequence within the $\alpha 3$ domain and the presence of a YXXZ motif (tyrosine-amino acid-amino acid-hydrophobic amino acid) in the cytoplasmic tail that controls protein movement to an endocytic compartment where MHC class II processing occurs. CD1d shares the YXXZ motif with CD1b and c and exhibits a narrow but deep hydrophobic pocket[45], suggesting a similar but unproven capability of binding and presenting exogenous and/or endogenous lipid antigens to T cells generated by a processing pathway that bisects MHC class II. In contrast to MHC class Ia molecules, however, CD1d is clearly stable in the absence of β_2m in transfected model systems and possibly in the absence of antigen, raising the possibility for other immunoregulatory functions of CD1d[46]. This may be especially relevant to CD1d function in epithelial cells. In AECs, CD1d transcription occurs within the lower zones of the crypt epithelium with protein expression predominantly on IECs within the upper crypts and villi[47]. Moreover, AEC CD1d is expressed as both a β_2m-associated, fully glycosylated molecule (R. S. Blumberg, unpublished observations) and as a form that is independent of β_2m and carbohydrate side chain modification[46]. CD8+ T cells recognize CD1d expressed on the cell surface of AECs[47]. Fully glycosylated, β_2m-associated CD1d appears to be a ligand for an invariant TCR-α chain expressed on double negative human T cells bearing NKR-P1A, a KIR[48]. Upon CD1d ligation, these double negative T cells secrete high quantities of γ-interferon and interleukin-4 suggesting an important immunoregulatory function. Whether epithelial cell CD1d performs a similar immunoregulatory function for local T cell functions in the sampling of luminal bacterial antigens for presentation to local T cells or other functions remains to be established[49].

The trophoblastic epithelium of human placenta, which is in direct contact with maternal tissues, lacks classical MHC class I and class II (HLA-DR, DP, and DQ) proteins, making it susceptible to lysis by maternal NK cells which are present in large numbers in human decidua. This problem may be remedied by the expression of HLA-G on syncytiotrophoblast. Although considered a non-classical MHC class I molecule that is linked to the MHC locus on chromosome 6, HLA-G exhibits a limited amount of allelic polymorphism in the $\alpha 1$ and $\alpha 2$ domains, exhibits prerequisite dependency on β_2m and contains $\alpha 1$ and $\alpha 2$

domains that fold into a groove competent to bind nonameric peptides[50]. Recent evidence also suggests that HLA-G is a relatively public receptor for KIRs specific for HLA-C[51]. Given the possibility that HLA-G is more widely expressed than originally believed, including possibly on other epithelial surfaces, it should be considered that these mechanisms of NK inhibition may be more generally applicable.

MICA is a recently described, MHC-linked, class Ib molecule that appears to exhibit relatively restricted expression to intestinal epithelium and, like CD1d, is somewhat indifferent to β_2m for cell surface expression[40,41]. Although the function of MICA remains unknown, a clue may be provided by the promoter region which exhibits functional heat shock response elements[41]. This suggests a possible functional role as a cell surface flag which provides a danger signal as a consequence of some ubiquitous stress signal. This would predict that local T cells expressing ligands for MICA may possibly be responsible for eliciting a cellular response to epithelial cell injury.

The newest member of the MHC class Ib group relevant to epithelial biology is the recently described HLA-H gene product, which has recently been renamed Hfe[52]. The *Hfe* gene product is widely expressed through the gastrointestinal epithelium with most prominent expression in the crypts of the small intestine[53]. Mutations of this protein have been linked to the iron overload disorder, haemochromatosis. Almost all haemochromatosis subjects manifest a cystine 282 $\rightarrow$ tyrosine (C282Y) mutation which disrupts association of Hfe with β_2m and, consequently, cell surface expression of this molecule, consistent with the observation that β_2m-deficient mice exhibit iron overload[54]. Of note, the *Hfe* gene also contains iron response elements. The specific relationship of this allelic variant to iron transport is unknown but may lie through intermolecular associations with recently described iron transporters. These iron transporters are multiple membrane spanners[58]. Interestingly, similar molecules, such as CD82, have been shown to associate with MHC class Ia molecules[56]. This raises the possibility that these newly described iron transporters may coassociate with Hfe/β_2m to somehow regulate intracellular iron levels. The specific ligand of Hfe remains to be determined and its crystal structure is presently unknown.

THE FcRn AND TRANSCYTOSIS OF IgG

The final MHC class I-related molecule expressed by AECs is the FcRn. It remains uncertain whether there is a single common transcellular pathway among all intestinal epithelial cell types or multiple pathways coupled to distinct cell surface receptors[12,14]. One potential transcellular pathway across absorptive enterocytes is related to the receptor–ligand interaction between an MHC class I-related Fc receptor and IgG[19,57,58]. This receptor, the neonatal Fc receptor (or FcRn) has been cloned from the rat[58] and mouse[59]. The designation as neonatal captures the historical connotation which suggests that expression of this molecule is limited to the neonatal period of life. This molecule has significant structural similarities to major histocompatibility complex class I molecules including the prerequisite functional relationship with β_2m[60,61]. In mice made deficient in β_2m expression by homologous recombination (β_2m$^{-/-}$ mice), the

FcRn is not expressed on the cell surface and is non-functional. The rodent FcRn preferentially binds IgG at acidic pH (pH < 6.5)[62,63]. This pH dependency of ligand binding may account for the vectorial transport (lumen to serosa) and passive acquisition of maternal IgG and IgG–immune complexes in the neonatal rodent (rats and mice)[64,65]. For example, it is currently thought that on the apical surface of the neonatal animal, the Fc portion of IgG is bound to the enterocyte receptor at the relatively acidic pH presumed to be present in the immediate microenvironment of the intestinal apical membrane (lumen). Following transcytosis to the basolateral plasma membrane, discharge of the immunoglobulin occurs at the relatively neutral pH of the interstitial fluids (in the lamina propria). The rodent neonatal Fc receptor (FcRn) therefore could be responsible for delivery of maternal IgG and IgG–immune complexes to the tissue spaces of the interstition[58,59,61–64,66]. As such, FcRn–IgG transport may be responsible for the passive acquisition of IgG during this period, and for stimulation of the naive immune system by delivery of luminal antigens[60].

In humans, maternal IgG is actively transported across the placenta. The receptor responsible for this transport has been sought for many years. Several IgG-binding proteins have been isolated from placenta. FcγRII was detected in placental endothelium[67] and FcγRIII in syncytiotrophoblasts[68]. Both of these receptors, however, showed a relatively low affinity for monomeric IgG. Recently, the isolation from placenta of a cDNA encoding a human homologue of the rat and mouse enterocyte receptor for IgG was reported by Simister and colleagues[69]. This Fc receptor for IgG may be responsible for the transport of maternal IgG to the human fetus (and possibly to the human neonate via putative transport across the intestine, see below), as the molecule is highly homologous over its open reading frame with the rat FcRn sequence (69% nucleotide identity and 65% predicted amino acid identity). As such, this so called passive immunization of the human fetus may now become better understood. In addition, the human FcRn was shown to be expressed in both fetal and neonatal intestinal epithelial cells. In the former case, available data indicate that the molecule may be functional[70].

The general paradigm for FcRn expression and function has been that it is limited to the neonatal period of life in mammals for the passive acquisition of IgG and/or IgG–antigen complexes. As described below, in recent work from our laboratories evidence has been provided that FcRn is expressed in adult human intestine, and that the receptor is functional. These data imply that FcRn may mediate transport of IgG, IgG–immune complexes, or both across the intestinal barrier *in vivo*.

Expression of FcRn in adult rodents

We have recently shown that the rat homologue of the FcRn is functionally expressed beyond the neonatal period on the canalicular cell surface of adult rat hepatocytes[77]. This report represented the first description of functional FcRn on an adult epithelial surface. We have also been able to detect evidence of FcRn transcription in adult rat lung, small intestine and large intestine by reverse transcriptase-polymerase chain reaction (RT-PCR) amplification of mRNA derived from these tissues. Cloning and sequencing of these PCR amplification products proved that they were indeed derived from the FcRn gene (data not shown). This transcription is, however, significantly less than that observed during neonatal rat life based upon Northern blot analysis[58]. Similar observations have also recently been made by Ward and colleagues in adult mice[72]. Using a quantitative RT-PCR assay, they estimated that transcription was 1000-fold lower in adult life yet functionally significant based upon the abnormally short serum half-life of IgG in $\beta_2 m^{-/-}$ mice[72]. Thus, FcRn continues to be expressed in adult rats and mice albeit at lower levels than in the neonate, and probably remains functional, making these species potential experimental models. This expression may not only be limited to AECs but also to endothelial cells which may function in the regulation of IgG levels in the host[73].

Expression of FcRn in adult humans

More recently, we have shown that the adult human AEC surface probably also represents an important site of FcRn expression. Adult human intestinal epithelial cells[74] as well as the intestinal epithelial cell lines CaCo-2, HT29 and T84 express significant levels of FcRn transcript by Northern blotting of total cellular RNA. Moreover, cloning and sequencing of these intestinal transcripts by RT-PCR amplification have shown that they are identical to the previously published sequences obtained from human placenta[74]. FcRn protein can also be identified by Western blotting of protein derived from purified human small and large intestinal epithelial cells as well as the intestinal epithelial cell lines CaCo-2, the CL19A clone of HT29 and T84 cells. Interestingly, whereas the molecular weight identified in small intestine and colon is approximately 40 kDa, the intestinal epithelial cell tumour lines express two forms (40 and 48 kDa; data not shown). Whether these represent posttranslational modifications or different structural, and possibly functionally distinct, isoforms remains to be determined. Similarly, in other studies, human FcRn protein has been detected in adult small intestinal epithelial cells by immunohistological analysis using an affinity purified anti-peptide antibody[74]. Thus, the FcRn is abundantly expressed at moderately high levels in AECs of adult humans.

Functional expression of human FcRn *in vitro*

Studies in epithelial cell lines suggest that the FcRn expressed by human intestinal epithelial cells is probably functional. Using normal human IgG coupled to Sepharose beads, a 12 kDa protein (consistent with the mobility of $\beta_2 m$) and a 40 kDa protein (consistent with the mobility of FcRn) can be immunoprecipitated from lysates of human HT29, T84, and CaCo2 cells containing cell surface proteins previously labelled with biotin. The immunoprecipitations of these bands are specific and display pH dependency characteristic of ligand binding to human FcRn (stronger at pH 6 and weaker at pH 8). Similarly, human IgG coupled to Sepharose beads can immunoprecipitate a $\beta_2 m$-associated 40 kDa protein from metabolically labelled CaCo2 cells at pH 6.0 but not pH 8.0.

To further show that intact protein (IgG) is transported across T84 monolayers, we have examined the transepithelial flux of biotin-labelled IgG (which is detected by SDS-PAGE and avidin blot). When biotin-labelled IgG is added to either the apical or basolateral reservoire, intact IgG heavy and light chains can be detected in the contralateral basolateral reservoirs at 37°C but not at 4°C, indicating that transport of IgG occurs via the transcellular but not the paracellular route. These studies further suggest that IgG transport is bidirectional and specific since transport is not observed for either chicken IgY or horseradish peroxidase which do not bind FcRn.

To determine whether this pathway is functional *in vivo*, we have further utilized wild-type (wt) β_2m$^{-/-}$ mice to examine the possibility that transport of luminal antigens across the epithelial barrier via IgG–FcRn transcytosis may affect the mucosal immune system. In preliminary experiments, we orally immunized wt or β_2m$^{-/-}$ mice with rhodamine–IgG or rhodamine-labelled cholera toxin B-subunit (CTB) as a positive control. All animals received cholera holotoxin as adjuvant. After 3 doses separated by 10 days, we assayed serum and bile for anti-rhodamine IgG antibodies. All wt mice receiving rhodamine-labelled cholera toxin B-subunit developed anti-rhodamine antibodies in serum and bile. The response of wt mice to rhodamine-labelled IgG was less strong than the CTB transfected animals but clearly more positive than the response of the β_2m$^{-/-}$ mice given the same antigen. Importantly, control experiments showed that β_2m$^{-/-}$ mice responded to rhodamine-labelled CTB subunit as well as wt animals, given recent results that serum IgG in β_2m$^{-/-}$ mice exhibited a shorter half-life than wt animals[72,73].

SUMMARY

A major function of the epithelial cells lining the mucosal surface of the intestine (and respiratory and genitourinary tracts) lies in the management of immune responses to luminal antigens. Luminal antigens are normally excluded from transport across the intestinal barrier. The microvillous cell (M cell) and absorptive enterocyte (AEC) represent two distinct cell types which may transport antigens into the subepithelial space by endocytosis and vesicular traffic in a process termed transcytosis. Such transport of antigen across the M cell is thought to play a key role in the inductive immune response of the mucosal immune system. We have recently found that adult human and rodent intestinal AEC express the major histocompatibility complex class I-related neonatal Fc receptor for IgG (FcRn). Murine FcRn mediates transport of IgG across the intestine of suckling rodents by entering a basolaterally directed transcytotic pathway, and human FcRn is presumed to mediate maternal–fetal transcytosis of IgG across the placenta. Whether FcRn can function in adult AECs to transport IgG, IgG-immune complexes, or both across the intestine, and whether such transport may regulate the host immune response to luminal antigen remain undefined. We are pursuing a model in which the mucosal immune response to luminal antigens depends in part on the bidirectional movement of intact IgG, or IgG-immune complexes, or both across intestinal epithelium by transcytosis.

References

1. Neutra MR, Frey A, Kraehenbuhl J-P. Epithelial M-cells: gateways for mucosal infection and immunization. Cell. 1996;43:389–390.
2. Kraehenbuhl J-P, Neutra MR. Molecular and cellular basis of immune protection of mucosal surfaces. Physiol Rev. 1992;72:853–880.
3. Mayer L. Antigen presentation in the intestine. Curr Opin Gastroenterol. 1991;7:446–449.
4. Kernéis C, Bogdanova A, Kraehenbuhl J-P, Pringault E. Conversion by Peyer's patch lymphocytes of human enterocytes into M cells that transport bacteria. Science. 1997;277: 949–952.
5. Allan CH, Mendrick DL, Trier JS. Rat intestinal M cells contain acidic endosomal-lysosomal compartments and express class II major histocompatibility complex determinants. Gastroenterology. 1993;104:698–708.
6. Madara JL. Epithelia: biologic principles of organization. In: Yamada T, Alpers DH, Owyang C, Powell DW, Silverstein FE (eds). Textbook of Gastroenterology. Philadelphia: JB Lippincott Co., 1991:102–118.
7. Neutra MR, Michetti P, Kraehenbuhl J-P. Secretory immunoglobulin A: induction, biogenesis, and function. In: Johnson LR (ed.) Physiology of the Gastrointestinal Tract. New York: Raven Press, 1994:685–708.
8. Lencer WI, Brown D, Ausiello DA, Verkman AS. Endocytosis of water channels in rat kidney: cell specificity and correlation with in vivo antidiuresis. Am J Physiol. 1990;259:C920–C932.
9. Lencer WI, Constable C, Moe S et al. Targeting of cholera toxin and E. coli heat labile toxin in polarized epithelia: role of C-terminal KDEL. J Cell Biol. 1995;131:951–962.
10. Lencer WI, de Almeida JB, Moe S, Stow JL, Ausiello DA, Madera JL. Entry of cholera toxin into polarized human intestinal epithelial cells: identification of an early brefeldin A sensitive event required for A1-peptide generation. J Clin Invest. 1993;92:2941–2951.
11. Lencer WI, Delp C, Neutra MR, Madara JL. Mechanism of cholera toxin action on a polarized human epithelial cell line: role of vesicular traffic. J Cell Biol. 1992;117: 1197–1209.
12. Lencer WI, Moe S, Rufo PA, Madara JL. Transcytosis of cholera toxin subunits across model human intestinal epithelia. Proc Natl Acad Sci USA. 1995;92:10094–10098.
13. Mostov KE, Simister NE. Transcytosis. Cell. 1985;43:389–390.
14. Mostov KE. Transepithelial transport of immunoglobulins. Annu Rev Immunol. 1994;12:63–84.
15. Mostov K, Apodaca G, Aroeti B, Okamoto C. Plasma membrane protein sorting in polarized epithelial cells. J Cell Biol. 1992;116:577–583.
16. Stafford J, Dharmsathaphorn K, Carlson S. Structural analysis of a human intestinal epithelial cell line. Gastroenterology. 1987;92:1133–1145.
17. Elson CO, Ealing W. Genetic control of the murine immune response to cholera toxin. J Immunol. 1985;135:930–932.
18. Elson CO, Ealing W. Generalized systemic and mucosal immunity in mice after mucosal stimulation with cholera toxin. J Immunol. 1984;132:2736–2741.
19. Dertzbaugh NM T, Elson CO. Cholera toxin as a mucosal adjuvant. In: Spriggs DR, Koff WC (eds). Topics in Vaccine Adjuvant Research. Boca Raton, FL: CRC Press, 1990:119–131.
20. Czerkinsky C, Russell MW, Lycke N, Lindblad M, Holmgren J. Oral administration of a streptococcal antigen coupled to cholera toxin B subunit evokes strong antibody responses in salivary glands and extramucosal tissues. Infect Immun. 1989;57:1072–1077.
21. Lencer WI, Strohmeier G, Moe S, Carlson SL, Constable CT, Madara JL. Signal transduction by cholera toxin: processing in vesicular compartments does not require acidification. Am J Physiol. 1995;269:G548–G557.
22. Madara JL. Loosening tight junctions. J Clin Invest. 1989;83:1089–1094.
23. Cassuto J, Jodal M, Lundgren O. On the role of intramural nerves in the pathogenesis of cholera toxin-induced intestinal secretion. Scand J Gastroenterol. 1981;16:377–384.
24. Holmgren J, Lycke N, Czerkinsky C. Cholera toxin and cholera B subunit as oral-mucosal adjuvant and antigen vector systems. Vaccine 1993;11:1179–1184.
25. Parham P. The rise and fall of great class I genes. Semin Immunol. 1994;6:373–382.
26. Engelhard VH. Structure of peptides associated with MHC class I molecules. Curr Opin Immunol. 1994;6:13–23.

27. Tysoe-Calnon A, Grundy JE, Perkins SJ. Molecular comparisons of the β_2-microglobulin-binding site in class I major-histocompatibility-complex α-chains and proteins of related sequences. Biochem J. 1991;277:359–369.
28. Bjorkman PJ, Saper MA, Samraoui B, Bennett WS, Strominger JL, Wiley DC. Structure of the human class I histocompatibility antigen. HLA-A2. Nature. 1987;329:506–518.
29. Blumberg RS, Simister N, Christ AD, Israel EJ, Colgan SP, Balk SP. MHC-like molecules on mucosal epithelial cells. In: Kagnoff MF, Kiyono H (eds). Essentials of Mucosal Immunology. San Diego: Academic Press, 1996:85–99.
30. Germain RN. MHC-dependent antigen processing and peptide presentation: providing ligands for T lymphocyte activation. Cell. 1994;76:287–299.
31. Blumberg RS, Balk SP. Intraepithelial lymphocytes and their recognition of non-classical MHC molecules. Int Rev Immunol. 1994;11:15–30.
32. Burgert H-G, Kvist S. The E3/19K protein of adenovirus type 2 binds to the domains of histocompatibility antigens required for CTL recognition. EMBO J. 1987;6:2019–2026.
33. Hill AB, Barnett BC, McMichael AJ, McGeoch DJ. HLA Class I molecules are not transported to the cell surface in cells infected with Herpes simplex virus types 1 and 2. J Immunol. 1994;152:2736–2741.
34. Browne H, Smith G, Beck S, Minson T. A complex between the MHC class I homologue encoded by human cytomegalovirus and b$_2$ microglobulin. Nature. 1990;346:770–772.
35. Moretta A, Biassoni R, Bottino C et al. Major histocompatibility complex class I-specific receptors on human natural killer and T lymphocytes. In: Parham P (ed.) Immunological Reviews. Copenhagen: Munksgaard, 1997:105–117.
36. Bicknell DC, Rowan A, Bodmer WF. β_2-microglobulin gene mutations: a study of established colorectal cell lines and fresh tumors. Proc Natl Acad Sci USA. 1994;91:4751–4755.
37. MacDonald HR. NK1.1$^+$ T cell receptor-α/β^+ cells: new clues to their origin, specificity, and function. Curr Opin Immunol. 1995;7:633–638.
38. Hashimoto K, Hirai M, Kurosawa Y. A gene outside the human MHC related to classical HAL class I genes. Science. 1995;269:693–695.
39. Sánchez LM, López-Orín C, Bjorkman PJ. Biochemical characterization and crystallization of human Zn-a$_2$-glycoprotein, a soluble class I major histocompatibility complex homolog. Proc Natl Acad Sci USA. 1997;94:46216–4630.
40. Bahram S, Bresnahan M, Geraghty DE, Spies T. A second lineage of mammalian major histocompatibility complex class I genes. Proc Natl Acad Sci USA. 1994;91:6259–6263.
41. Groh V, Bahram S, Bauer S, Herman A, Beauchamp M, Spies T. Cell stress-related human major histocompatibility complex class I gene expressed in gastrointestinal epithelium. Proc Natl Acad Sci USA. 1996;93:12445–12450.
42. Blumberg RS, Gerdes D, Chott A, Porcelli SA, Balk SP. Structure and function of the CD1 family of MHC-like cell surface proteins. In: Möller G (ed.) Immunological Reviews. Copenhagen: Munksgaard, 1995:1–29.
43. Jullien D, Stenger S, Ernst WA, Modlin RL. CD1 presentation of microbial nonpeptide antigens to T cells. J Clin Invest. 1997;99:2071–2074.
44. Sugita M, Jackman RM, van Donselaar E et al. Cytoplasmic tail-dependent localization of CD1b antigen-presenting molecules to MIICs. Science. 1996;273:349–352.
45. Zang Z-H, Castaño AR, Segelke BW, Sturn EA, Peterson PA, Wilson IA. Crystal structure of mouse CD1: an MHC-like fold with a large hydrophobic binding groove. Science. 1997;277:339–345.
46. Balk SP, Burke S, Polischuk JE et al. β_2-microglobulin-independent MHC class 1b molecule expressed by human intestinal epithelium. Science. 1994;265:259–262.
47. Kasai K, Matsuura A, Kikuchi K, Hashimoto Y, Ichimiya S. Localization of rat CD1 transcripts and protein in rat – an analysis of rat CD1 expression by in situ hybridization and immuno-histochemistry. Clin Exp Immunol. 1997;109:317–322.
48. Exley M, Garcia J, Balk SP, Porcelli S. Requirements for CD1d recognition by human invariant Vα24$^+$ CD4$^-$ CD8$^-$ T cells. J Exp Med. 1997;186:1–11.
49. Blumberg RS, Colgan SP, Balk SP. CD1d: outside-in antigen presentation in the intestinal epithelium? Clin Exp Immunol. 1997;109:223–225.
50. Lee N, Malacko AR, Ishitani A et al. The membrane-bound and soluble forms of HLA-G bind identical sets of endogenous peptides but differ with respect to TAP association. Immunology. 1995;3:591–600.

51. Pazmany L, Mandelboim O, Valés-Gómez M, Davis DM, Reyburn HT, Strominger JL. Protection from natural killer cell-mediated lysis by HLA-G expression on target cells. Science. 1996;274:792–795.
52. Feder JN, Gnirke A, Thomas W et al. A novel MHC class I-like gene is mutated in patients with hereditary haemochromatosis. Nature Genet. 1996;13:399–408.
53. Parkkila S, Waheed A, Britton RS et al. Immunohistochemistry of HLA-H, the protein defective in patients with hereditary hemochromatosis, reveals unique pattern of expression in gastrointestinal tract. Proc Natl Acad Sci USA. 1997;94:2534–2539.
54. Feder JN, Tsuchihashi Z, Irrinki A et al. The hemochromatosis founder mutation in HLA-H disrupts β2-microglobulin interaction and cell surface expression. J Biol Chem. 1997;272: 14025–14028.
55. Gunshin H, Mackenzie B, Berger UV et al. Cloning and characterization of a mammalian proton-coupled metal-ion transporter. Nature. 1997;388:482–488.
56. Lagaudrière-Gesbert C, Lebel-Binay S, Wiertz E, Ploegh HL, Fradelizi D, Conjeaud H. The tetraspanin protein CD82 associates with both free HLA class I heavy chain and heterodimeric β_2-microglobulin complexes. J Immunol. 1997;158:2790–2797.
57. Abrahamson DR, Powers A, Rodewald R. Intestinal absorption of immune complexes by neonatal rats: transfer of antigen from mother to young. Science. 1979;206:567–569.
58. Rodewald R, Kraehenbuhl J-P. Receptor-mediated transport of IgG. J Cell Biol. 1984;99: 159S–164S.
59. Rodewald R. Intestinal transport of antibodies in the newborn rat. J Cell Biol. 1973;58:189–211.
60. Israel EJ, Patel VK, Taylor SF, Marshak-Rothstein A, Simister NE. Requirement for a β2-microglobulin-associated Fc receptor for acquisition of maternal IgG by fetal and neonatal mice. J Immunol. 1995;154:6246–6251.
61. Zijlstra M, Bix M, Simister NE, Loring JM, Raulet DH, Jaenisch R. β2-microglobulin deficient mice lack CD4$^-$8$^+$ cytolytic T cells. Nature. 1990;344:742–746.
62. Jones EA, Waldman TA. The mechanism of intestinal uptake and transcellular transport of IgG in the neonatal rat. J Clin Invest. 1972;51:2916–2927.
63. Rodewald R. pH-dependent binding of immunoglobulins to intestinal cells of the neonatal rat. J Cell Biol. 1976;71:666–670.
64. Abrahamson DR, Rodewald R. Evidence for sorting of endocytic vesicle contents during the receptor-mediated transport of IgG across the newborn rat intestine. J Cell Biol. 1981;91: 270–280.
65. Martin MG, Wu V, Ohning G, Wong H, Walsh JH. Parenterally or enterally administered anti-somatostatin antibody induce increased gastrin in suckling rats. Am J Physiol. 1994;29: G417–G424.
66. Rodewald R. Distribution of immunoglobulin G receptors in the small intestine of the young rat. J Cell Biol. 1980;85:18–32.
67. Kristoffersen EK, Ulvestad E, Vedeler CA, Matre R. Fcγ receptor heterogeneity in the human placenta. Scand J Immunol. 1990;32:561–565.
68. Wainwright SD, Holmes CH. Distribution of Fcγ receptors on trophoblast during human placental development: an immunohistochemical and immunoblotting study. Immunology. 1993;80:343–340.
69. Story CM, Mikulska JE, Simister NE. A major histocompatibility complex class I-like Fc receptor cloned from human placenta: possible role in transfer of Immunoglobulin G from mother to fetus. J Exp Med. 1994;180:2377–2381.
70. Israel EJ, Simister N, Freiber E, Caplan A, Walker WA. Immunoglobulin G binding sites on the human foetal intestine: a possible mechanism for the passive transfer of immunity from mother to infant. Immunology. 1993;79:77–81.
71. Blumberg RS, Koss T, Story CM et al. A major histocompatibility complex class I-related Fc receptor for IgG on rat hepatocytes. J Clin Invest. 1995;95:2397–2402.
72. Ghetie V, Hubbard JG, Kim J-K, Tsen M-F, Lee Y, Ward ES. Abnormally short serum half-lives of IgG in β2-microglobulin-deficient mice. Eur J Immunol. 1996;26:690–696.
73. Junghans RP. Finally! The Branbell receptor (FcRB): mediator of transmission of immunity and protection from catabolism for IgG. Immunol Res. 1997;16:29–57.
74. Israel EJ, Taylor S, Wu Z et al. Expression of the neonatal Fc receptor, FcRn, on human intestinal epithelial cells. Immunology. 1997;92:69–74.

6
The intestinal epithelial cell proinflammatory programme: integral role of human intestinal epithelial cells in innate and acquired mucosal immunity

M. F. KAGNOFF and L. ECKMANN

Intestinal mucosal surfaces are a common route of entry of microbial pathogens into the host. Epithelial cells that line the intestinal mucosa form an important mechanical barrier that separates the host's internal milieu from the external environment. The apical surface of the intestinal epithelium is bathed in nutrients essential for host survival, but concurrently encounters commensal and pathogenic microbes. Many microbes, including commensals in the large bowel, do not invade epithelial cells. However, for those microbial pathogens that invade, epithelial cells are the first site of contact with the host. The host's mucosal response to infection with many pathogenic microbes is characterized by an acute inflammatory response with a rapid influx of neutrophils, monocytes, and other inflammatory cells that play a significant role in host defence and microbial destruction.

Recent studies have clearly shown the integral role that intestinal epithelial cells play in generating and transmitting signals between microbial pathogens and adjacent and underlying cells in the intestinal mucosa. This has led to the concept of epithelial cells as an integral component of a communications network that involves interactions between epithelial cells, luminal microbes and host immune and inflammatory cells (Fig. 1).

This chapter focuses on the repertoire of mediators produced by human intestinal epithelial cells in response to microbial infection and presents data that strengthen the concept that intestinal epithelial cells act as sensors of the intestinal microflora and provide signals to the host that initiate and regulate key aspects of mucosal inflammatory and immune responses. Although, by virtue of its brevity and focus, we describe mainly work from this laboratory, we also recognize at the outset the many significant contributions of other investigators to the field.

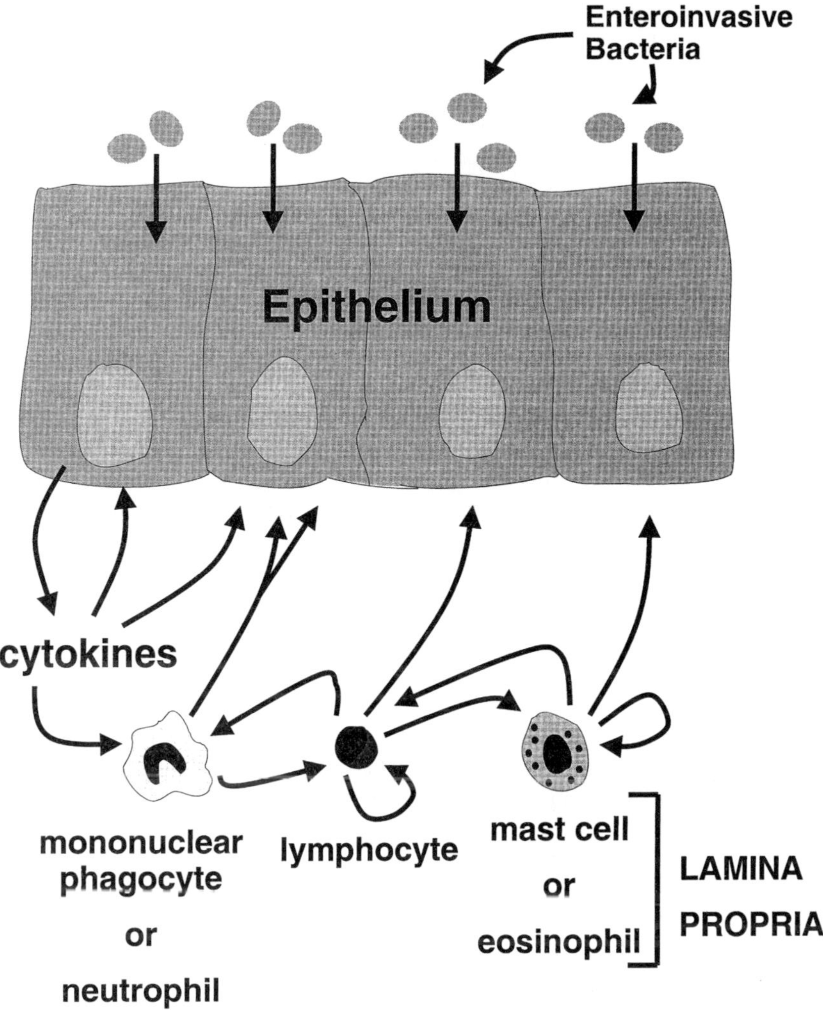

Figure 1 Epithelial cells as a component of a communications network. Infection of human colon epithelial cells with enteroinvasive bacteria results in the up-regulated expression of a proinflammatory gene programme, which is characterized in part by the increased production and release of proinflammatory cytokines. These cytokines can result in the activation and chemo-attraction of adjacent and underlying immune and inflammatory cells in the lamina propria, which, in turn, also can release mediators with autocrine and paracrine activities

MODEL SYSTEMS TO STUDY EPITHELIAL CELL–MICROBIAL INTERACTIONS

Epithelial cell interactions with intestinal bacterial and parasitic microbes can be studied using complementary *in vitro* and *in vivo* systems, as demonstrated by several reports from this laboratory[1-8]. The simplest approach utilizes cultured monolayers of long-term human intestinal epithelial cell lines to ask fundamental questions regarding epithelial cell responses. Transformed cell lines are used, since non-transformed human epithelial cell lines are not readily available[1-9]. In order to identify conserved functions that are independent of the transformation process, and have an *in vivo* correlate, it is essential that studies are performed in several different cell lines. Moreover, when interpreting data from such systems, it is important to recognize differences in the origin and receptor repertoire of the different cell lines, and differences among sublines of cells that have been maintained in different laboratories for long periods.

Epithelial cells that line the mucosa are polarized *in vivo* and, consequently, have structural and functional differences in their apical and basolateral domains. The availability of human intestinal epithelial cell lines that can be grown as polarized monolayers on microporous supports in transwell culture (i.e., the 'reductionist gut') has provided a second important model for studies of epithelial microbial interactions since one can assess the polarity of the epithelial cell response (e.g. the polarized secretion of chemokines in the physiological basolateral direction)[1,4,8-10].

Freshly isolated human intestinal epithelial cells can be obtained reasonably pure and with acceptable short-term viability. Such cells are suitable for addressing a limited number of questions regarding the regulated expression of proinflammatory mediators. Nonetheless, such cells currently have limited usefulness in studies of host–microbial interactions since they are viable for only short periods of time (24–48 h), proinflammatory genes often are activated by the manipulations associated with their isolation and, thus far, such cells have not been grown as polarized epithelial monolayers with functional tight junctions[2,7,9].

Human fetal intestinal xenografts implanted subcutaneously onto the backs of immunodeficient mice[11] provide a powerful tool for examining epithelial cell–microbe interactions[4,5,8,12,13]. By 10–12 weeks after transplantation, these xenografts contain an epithelium that is strictly of human origin and the xenograft lumen can be infected with pathogenic bacteria and parasites. Importantly, the earliest epithelial cell events that follow acute infection with enteric pathogens can be easily studied, whereas this is rarely possible in patients. Finally, mice with targeted gene 'knock outs' can provide useful models to study mucosal infection, although there can be fundamental differences in human and mouse pathogens and the host response to those pathogens.

THE EPITHELIAL CELL PROINFLAMMATORY PROGRAMME

Proinflammatory cytokines expressed by human intestinal epithelial cells

The potential of intestinal epithelial cells to activate or regulate mucosal inflammation has been studied extensively using conditions that maximally stimulate a set of epithelial cell responses related to the initiation or maintenance of mucosal inflammation (e.g. stimulation with agonists such as tumour necrosis factor-α (TNF-α) or interleukin-1 (IL-1), infection with invasive bacteria). Whereas the proinflammatory agonists TNF-α and IL-1 stimulate epithelial cells mainly via receptors on the basolateral membrane, invasive bacteria like *Salmonella* activate epithelial cell responses following entry through the apical cell membrane[1,14].

Stimulation of human intestinal epithelial cells with TNF-α or IL-1, or infection with enteroinvasive bacteria such as *Salmonella*, results in the increased expression and secretion of an array of cytokines with chemoattractant and proinflammatory activities[1,2,7,9]. Many of these cytokines (e.g. IL-8, GROα, GROβ, GROγ, ENA-78 and IP-10) belong to the C-X-C family of chemokines and, except for IP-10, are characterized by their ability to chemoattract and activate neutrophils. This suggests that an important function of intestinal epithelial cells is to initiate the mucosal influx of neutrophils, a hallmark of the initial acute inflammatory response. Activated human colon epithelial cells also produce a limited array of C-C chemokines, especially MCP-1, although MIP-1β, MIP-α, and RANTES are also expressed at lower levels[2,7,15]. C-C chemokines, in contrast to the C-X-C chemokines, act as chemoattractants of monocytes/macrophages, eosinophils and subpopulations of T cells. This suggests that activated intestinal epithelial cells, in addition to providing signals associated with an acute influx of PMN, may play a role in orchestrating the initiation of mucosal inflammatory and immune responses in which a number of different immune and inflammatory cell types participate.

In addition to the chemokines, agonist-stimulated (e.g. TNF-α, IL-1) or bacteria-infected human intestinal epithelial cells can express and secrete other proinflammatory cytokines, including TNF-α and GM-CSF, although secretion of those cytokines is lower than that of the major chemokines[2,7]. In contrast to the expression of proinflammatory cytokines, intestinal epithelial cells do not appear to express cytokines that are more commonly associated with antigen-specific acquired immune responses (e.g. IL-2, IL-4, IL-5, IL-12 p40, or interferon-γ (IFN-γ))[2,9]. Thus, the array of cytokines produced by intestinal epithelial cells suggests a more major role in initiating and regulating the host's innate mucosal inflammatory response than in antigen-specific immunity. Nonetheless, epithelial cells can probably also act as a bridge between the activation of innate and acquired mucosal immune responses. This may occur, for example, through the direct epithelial cell delivery and/or presentation of antigen to adjacent and underlying lymphoid cells[16] or dendritic cells in the intestinal mucosa or indirectly by the actions of epithelial cell cytokines and other mediators on adjacent mucosal lymphoid cells.

Up-regulated expression of proinflammatory cytokines in human intestinal epithelial cells occurs rapidly after stimulation with agonists such as TNF-α or IL-1, or after infection with invasive bacteria. Increased expression of most cytokines occurs within 90 min of infection, peaks by 3 h, and returns towards baseline by 6 h post-infection[1,7,9,15]. The increased release of proinflammatory cytokines by intestinal epithelial cells follows a parallel but delayed course, with maximal secretion occurring 4–6 h after stimulation, with a return towards baseline by 12 h[7,9]. This rapid but transient increase in epithelial proinflammatory signals suggests an important role for these mediators in activating the onset of the inflammatory response in response to infection with enteroinvasive microbes. Later during the course of the inflammatory response, signals important for maintaining chronic immune and inflammatory reactions likely are provided by monocytes/macrophages and/or other cellular components of the intestinal mucosa.

Although intestinal epithelial cells appear to play a major role in signalling inflammatory responses in the early period after microbial infection, it is noteworthy that increased epithelial cell expression of the C-X-C chemokine ENA-78 is delayed for several hours after bacterial infection or agonist stimulation[7]. Moreover, the up-regulated expression and secretion of ENA-78 continues for longer than the other C-X-C chemokines[7]. Differences in the kinetics of production of two neutrophil chemoattractants IL-8 and ENA-78, coupled with quantitative differences in their production and potency (i.e., IL-8 is produced in larger quantities and is more potent than ENA-78) supports the notion that human intestinal epithelial cells may play a more complex role in regulation of mucosal inflammation than initially appreciated. As shown in Figure 2, the differential expression of IL-8 and ENA-78 may result in different temporal and spatial chemotactic gradients for leukocytes in the intestinal mucosa[7]. Intestinal epithelial cells also produce the T cell and eosinophil chemoattractant RANTES at relatively low levels and with delayed kinetics in response to agonist stimulation or bacterial infection[7]. In contrast to the proinflammatory cytokines, less is known about the production and regulation of anti-inflammatory cytokines by epithelial cells during enteric infection (e.g. transforming growth factor-β1

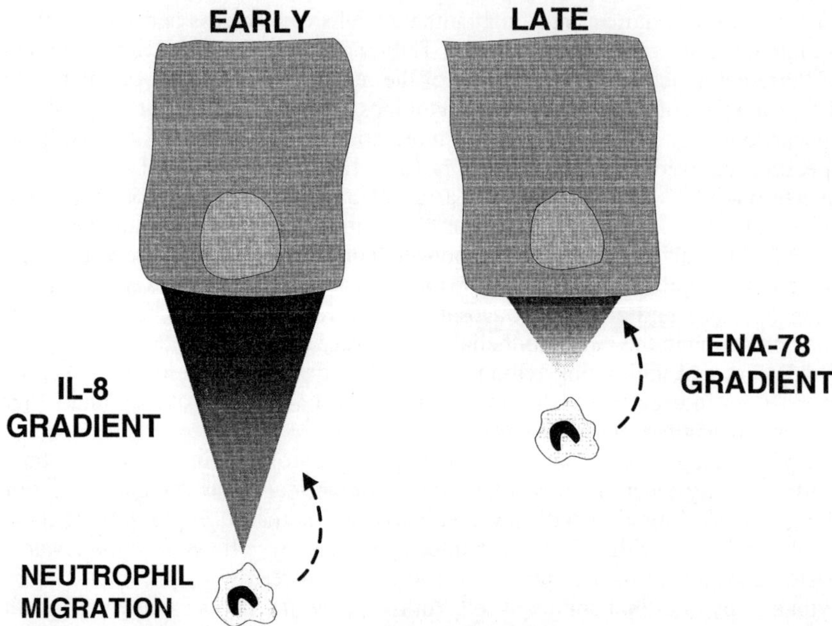

Figure 2 Temporal and spatial epithelial chemokine gradients. The C-X-C chemokine IL-8 is up-regulated earlier than the C-X-C chemokine ENA-78 following infection of intestinal epithelial cells with enteroinvasive bacteria. IL-8 is released from epithelial cells in larger quantities than ENA-78, and is a more potent neutrophil chemoattractant than ENA78, but ENA78 is produced over a longer period than is IL-8. This suggests a model in which IL-8 temporal and spatial haplotactic gradients are established in the mucosa. IL-8 released by epithelial cells may play an important role in the early chemoattraction of neutrophils at a greater distance from epithelial cells. ENA-78, in contrast, may be more important later in attracting neutrophils into close proximity with epithelial cells. Unknowns in such a model include the *in vivo* rate of degradation of IL-8 relative to ENA-78 and the respective binding of these chemokines to the mucosal proteoglycan matrix

(TGF-β1), IL-10, and IL-1 receptor antagonist) and the possible role those mediators play in down-regulating mucosal immune and inflammatory responses.

Epithelial gene products expressed at the cell membrane

The repertoire of cytokines produced by human intestinal epithelial cells suggests that they have an important function in orchestrating the onset of the innate mucosal inflammatory response and perhaps also serve as a bridge between innate and acquired immune responses. The spectrum of membrane molecules expressed by epithelial cells suggests that they can also contribute to antigen-specific mucosal immune responses. Thus, intestinal epithelial cells constitutively express or can be induced to express MHC class II molecules, can present protein antigens to T lymphocytes *in vitro*, and express classical MHC class I molecules and non-classical MHC-related molecules[16]. Furthermore, intestinal epithelial cells can respond to a range of signals from the underlying mucosa, as suggested by the expression of receptors for several cytokines including IFN-γ, IL-1, TNF-α, and TGF-β1, as well as IL-2, IL-4, IL-7, and IL-9[17].

Adhesion molecules are another important class of membrane molecules which play a central role in regulating the entry and passage of immune and inflammatory cells through tissues. ICAM-1 is a cell surface glycoprotein that serves as a counter receptor for β2 integrins expressed on neutrophils and lymphocytes. Intestinal epithelial cells up-regulate ICAM-1 expression in response to co-culture with invasive bacteria or after agonist stimulation[4,18]. When polarized monolayers of human intestinal epithelial cells or human intestinal xenografts in SCID mice were infected with invasive bacteria, ICAM-1 was shown to be expressed in a polarized distribution on the apical surface of intestinal epithelial cells after bacteria infection, its density being greatest in the area of the paracellular junctions[4]. Others have shown increased ICAM-1 expression on intestinal epithelial cells in chronically inflamed areas of intestinal mucosa[19]. Although colon epithelial cells expressing increased ICAM-1 can bind neutrophils and lymphocytes *in vitro*[4,18], a physiological role for increased ICAM-1 expression on epithelial cells following microbial infection *in vivo* has not yet been shown. However, the possibility exists that ICAM-1 expression on the apical surface of intestinal epithelial cells functions to maintain neutrophils that have transmigrated across the epithelium into the intestinal crypts within that site, thereby reducing further invasion of the mucosa by the enteric pathogen[4,19,20].

Gene products expressed within epithelial cells

Increased fluid secretion is initiated rapidly after infection of the intestinal tract with invasive bacteria. Following infection with enteroinvasive bacteria, human epithelial cells up-regulate the expression of one of the crucial rate-limiting enzymes for prostaglandin formation, prostaglandin H synthase (PGHS)-2 (also known as COX2), and PGE_2, and $PGF_{2\alpha}$ production, as shown in studies using colon epithelial cell lines or human intestinal xenografts in SCID mice[5]. These findings may explain the rapid onset of acute diarrhoea after enteroinvasive bacterial infection, since PGE_2 produced by infected intestinal epithelial cell lines can directly stimulate uninfected epithelial cells to increase chloride secretion[5], and can act indirectly by stimulating enteric nerves to release neuro-transmitters that activate epithelial ion transport processes[21]. Increased expression of PGHS-2 following microbial infection may also play a role in the altered growth regulation of the epithelium noted after bacterial infection. Thus, in addition to proinflammatory cytokines, epithelial cells have the capacity to produce additional physiological mediators that can act in an autocrine/paracrine function on neighbouring intestinal epithelial cells and other mucosal cells.

Nitric oxide (NO) is produced by NO synthases and affects multiple gastro-intestinal functions, including blood flow, barrier function and mucosal inflammation. Increased expression of inducible NO synthase (iNOS) is found in intestinal epithelial cells during the course of intestinal inflammation[22] and in response to stimulation of epithelial cell lines with a combination of cytokines (e.g. IL-1 and IFN-γ)[23]. We have shown that enteroinvasive bacteria can act as potent inducers of epithelial iNOS expression and NO production[10]. Further, in contrast to findings in a recent report[24], up-regulation of iNOS and NO production by enteroinvasive bacteria can occur independent of proinflammatory mediators known to stimulate iNOS expression (e.g. IFN-γ)[10]. These studies suggest that the up-regulated expression of iNOS and NO may play a role in epithelial microbial defence. In addition, our studies using NOS inhibitors suggest that increased NO production, which is part of the early epithelial cell response to bacterial infection, contributes to the later apoptosis of those cells[13].

INTERACTIONS OF INTESTINAL EPITHELIAL CELLS WITH ENTEROINVASIVE PATHOGENS, MINIMALLY INVASIVE PATHOGENS, NON-INVASIVE PATHOGENS AND THE COMMENSAL FLORA

Enteroinvasive pathogens

Microbial pathogens can be highly invasive, minimally invasive (i.e. reside in epithelial cells) or non-invasive. The mechanisms used by highly invasive bacteria such as *Salmonella*, *Yersinia*, *Shigella*, and *Listeria* to invade host epithelial cells have been studied extensively. Although these bacteria induce their own uptake into epithelial cells, the uptake processes involve different host receptors and cell signalling pathways[25]. Moreover, these organisms have different intra-cellular localizations (e.g. after entry, *Salmonella* and *Yersinia* reside in mem-brane-bound vesicles, whereas *Listeria* and *Shigella* rapidly lyse such vesicles and move freely within the cytoplasm). Nonetheless, entry of these bacteria requires rearrangement of the epithelial cell actin cytoskeleton, and is impaired by inhibitors of actin polymerization (e.g. cytochalasin D). Infection with such organisms results in a qualitatively similar host response with respect to the up-regulated expression of proinflammatory genes in epithelial cells and the increased production of proinflammatory cytokines[1,2], PGHS-2 and prosta-glandins[5], NOS2 and NO[10], and ICAM-1[4]. Thus, intestinal epithelial cells appear to have evolved a conserved set of functions that are activated in response to a broad array of different invasive bacterial pathogens, seemingly irrespective of the particular bacterial invasion strategy. The conserved nature of this response suggests that these epithelial functions are likely important for host survival.

Minimally invasive pathogens

Cryptosporidium parvum is a protozoan parasite that invades intestinal epithelial cells and, in the case of severe infections, is associated with an inflammatory response in the underlying mucosa. *C. parvum* undergoes a life cycle that results in lysis of epithelial cells 3–5 days after infection, releasing infective life stages of *C. parvum* which can infect previously uninfected neighbouring cells. Co-culture of *C. parvum* with human colon epithelial cell lines results in up-regulated expression and release of epithelial cell proinflammatory cytokines, including IL-8 and GROα, as well as PGHS-2[8,26]. Moreover, cytokine gene expression and PGHS expression by epithelial cells in response to *C. parvum* is delayed for 18–24 h post-infection, and increased levels of proinflammatory cytokine production persist for at least 72 h post-infection[8,26]. Although *Cryptosporidium* ultimately lyses intestinal epithelial cells at the apical surface, proinflammatory cytokine secretion occurs predominantly from the basolateral surface[8], underlining that the relevant target cells of these epithelial mediators are located in the underlying mucosa. Further, studies of *C. parvum* infection of epithelial cells in human intestinal xenografts in SCID mice have revealed that increased IL-8 expression in this model system is accompanied by a mucosal influx of neutrophils that are mostly of host origin[8].

These studies with *C. parvum*, and parallel observations with another minimally invasive mucosal pathogen *Chlamydia trachomatis* that invades epithelial cells but not deeper layers of the mucosa, have provided new insights into mechanisms by which intestinal epithelial cells may orchestrate a more prolonged mucosal inflammatory response than that seen after acute infection with enteroinvasive bacteria, by directly activating proinflammatory cytokine production by infected cells. Although the life span of the infected intestinal epithelial cells is limited due to their turnover every 3–5 days, these intracellular pathogens can maintain an ongoing inflammatory response in the host by virtue of their ability to lyse host epithelial cells and repeatedly infect newly generated healthy epithelial cells.

Non-invasive pathogens

Proinflammatory cytokine genes can be activated in uroepithelial cells following infection of these cells with non-invasive uropathogenic *Escherichia coli*. The latter bind to and interact with cell surface molecules, but do not appear to enter the epithelial cell or activate it by extracellular lipopolysaccharide[27]. Thus, colon epithelial cells, which are normally exposed to abundant flora, and uroepithelial cells, which normally reside in a sterile environment, respond in different ways to the bacteria–host interaction. Epithelial cells within the human stomach, like those in the urinary tract, reside in a relatively germ-free environment, and here too, interactions with a non-invasive bacterial pathogen, *Helicobacter pylori*, result in up-regulated IL-8 gene expression in the apparent absence of bacterial entry[28]. Finally, enteropathogenic *E. coli*, which bind to the epithelial cell surface and induce actin reorganization and membrane pedestal formation, can also stimulate low level epithelial cell IL-8 responses[29]. Whether this reflects the fact that this microorganism is minimally invasive or whether other membrane signalling events are involved is not known.

Resident commensal flora

Recent studies using models in which germ-free mice are associated with a single bacterial species indicate that commensal luminal bacteria, which are components of the conventional flora, can influence epithelial cell gene expression[30]. It is tempting to speculate that components of the commensal bacterial flora play a key role in determining the normal physiological inflammation of the intestinal mucosa via signalling through epithelial cells. Moreover, extending that notion, it is possible to envision that alterations in intestinal epithelial cell signalling may result in abnormal mucosal inflammation and that epithelial cells may serve as a therapeutic target for altering mucosal inflammatory responses.

CONCLUSION

Epithelial cells that line mucosal surfaces are a critical component of a communications network that links luminal and invasive microbes to immune and inflammatory cells in the underlying mucosa. The epithelial cell has evolved a series of conserved responses by which it interacts with invasive, minimally invasive and non-invasive mucosal microbial pathogens and host commensal microbes. We have termed the most extensively studied set of these responses the epithelial cell inflammatory gene programme. This programme includes, but is probably not limited to, the regulated expression and production of proinflammatory cytokines, PGHS-2 and prostaglandins, NOS2 and nitric oxide, and increased cell surface expression of ICAM-1[1–8,10]. Each of the up-regulated genes in this proinflammatory programme is a target gene of the transcription factor NF-κB, and we have found more recently that infection of epithelial cells with different enteroinvasive bacteria activates the NF-κB transcription factor complex. Each of the products encoded or produced as a result of up-regulated expression of these genes probably plays a role in the host's resistance to intestinal microbes and in host mucosal defence. For example, chemokines produced by epithelial cells in response to microbial infection can provide signals essential for the initiation and, in the case of intraepithelial pathogens, maintenance of the mucosal inflammatory response. PGHS-2, on the other hand, is responsible for increased epithelial prostaglandin production, and thereby may contribute to infection-related diarrhoea[5]. PGHS-2 may also influence epithelial cell growth and apoptosis[13] following microbial infection and may act to dampen mucosal inflammation through the action of prostaglandins on other mucosal cell types. Recent studies suggest that epithelial cells in the intestinal tract can also sense the conventional microbial flora[30]. Thus, it is tempting to speculate that communication between the normal resident microbial flora and intestinal epithelial cells may play a role in regulating normal epithelial cell growth and development as well as lymphoid cell development and 'physiological inflammation' in the intestine. It now also seems clear that intestinal epithelial cells maintain a dialogue with immune cells in the adjacent and underlying mucosa through the production of growth factors (e.g. IL-7 and stem cell factor) and perhaps also through local hormone networks, as reported for thyroid stimulating hormone[31]. Definition of the signal transduction and regulatory mechanisms that govern interactions between epithelial cells, mucosal microbes, and inflammatory and immune cells in the adjacent mucosa may lead to new therapeutic approaches for manipulating and regulating inflammatory and immune responses at mucosal surfaces and for regulating the growth and development of epithelial cells and other cell types in these tissues.

ACKNOWLEDGEMENTS

The authors acknowledge the contribution of former postodoctoral fellows, especially Drs S. K. Yang, F. Laurent, T. Witthoeft, J. M. Kim, H. C. Jung, and G. T. Huang, and many valued collaborators at USCD and other Institutions in the U.S. and abroad. The authors thank Roslyn Lara for preparation of the manuscript. This work was supported by NIH grant DK-35108. L. Eckmann is supported by a Research Career Development Award from the Crohn's and Colitis Foundation of America.

References

1. Eckmann L, Kagnoff MF, Fierer J. Epithelial cells secrete the chemokine interleukin-8 in response to bacterial entry. Infect Immun. 1993;61:4569–4574.
2. Jung HC, Eckmann L, Yang SK et al. A distinct array of proinflammatory cytokines is expressed in human colon epithelial cells in response to bacterial invasion. J. Clin Invest. 1995;95:55–65.
3. Eckmann L, Reed SL, Smith JR, Kagnoff MF. *Entamoeba histolytica* trophozoites induce an inflammatory cytokine response by cultured human cells through the paracrine action of cytolytically released interleukin-1 alpha. J. Clin Invest. 1995;96:1269–1279.
4. Huang GT, Eckmann L, Savidge TC, Kagnoff MF. Infection of human intestinal epithelial cells with invasive bacteria upregulates apical intercellular adhesion molecule-1 (ICAM)-1 expression and neutrophil adhesion. J Clin Invest. 1996;98:572–583.
5. Eckmann L, Stenson WF, Savidge TC et al. Role of intestinal epithelial cells in the host secretory response to infection by invasive bacteria: bacterial entry induces epithelial prostaglandin H synthase-2 expression, and prostaglandin E_2 and $F_{2\alpha}$ production. J. Clin Invest. 1997;100:296–309.
6. Rasmussen SJ, Eckmann L, Quayle AJ et al. Secretion of proinflammatory cytokines by epithelial cells in response to *Chlamydia* infection suggests a central role for epithelial cells in chlamydial pathogenesis. J Clin Invest. 1997;99:77–87.
7. Yang SK, Eckmann L, Panja A, Kagnoff MF. Differential and regulated expression of C-X-C, C-C and C-chemokines by human colon epithelial cells. Gastroenterology. 1997;113:1214–1223.
8. Laurent F, Eckmann L, Savidge TC, Morgan G, Theodos C, Naciri M, Kagnoff MF. Infection of human intestinal epithelial cells induces the polarized secretion of C-X-C chemokines. Infect Immun. 1997;65:5067–73.
9. Eckmann L, Jung HC, Schurer-Maly C, Panja A, Morzycka-Wroblewska E, Kagnoff MF. Differential cytokine expression by human intestinal epithelial cell lines: regulated expression of interleukin 8. Gastroenterology. 1993;105:1689–1697.
10. Witthöft T, Eckmann L, Kim JM, Kagnoff MF. Enteroinvasive bacteria directly activate expression of iNOS and NO production in human colon epithelial cells. Am. J. Physiol. 1998;275:G564–G571.
11. Savidge TC, Morey AL, Ferguson DJ, Fleming KA, Shmakov AN, Phillips AD. Human intestinal development in a severe-combined immunodeficient xenograft model. Differentiation. 1995;58:361–371.
12. Seydel KB, Li E, Swanson PE, Stanely SL Jr. Human intestinal epithelial cells produce proinflammatory cytokines in response to infection in a SCID mouse-human intestinal xenograft model of amebiasis. Infect Immun. 1997;65:1631–1639.
13. Kim JM, Eckmann L, Savidge TC, Lowe DC, Witthoeft T, Kagnoff MF. Apoptosis of human intestinal epithelial cells in response to bacterial invasion and replication. J Clin Invest., in press.

14. McCormick BA, Colgan SP, Delp-Archer C, Miller SI, Madara JL. *Salmonella typhimurium* attachment to human intestinal epithelial monolayers: transcellular signalling to subepithelial neutrophils. J Cell Biol. 1993;123:895–907.

15. Reinecker HC, Loh EY, Ringler DJ, Mehta A, Rombeau JL, MacDermott RP. Monocyte-chemoattractant protein 1 gene expression in intestinal epithelial cells and inflammatory bowel disease mucosa. Gastroenterology. 1995;108:40–50.

16. Panja A, Blumberg RS, Balk SP, Mayer L. CD1d is involved in T cell–intestinal epithelial cell interactions. J Exp Med. 1993;178:1115–1119.

17. Reinecker HC, Podolsky DK. Human intestinal epithelial cells express functional cytokine receptors sharing the common γc chain of the interleukin 2 receptor. Proc Natl Acad Sci USA. 1995;92:8353–8357.

18. Kelly CP, O'Keane JC, Orellana J et al. Human colon cancer cells express ICAM-1 in vivo and support LFA-1-dependent lymphocyte adhesion in vitro. Am J Physiol. 1992;263:G864–G870.

19. Parkos CA, Colgan SP, Diamond MS et al. Expression and polarization of intercellular adhesion molecule-1 on human intestinal epithelia: consequences for CD11b/CD18-mediated interactions with neutrophils. Mol Med. 1996;2:489–505.

20. Parkos CA, Colgan SP, Madara JL. Interactions of neutrophils with epithelial cells: lessons from the intestine. J Am Soc Nephrol. 1994;5:138–152.

21. Eberhart CE, Dubois RN. Eicosanoids and the gastrointestinal tract. Gastroenterology. 1995;109:285–301.

22. Ribbons KA, Zhang XJ, Thompson JH et al. Potential role of nitric oxide in a model of chronic colitis in rhesus macaques. Gastroenterology. 1995;108:705–711.

23. Salzman A, Denenberg AG, Ueta I, O'Connor M, Linn SC, Szabo C. Induction and activity of nitric oxide synthase in cultured human intestinal epithelial monolayers. Am J Physiol. 1996;270:G565–G573.

24. Salzman AL, Pyles-Eaves T, Linn SC, Denenberg AG, Szabo C. Bacterial induction of inducible nitric oxide synthase in cultured human intestinal epithelial cells. Gastroenterology. 1998;114:93–102.

25. Galan JE, Bliska JB. Cross-talk between bacterial pathogens and their host cells. Annu Rev Cell Dev Biol. 1996;12:221–255.

26. Laurent F, Kagnoff MF, Savidge TC, Naciri M, Eckmann L. Human intestinal epithelial cells respond to *Cryptosporidium parvum* infection with increased prostaglandin H synthase 2 expression and prostaglandin E_2 and $F_{2\alpha}$ production. Infect Immun. 1998;66:1789–1790.

27. Svanborg C, Hedlund M, Connell H et al. Bacterial adherence and mucosal cytokine responses. Receptors and transmembrane signalling. Ann NY Acad Sci. 1996;797:177–190.

28. Crowe SE, Alvarez L, Dytoc M et al. Expression of interleukin 8 and CD54 by human gastric epithelium after *Helicobacter pylori* infection in vitro. Gastroenterology. 1995;108:65–74.

29. Savkovic SD, Koutsouris A, Hecht G. Attachment of a noninvasive enteric pathogen, enteropathogenic *Escherichia coli*, to cultured human intestinal epithelial monolayers induces transmigration of neutrophils. Infect Immun. 1996;64:4480–4487.

30. Bry L, Falk PG, Midtvedt T, Gordon JI. A model of host–microbial interactions in an open mammalian ecosystem. Science. 1996;273:1380–1383.

31. Wang J, Whetsell M, Klein JR. Local hormone networks and intestinal T cell homeostasis. Science. 1997;275:1937–1939.

Section II
Origin, phenotype and function of intestinal T cells

7
Finding the source: continuing controversies regarding the origin of intraepithelial lymphocytes

M. KRONENBERG, L. GAPIN, V. CAMERINI, D. CRUZ,
C. PANWALA, B. C. SYDORA and H. CHEROUTRE

INTRODUCTION

Resident lymphocytes of the intestine may be important for the local regulation of immune responses and the prevention of uncontrolled inflammatory responses. In addition to lymphocytes found in organized lymphoid tissues, such as Peyer's patches and lymphoid aggregates, numerous lymphocytes also reside in the small and large intestine outside such organized lymphoid tissues, in the lamina propria tissue and in the epithelial layer. A better understanding of the origin, trafficking, and specificity of these lamina propria lymphocytes (LPL) and intraepithelial lymphocytes (IEL) will aid in understanding the homeostasis of the mucosal immune response.

Most studies of the development of the mucosal immune system have focused on the small intestine IEL (sIEL) of the mouse: it is primarily these studies which will be reviewed here. It should be noted, however, that the IEL of the mouse large intestine are different from those in the small intestine[1], IEL and LPL also are quite distinct from one another, and that there are likely to be very significant differences between mice and other species. Therefore caution must be exercised in any attempt to generalize from mouse sIEL to mucosal lymphocytes in other locations or in other species.

sIEL are T lymphocytes, but the pattern of cell surface molecules they express is unlike those expressed by thymus derived, TCR $\alpha\beta^+$, CD4 and CD8 single positive T cells found in spleen and lymph node. These thymus derived lymphocytes are hereafter called mainstream T cells. Many sIEL in the mouse are TCR $\gamma\delta^{+}$[2] and, ignoring the small population of double-negative cells, the TCR $\alpha\beta^+$ IEL have one of four patterns of co-receptor expression: either CD4$^+$, CD4$^+$ CD8$\alpha\alpha^+$, CD8$\alpha\alpha^+$ or CD8$\alpha\beta^+$[3-6]. A complete description of mouse sIEL differentiation therefore must account for the presence of these five major T cell populations, four TCR $\alpha\beta^+$, and one TCR $\gamma\delta^+$, classified by TCR and co-receptor expression.

Differential effect of gene knockouts on IEL subpopulations

Table 1 shows the effects of a selected set of null mutations, or gene knockouts, on the differentiation of different mouse sIEL and mainstream T cell populations. The data summarized in the table demonstrate the heterogeneity of the sIEL populations. With the exception of the deficiency in the $\beta7$ integrin[7], all of the other mutations have differential effects on subsets of sIEL. Not surprisingly, the effects of the different mutations on TCR $\alpha\beta^+$ CD4$^+$ and TCR $\alpha\beta^+$ CD8$^+$ are most similar to the reported effects on mainstream T cells, particularly with regard to the absence of components of the CD3 complex, and of cytokines and cytokine receptors. Such heterogeneity among sIEL certainly complicates any analysis of their differentiation.

IEL Differentiation in athymic mice

The possible extrathymic origin of sIEL in the mouse is a long-standing controversy with the results from several studies resulting in conflicting conclusions[8–12]. While it is safe to assert that there are sIEL that differentiate via an extrathymic pathway, in some subpopulations, such as TCR $\alpha\beta^+$ CD4$^+$ cells, there is controversy over the existence of any extrathymic component, and in other subpopulations, such as TCR $\gamma\delta^+$ sIEL, the size of the extrathymic versus the thymus-derived population remains open to dispute. Table 2 summarizes the results of some of these studies, with the populations most consistently found to be extrathymic located in the more left hand columns. For example, TCR $\gamma\delta^+$ IEL are found in congenitally athymic *nu/nu* (nude mice)[13], albeit in reduced numbers compared with wild type controls, and in irradiated thymectomized mice given a source of stem cells (athymic chimeras)[5,14,15], indicating their more thymic independent nature. All the studies agree that TCR $\alpha\beta^+$ CD8$\alpha\alpha^+$ sIEL

Table 1 Subpopulations of IEL have different developmental requirements

Genetic deficiency	$\gamma\delta$	TCR $\alpha\beta$ CD8$\alpha\alpha$	TCR $\alpha\beta$ CD8$\alpha\beta$	TCR $\alpha\beta$ CD4 or CD4 CD8$\alpha\alpha$	Ref.
CD3 $\zeta\eta$	+[a]	+	–	–	41–45
syk	–	ND[b]	ND[b]	ND[b]	46
lck	↓	–	+	+	47
Fyn	+	↓	+	+	47
lck/Fyn	–	–	–	–	47
FcεRIγ	+	+	+	+	48,49
IL-7/IL-7R	–	+	+	+	50–53
IL-2R β	–	–	+	+	54
β_7 integrin	–	–	–	–	7
β_2m	+	–	–	+	55,56
TAP	+	↓	↓	+	56
Class II	+	+	+	–	57
Class II/β_2m	+	–	–	–	57
IRF1	–	–	↓	ND	58

[a] + = no effect, ↓ = some decrease, – = marked decrease or absent, ND = no data.
[b] $\alpha\beta$ T-cell are still present, but not analysed according to subpopulations.

Table 2 Experiments suggestive of a thymus-independent origin at IEL

	TCR $\gamma\beta$	TCR $\alpha\beta$ CD4CD8$\alpha\alpha$	TCR $\alpha\beta$ CD4$\alpha\alpha$	TCR $\alpha\beta$ CD4	TCR $\alpha\beta$ CD8$\alpha\beta$	Ref.
Young *nu/nu* (nude)	+	–	–	–	–	13
Irrad, tx. stem cell reconstituted[a]	+	+	C[b]	C	C	5,8–12, 14,15
RAG$^{-/-}$, tx. stem cell reconstituted[c]	+	+	–	–	–	16
tx. stem cell reconstituted[d]	+	+	–	–	–	17

[a] T cell-depleted adult bone marrow or fetal liver used as a source of stem cells. Irrad., irradiated; tx., thymectomized.
[b] C, conflicting data from different reports.
[c] Thymectomized RAG 2$^{-/-}$ mice given bone marrow from athymic mice without irradiation.
[d] W^v/W or c-kit deficient rather than irradiated recipients used.

are present in athymic chimeras, although these cells are undetectable in young nude mice. There is less agreement on the presence of TCR $\alpha\beta^+$ CD4$^+$ and TCR $\alpha\beta^+$ CD8$\alpha\beta^+$ sIEL in athymic chimeras.

A concern with the athymic chimera experiments is that irradiation of the thymectomized recipients leads either to abnormal pathways of cell differentiation or augmentation of a minor pathway. To address this issue, in several more recent studies, thymectomized RAG deficient mice[16] or thymectomized W^v/W (c-kit) mutant animals[17] were used recently as recipients for stem cells. In both cases, IEL in these animals could be reconstituted without irradiation, and the resulting donor-derived T cell populations were mostly TCR $\gamma\delta^+$ and TCR $\alpha\beta^+$ CD8$\alpha\alpha^+$. In summary, while there are data in favour of an extrathymic origin for all sIEL subpopulations, the most consistent data favour an extrathymic source for TCR $\gamma\delta^+$ and, to some extent, for TCR $\alpha\beta^+$ CD8$\alpha\alpha^+$ T cells.

Evidence that the thymus contributes to all IEL subpopulations

Despite the results from many experiments outlined above, data from a different set of investigations, summarized in Table 3, indicate that all subpopulations of sIEL can be thymic derived. For example, transplant of thymus tissue into SCID, nude or irradiated mice gives rise to thymus donor-derived sIEL, including those

Table 3 Experiments suggestive of a thymus-dependent origin at IEL

	TCR $\gamma\delta$	TCR $\alpha\beta$ CD8$\alpha\alpha$	TCR $\alpha\beta$ CD4$\alpha\alpha$	TCR $\alpha\beta$ CD4	TCR $\alpha\beta$ CD8$\alpha\beta$	Ref.
Neonatal tx.	↓[a]	↓	↓	↓	↓	18,19,21
Thymus transplant	+	+	+	+	+	18–20

[a] Populations were present, but decreased.

with the most 'extrathymic' TCR $\gamma\delta^+$ and TCR $\alpha\beta^+$ CD8$\alpha\alpha^+$ phenotypes[18–20]. It is not known whether the thymus-derived sIEL precursor in these cases is a relatively undifferentiated TCR negative cell or a fully differentiated and selected TCR-positive lymphocyte. Consistent with an important role for the thymus, neonatal thymectomy in most cases results in a significant decrease in all sIEL subpopulations including TCR $\gamma\delta^+$ IEL[18,19,21]. This has led some investigators to conclude that the extrathymic contribution to the sIEL population is minor compared to the thymus-derived contribution, although these experiments do not rule out an extrathymic differentiation pathway.

The neonatal thymectomy experiments also do not determine whether the thymus is required for sIEL differentiation because it supplies thymus-derived T cells, stem cells and/or differentiated cells, or because of some other effect of this organ. Klein and colleagues hypothesized that the thymus is needed to generate a neuroendocrine signal, required only early in life, which is needed to make the intestine receptive to extrathymic sIEL differentiation[22]. Their published data consistent with this intriguing and provocative hypothesis include the facts that neonatally thymectomized mice treated with thyrotropin releasing hormone or thyroid stimulating hormone develop normal numbers of sIEL, including CD4$^+$ and CD8$\alpha\beta^+$ cells[23,24], and that intestinal epithelial cells make thyroid stimulating hormone and sIEL have receptors for thyroid stimulating hormone. Furthermore, mice with a mutation in the thyroid stimulating hormone receptor do not develop normal numbers of sIEL[25]. The details of this postulated thymus-dependent neurocrine network remain to be worked out.

It is not easy to make a coherent picture on the role of the thymus in mouse sIEL differentiation from all of these data. sIEL are likely to arise from both thymus-dependent and thymus-independent pathways. Data from a variety of experiments show that thymus-derived, mainstream T cells can migrate to the intestine, and that this migration is associated with T cell activation, which may occur in the intestine or elsewhere. Our own experiments show that thymus-derived, mainstream T cells that reside in the intestine acquire a mucosal phenotype, including expression of the mucosal-specific integrin $\alpha_E\beta_7$[26,27], cytolytic capability[27], and a poor TCR-mediated proliferative response[27], all properties similar to normal sIEL. Furthermore, mainstream T cells that reside in the intestinal epithelium have a tendency to re-home specifically to the intestine upon adoptive transfer[27,28]. Therefore, it is clear that the systemic and intestinal immune systems are not likely to be separate, but they are more likely to be interconnected in various ways, including the migration of activated mainstream T cells to the intestine. We cannot conclude, however, that all sIEL with a mainstream phenotype, namely TCR $\alpha\beta^+$ CD4$^+$ and TCR $\alpha\beta^+$ CD8$\alpha\beta^+$, have migrated from the periphery. In addition to supplying thymus-derived mainstream T cells that become sIEL, the thymus may also contribute to the extrathymic pathway of sIEL differentiation in two ways. First, it may export either undifferentiated or partially differentiated sIEL precursors. Second, the thymus may contribute by an indirect mechanism, which may involve the regulation of the secretion of neuroendocrine hormones required to make the intestine receptive to extrathymic T cell differentiation.

Does extrathymic IEL differentiation take place in the intestine?

The putative extrathymic T cell differentiation process for sIEL could take place in one or more sites, including the bone marrow, the liver and the intestine itself. According to one view, a thymus-like differentiation process might take place within the intestinal epithelium, in which TCR$^+$ double-positive precursors give rise initially to CD8$\alpha\alpha$ single-positive and eventually also to CD8$\alpha\beta$ single-positive sIEL. More data in favour of an intestinal location for T cell differentiation are summarized in Table 4. The mouse IEL population contains variable numbers of CD3 negative lymphocytes which could be intraintestinal precursors. This population contains mRNA for components of the V-J recombination machinery[5,29,30]. There also is evidence for intermediates in the V-J rearrangement process in IEL, including the presence of V-J rearrangement excision products. Furthermore, there is pre Tα mRNA, in mouse sIEL[31], and in fetal human sIEL, TCR β mRNA is present along with germline α locus TEA transcripts[32]. Both of these phenomena are suggestive of TCR β rearrangement and expression in the absence of TCR α expression, as occurs normally during thymocyte differentiation. Furthermore, we have found Vγ gene rearrangements in sorted CD3$^-$ sIEL from TCR $\delta^{-/-}$ mice, suggestive of the presence of blocked $\gamma\delta$ precursors in the intestine (Panwala et al., manuscript in preparation). The co-expression of CD4 and CD8, as well as the expression of forbidden or autoreactive Vβ TCR, also have been taken as evidence for an intraintestinal T cell differentiation process[9].

It should be noted that the double-positive stage does not seem to be required for the development of CD8$\alpha\alpha^+$ IEL, because in TCR transgenic mice differentiation CD8$\alpha\alpha$ IEL can occur in the absence of a detectable double-positive intermediate[33]. Although the presence of double-positive IEL is suggestive for an intraintestinal pathway, however, it is not a direct proof. Some of the double-positive IEL derive from mainstream CD4 cells which have acquired CD8$\alpha\alpha$ upon residing in the intestine. Therefore it is not known whether this double-positive stage is a transient or end stage of differentiation.

The results from two other types of experiments more directly implicate the intestine in sIEL differentiation. Irradiated, thymectomized mice were reconstituted with T cell depleted bone marrow and transplanted with a fragment of fetal intestine under the kidney capsule[34]. In some successful transplants of the recipients, the fetal intestine acted as a surrogate thymus, in that it stimulated the differentiation of mainstream T cells located in spleen and lymph node as well as

Table 4 Evidence that has been cited in favour of the intestine as a site of extrathymic T cell development

1. The expression, by CD3$^-$ IEL, of RAG 1, RAG 2, TdT, and pre Tα mRNA in normal mice, germ line α transcripts in humans, and the presence of V-J rearrangement excision products and rearranged Vγ genes in TCR $\delta^{-/-}$ mice[29-32] Panwala *et al.*, manuscript in preparation).
2. Presence of CD4, CD8 double-positive IEL[3,4,9].
3. Presence of IEL with forbidden or autoreactive TCR[5,6,9].
4. In thymectomized, irradiated and bone marrow reconstituted mice, ectopic transplant of the neonatal intestine can lead to peripheral T cell reconstitution[35].
5. Transfer of CD3$^-$ IEL or cryptopatch cells leads to the development of CD3$^+$ IEL in the recipients[36,37].

sIEL derived from precursors in the bone marrow inoculum. This T cell differentiation did not occur in all the recipients, it has not been repeated by several other laboratories, and it needs to be confirmed using a nude mouse or some other recipient in which irradiation is not required. Second, transfer of CD3⁻ sIEL to SCID recipients led to the generation of donor derived CD3⁺ sIEL[35]. In our hands, however, sorted CD3⁺ IEL were more effective at populating the intestine of a SCID host than CD3⁻ sIEL, and we therefore cannot exclude the possibility that the CD3⁺ sIEL derived from the CD3⁻ cell transfer in our experiment were derived from a few contaminating CD3⁺ cells.

An extrathymic site for T cell differentiation, by analogy with the thymus and the bone marrow, is likely to be composed of clusters of proliferating lymphocytes in contact with a stromal cell network. By these criteria, the epithelial compartment, which consists mostly of solitary, non-cycling lymphocytes dispersed among the epithelial cells, does not appear to be a likely site for T cell differentiation. There was therefore great interest in the recent discovery of the so-called cryptopatches[36]. Cryptopatches are small (approximately 10^3 cells) aggregates of lymphocytes located below the epithelium at the base of the intestinal villi in the mouse small and large intestine. Many cryptopatch cells have markers characteristic of immature lymphocytes such as the IL-7 receptor and CD117 (c-kit). From an anatomical point of view, cryptopatches are an attractive possible location for intraintestinal sIEL differentiation, and a very recent and compelling study has demonstrated that CD3⁻ CD117⁺ cryptopatch cells give rise to TCR $\alpha\beta^+$ and TCR $\gamma\delta^+$ IEL upon transfer to an irradiated SCID recipient[37]. Cryptopatches are also present in immune deficient (SCID, Rag 2⁻/⁻) mice, where they contain predominantly cycling cells. It therefore appears that TCR expression does not occur in the cryptopatch. It therefore is possible that CD3⁻, CD117⁺ cryptopatch cells give rise to CD3⁻ sIEL, which in turn may eventually give rise to CD3⁺ sIEL. Alternatively, IEL preparations could be routinely contaminated with cryptopatch cells, in which case the hypothesized intraepithelial T cell precursor could in fact be a contaminant from below the epithelium.

The TCR selected in the thymus may not be selected in IEL

To make further progress in analysing the differentiation of sIEL, we have undertaken an analysis of T cell monoclonal mice by breeding TCR transgenic mice on to the RAG 2⁻/⁻ background. Two well studied systems have been analysed so far, as summarized in Table 5. The first is a TCR transgene specific for a male-derived peptide (H-Y) presented by D^b. In male D^{b+} mice, TCR transgene-positive, CD8⁺ T cells are deleted in the thymus[38,39]. In female mice, CD8⁺ TCR transgene-positive T cells are positively selected, presumably due to the expression in females of a peptide or peptides which can interact with the appropriate avidity with this TCR. The second system is the AND transgenic mouse, which has a TCR transgene specific for a carboxyl terminal peptide of pigeon cytochrome c presented by the E^k class II molecule. This TCR is positively selected in mouse strains that express either E^k, E^{d/b}, or A^b class II molecules[39].

There have been several previous analyses of IEL in TCR transgenic mice. With one exception, in which only small intestine LPL but not IEL were

Table 5 TCR selected in the thymus are not selected in IEL

TCR transgene[a]	Phenotype selected in the thymus	Genetic background of transgene	Presence of CD4 or CD8$^+$ single-positive TCR$^+$ T cells	
			Thymus	IEL
H-Y(Vβ8/Vα3)	CD8$\alpha\beta^+$	Female D^b	+	−
H-Y(Vβ8/Vα3)	CD8$\alpha\beta^+$	Male D^b	−	+[b]
H-Y(Vβ8/Vα3)	CD8$\alpha\beta^+$	Male or Female TAP-1$^{-/-}$	−	−
AND(Vβ3/Vα11)	CD4	I-A^b	+	−

[a] All TCR transgenes on the RAG 2$^{-/-}$ background.
[b] IEL are mostly CD8$\alpha\alpha^+$ with some CD8α^+ β^{low}.

analysed[40], none of these studies has used transgenic mice on a recombination deficient (RAG2$^{-/-}$), or SCID genetic background. On account of rearrangement and expression of endogenous TCR genes and the expression of more than one TCR by many T cells in TCR transgenic mice, it therefore is difficult to determine in such mice whether a mature T cell has been selected on the basis of expression of the TCR transgene or some other endogenous, rearranged TCR. Expression of inappropriate CD4 or CD8 coreceptors, which are not matched to the MHC class I or class II specificity of the TCR, is one indication of endogenous TCR rearrangement and expression. For example, sIEL of H-Y/D^b TCR transgenic mice on the RAG 2$^{+/-}$ background contain CD4$^+$ cells, while AND TCR transgenic RAG-2$^{+/-}$ mice contain numerous CD8$^+$ sIEL. Detectable levels of the TCR transgenic α and β chains can be found on the AND TCR$^+$ sIEL that express the inappropriate CD8 co-receptor. These sIEL must also express an endogenous α chain, however, as the AND TCR$^+$ CD8$^+$ sIEL are not present when this TCR transgene is crossed to the RAG 2$^{-/-}$ background.

H-Y/D^b TCR$^+$ RAG 2$^{-/-}$ transgenic mice on the nonselecting TAP 1$^{-/-}$ background (Table 5) or the nonselecting D^d background did not have detectable TCR sIEL[33], consistent with other data suggesting that TCR $\alpha\beta^+$ sIEL require positive selection. Surprisingly, TCR transgenes selected in the thymus are not found in sIEL. AND TCR transgenic$^+$ RAG 2$^{-/-}$ mice on the positively selecting A^b background have numerous TCR$^+$ transgene CD4$^+$ T cells in the spleen and lymph node, but virtually no detectable TCR$^+$ sIEL. Similarly, female H-Y/D^b specific TCR transgenic$^+$ RAG 2$^{-/-}$ mice that are on the selecting D^{b+} background also do not have TCR$^+$ sIEL, despite the positive selection of these T cells in the thymus of these mice. By contrast to the female transgenic mice, male H-Y/D^b TCR transgenic$^+$ RAG 2$^{-/-}$ mice have numerous TCR transgene positive CD8$\alpha\alpha^+$ sIEL[33]. The origin of these IEL in male TCR transgenic mice currently is under investigation, but the data suggest that the expression of CD8$\alpha\alpha$ homodimers may permit positive selection of the H-Y/D^b specific TCR in male mice.

In summary, these data show that two TCR that are positively selected in the thymus, and which give rise to numerous, circulating, TCR transgene positive

T cells in spleen and lymph node, are not found in any appreciable number in sIEL. One of these is CD8[+], class I-specific TCR, and the other is CD4[+] and class II reactive. These data have two important implications for the thymus dependent and independent origins of sIEL that we have discussed. First, in both types of TCR transgenic mice, mainstream T cells do not reside long term in the intestinal epithelium, despite the numerous transgene-positive cells in the lymph node, spleen and circulation. This indicates that peripheral T cells do not randomly enter the intestinal mucosal compartments, and this is consistent with other suggestions that such entry requires antigen activation. Second, if there is an sIEL differentiation pathway that is centred in the intestine, which appears likely based upon the analysis of cryptopatch cells and our own *in vitro* studies, then the absence of sIEL in the two types of TCR transgenic mice is consistent with a failure of positive selection in the intestine, while positive selection of the same TCR is occurring in the thymus. This demonstrates that the TCR repertoire selected in the intestine for sIEL is distinct from the repertoire selected in the thymus. Our current studies are directed towards understanding the conditions and circumstances in these two models that will permit the entry of mainstream TCR transgene-positive cells into the epithelium of the intestine.

ACKNOWLEDGEMENTS

This work was supported by NIH grant DK46763 (M.K.), a Medical Scientist Training Grant (GM08042) to UCLA, and grants from l'Association pour la recherche contre le Cancer (L.G.), the Crohn's & Colitis Foundation of America (B.C.S.), and the R. W. Johnson Foundation (V.C.). We thank Ms Nancy Houghton for assistance with the preparation of this manuscript. This is manuscript number 239 from the La Jolla Institute for Allergy & Immunology.

References

1. Camerini V, Panwala C, Kronenberg M. Regional specialization of the mucosal immune system. Intraepithelial lymphocytes of the large intestine have a different phenotype and function than those of the small intestine. J Immunol. 1993;151:1765–1776.
2. Goodman T, Lefrancois L. Expression of the gamma-delta T-cell receptor on intestinal CD8[+] intraepithelial lymphocytes. Nature. 1988;333:855–858.
3. Mosley RL, Styre D, Klein JR. CD4[+] CD8[+] murine intestinal intraepithelial lymphocytes. Int Immunol. 1990;2:361–365.
4. Lefrancois L. Phenotypic complexity of intraepithelial lymphocytes of the small intestine. J Immunol. 1991;147:1746–1751.
5. Guy-Grand D, Cerf-Bensussan N, Malissen B, Malassis-Seris M, Briottet C, Vassalli P. Two gut intraepithelial CD8[+] lymphocyte populations with different T cell receptors: a role for the gut epithelium in T cell differentiation. J Exp Med. 1991;173:471–481.
6. Guy-Grand D, Vassalli P. Gut intraepithelial T lymphocytes. Curr Opin Immunol. 1993;5:247–252.
7. Wagner N, Lohler J, Kunkel EJ et al. Critical role for beta 7 integrins in formation of the gut-associated lymphoid tissue. Nature. 1996;382:366–370.
8. Poussier P, Julius M. Intestinal intraepithelial lymphocytes: the plot thickens. J Exp Med. 1994;180:1185–1189.
9. Poussier P, Julius M. T-cell development and selection in the intestinal epithelium. Semin Immunol. 1995;7:321–334.
10. Rocha B, Guy-Grand D, Vassalli P. Extrathymic T cell differentiation. Curr Opin Immunol. 1995;7:235–242.

with the oligonucleotides 5′-GGATATGTTTTTACCTCAATT-3′ and 5′-GAT-GAACAAAAAGTTTCTGCT-3′ for the substitution of serine by phenylalanine at position 61 (S61F) and glutamate by lysine at position 112 (E112K), respectively (Fig. 1). These amino acid mutation sites are located in the CT-A subunit. Similar substitutions in LT completely inactivate ADP-ribosyltransferase activity and enterotoxicity[29,30]. The efficiency of these mutations was evaluated *in vitro* by measuring the toxicity in cultured Chinese hamster ovary (CHO) cells and by assessing ADP-ribosyltransferase activity. *In vivo* characterization was performed by analysing the toxicity in mouse ileal loops. While native CT (nCT) increased cAMP and induced spindle cell formation in CHO cell cultures, none of these effects were observed with mutant CT (mCT)[31]. The mCT also failed to induce fluid accumulation in ligated intestinal loop assays[31].

Several antigens (i.e., tetanus toxoid, influenza virus, ovalbumin and PspA) have been co-administered with mCTs by the systemic (i.e., subcutaneously) and the mucosal routes to test the ability of mCTs to boost the immune response to co-administered protein antigens[31–33]. To help delineate the effect of CT-B on the adjuvanticity of mCTs, recombinant CT-B (rCT-B) was tested under the same conditions as native CT (nCT) and mCT. No significant enhancement of systemic immunity to co-administered antigens was measured after either systemic or mucosal administration of rCT-B. In contrast, both S61F and E112K mCTs significantly enhanced antigen-specific serum Ig isotypes and mucosal IgA Ab responses to the co-administered protein antigen[31–33]. The immune-enhancing effects of mCT were observed regardless of the route of administration: 10 μg mCT induced Ab titers comparable to those achieved with 1 μg nCT administered by the same route[31–33].

The adjuvant effect of nCT is known to induce serum IgG1 followed by IgG2b subclasses and IgE Abs[3,34]. Interestingly, this pattern of IgG subclass and IgE Ab responses was also observed with the E112K and S61F mCT obtained by site-directed mutagenesis in the A subunit. Further, the adjuvant effect of the mCT on the induction of S-IgA Ab responses to co-administered protein antigens was comparable to that of nCT[32,33]. It has been postulated that the adjuvant effect of nCT involves the ADP ribosyltransferase activity associated with the A subunit[35,36]. Since these pharmacological effects may influence the pattern of cytokines secreted by CD4$^+$ T cells, antigen-specific T_H responses induced by mCT were analysed. Co-administration of mCT with protein antigen by either parenteral, nasal or oral routes stimulated antigen-specific CD4$^+$ T cells secreting IL-4, IL-S, IL-6 and IL-10, while T_H1-type cytokines (i.e., IL-2 and IFN-γ) were not significantly enhanced[31–33] (Fig. 2). Finally, both nCT and mCT enhanced the expression of co-stimulatory molecules of the B7 family and their correspondent receptors[37,38].

Others have also reported the engineering of mCT which display little or no toxicity and retain mucosal adjuvant effects[39]. These mutants, CTS106 and CTK63, were obtained by single amino acid substitution at position 106 and 63 around the NAD binding cleft of the A subunit, respectively, and both mutants generated mucosal and systemic immune responses to co-nasally administered protein antigens[39] (Fig. 1). The T_H cell responses induced by these CT derivatives were not specifically addressed in this study; however, indirect evidence provided by the profile of IgG subclasses suggested that the same pattern of

11. Klein JR. T-lymphopoietic capacity of the mouse intestinal epithelium. Semin Immunol. 1995;7:291–297.

12. Klein JR. Whence the intestinal intraepithelial lymphocyte? J Exp Med. 1996;184: 1203–1206.

13. De Geus B, Van den Enden M, Coolen C, Nagelkerken L, Van der Heijden P, Rozing J. Phenotype of intraepithelial lymphocytes in euthymic and athymic mice: implications for differentiation of cells bearing a CD3-associated gamma delta T cell receptor. Eur J Immunol. 1990;20:291–298.

14. Mosley RL, Styre D, Klein JR. Differentiation and functional maturation of bone marrow-derived intestinal epithelial T cells expressing membrane T cell receptor in athymic radiation chimeras. J Immunol. 1990;145:1369–1375.

15. Bandeira A, Itohara S, Bonneville M et al. Extrathymic origin of intestinal intraepithelial lymphocytes bearing T-cell antigen receptor gamma delta. Proc Natl Acad Sci USA. 1991;88:43–47.

16. Rocha B, Vassalli P, Guy-Grand D. Thymic and extrathymic origins of gut intraepithelial lymphocyte populations in mice. J. Exp Med. 1994;180:681–686.

17. Lefrancois L, Olson S. Reconstitution of the extrathymic intestinal T cell compartment in the absence of irradiation. J Immunol. 1997;159:538–541.

18. Lin T, Matsuzaki G, Kenai H, Nomoto K. Progenies of fetal thymocytes are the major source of CD4-CD8+ alpha alpha intestinal intraepithelial lymphocytes early in ontogeny. Eur J Immunol. 1994;24:1785–1791.

19. Lefrancois L, Olson S. A novel pathway of thymus-directed T lymphocyte maturation. J Immunol. 1994;153:987–995.

20. Lin T, Matsuzaki G, Yoshida et al. Thymus ontogeny and the development of TCR alpha beta intestinal intraepithelial lymphocytes. Cell Immunol. 1996;171:132–139.

21. Lin T, Matsuzaki G, Kenai H, Nakamura T, Nomoto K. Thymus influences the development of extrathymically derived intestinal intraepithelial lymphocytes. Eur J Immunol. 1993;23: 1968–1974.

22. Klein JR. T cell development within the intestinal mucosa: clues to a novel immune-endocrine network? Adv Neuroimmunol. 1996;6:397–405.

23. Wang J, Klein JR. Hormonal regulation of extrathymic gut T cell development: involvement of thyroid stimulating hormone. Cell Immunol. 1995;161:299–302.

24. Wang J, Klein JR. Thymus-neuroendocrine interactions in extrathymic T cell development. Science 1994;265:1860–1862.

25. Wang J, Whetsell M, Klein JR. Local hormone networks and intestinal T cell homeostasis. Science. 1997;275:1937–1939.

26. Aranda R, Sydora BC, McAllister PL et al. Analysis of intestinal lymphocytes in mouse colitis mediated by transfer of CD4+, CD45RBhigh T cells to SCID recipients. J Immunol. 1997;158: 3464–3473.

27. Camerini V, Sydora BC, Aranda R et al. Generation of intestinal mucosal lymphocytes in SCID mice reconstituted with mature, thymus-derived T cells. J Immunol. 1998;160:2608–2618.

28. Sydora BC, Habu S, Taniguchi M. Intestinal intraepithelial lymphocytes preferentially repopulate the intestinal epithelium. Int Immunol. 1993;5:743–751.

29. Guy-Grand D, Vanden Broecke C, Briottet C, Malassis-Seris M, Selz F, Vassalli P. Different expression of the recombination activity gene RAG-1 in various populations of thymocytes, peripheral T cells and gut thymus-independent intraepithelial lymphocytes suggests two pathways of T cell receptor rearrangement. Eur J Immunol. 1992;22:505–510.

30. Lin T, Matsuzaki G, Yoshida H et al. CD3⁻ CD8⁺ intestinal intraepithelial lymphocytes (IEL) and the extrathymic development of IEL. Eur J Immunol. 1994;24:1080–1087.

31. Bruno L, Rocha B, Rolink A, von Boehmer H, Rodewald HR. Intra- and extra-thymic expression of the pre-T cell receptor alpha gene. Eur J Immunol. 1995;25:1877–1882.

32. Koningsberger JC, Chott A, Logtenberg T et al. TCR expression in human fetal intestine and identification of an early T cell receptor beta-chain transcript. J Immunol. 1997;159: 1775–1782.

33. Cruz D, Sydora BC, Hetzel K, Yakoub G, Kronenberg M, Cheroutre H. An opposite pattern of selection of a single T cell antigen receptor in the thymus and among intraepithelial lymphocytes. J Exp Med. 1998;188:255–265.

34. Hamad M, Whetsell M, Wang J, Klein JR. T cell progenitors in the murine small intestine. Dev Comp Immunol. 1997;21:435–442.

35. Mosley RL, Klein JR. Peripheral engraftment of fetal intestine into athymic mice sponsors T cell development: direct evidence for thymopoietic function of murine small intestine. J Exp Med. 1992;176:1365–1373.

36. Kanamori Y, Ishimaru K, Nanno M et al. Identification of novel lymphoid tissues in murine intestinal mucosa where clusters of c-kit⁺ IL-7R⁺ Thy 1⁺ lympho-hemopoietic progenitors develop. J Exp Med. 1996;184:1449–1459.

37. Saito H, Kanamori Y, Takemori T et al. Generation of intestinal T cells from progenitors residing in gut cryptopatches. Science. 1998;280:275–278.

38. Bluthmann H, Kisielow P, Uematsu Y et al. T-cell-specific deletion of T-cell receptor transgenes allows functional rearrangement of endogenous alpha- and beta-genes. Nature. 1988;334:156–159.

39. Kaye J, Vasquez NJ, Hedrick SM. Involvement of the same region of the T cell antigen receptor in thymic selection and foreign peptide recognition. J Immunol. 1992;148:3342–3353.

40. Hurst SD, Sitterding SM, Ji S, Barrett TA. Functional differentiation of T cells in the intestine of T cell receptor transgenic mice. Proc Natl Acad Sci USA. 1997;94:3920–3925.

41. Malissen M, Gillet A, Rocha B et al. T cell development in mice lacking the CD3-zeta/eta gene. EMBO J. 1993;12:4347–4355.

42. Ohno H, Ono S, Hirayama N, Shimada S, Saito T. Preferential usage of the Fc receptor gamma chain in the T cell antigen receptor complex by gamma/delta T cells localized in epithelia. J Exp Med. 1994;179:365–369.

43. Guy-Grand D, Rocha B, Mintz P et al. Different use of T cell receptor transducing modules in two populations of gut intraepithelial lymphocytes are related to distinct pathways of T cell differentiation. J Exp Med. 1994;180:673–679.

44. Khattri R, Sperling AI, Qian D et al. TCR-gamma delta cells in CD3 zeta-deficient mice contain Fc epsilon RI gamma in the receptor complex but are specifically unresponsive to antigen. J Immunol. 1996;157:2320–2327.

45. She J, Simpson SJ, Gupta A et al. CD16-expressing CD8alpha alpha⁺ T lymphocytes in the intestinal epithelium: possible precursors of Fc gammaR⁻ CD8alpha alpha⁺ T cells. J Immunol. 1997;158:4678–4687.

46. Mallick-Wood CA, Pao W, Cheng AM et al. Disruption of epithelial gamma delta T cell repertoires by mutation of the Syk tyrosine kinase. Proc Natl Acad Sci USA. 1996;93:9704–9709.

47. Page ST, van Oers NS, Perlmutter RM, Weiss A, Pullen AM. Differential contribution of Lck and Fyn protein tyrosine kinases to intraepithelial lymphocyte development. Eur J Immunol. 1997;27:554–562.

48. Park SY, Arase H, Wakizaka K et al. Differential contribution of the FcR gamma chain to the surface expression of the T cell receptor among T cells localized in epithelia: analysis of FcR gamma-deficient mice. Eur J Immunol. 1995;25:2107–2110.

49. Heiken H, Schulz RJ, Ravetch JV, Reinherz EL, Koyasu S. T lymphocyte development in the absence of Fc epsilon receptor I gamma subunit: analysis of thymic-dependent and independent alpha beta and gamma delta pathways. Eur J Immunol. 1996;26:1935–1943.

50. He YW, Malek TR. Interleukin-7 receptor alpha is essential for the development of gamma delta⁺ T cells, but not natural killer cells. J Exp Med. 1996;184:289–293.

51. Maki K, Sunaga S, Komagata Y et al. Interleukin 7 receptor-deficient mice lack gammadelta T cells. Proc Natl Acad Sci USA. 1996;93:7172–7177.

52. Moore TA, von Freeden-Jeffry U, Murray R, Zlotnik A. Inhibition of gamma delta T cell development and early thymocyte maturation in IL-7⁻/⁻ mice. J Immunol. 1996;157:2366–2373.

53. Fujihashi K, McGhee JR, Yamamoto M, Peschon JJ, Kiyono H. An interleukin-7 internet for intestinal intraepithelial T cell development: knockout of ligand or receptor reveal differences in the immunodeficient state. Eur J Immunol. 1997;27:2133–2138.

54. Suzuki H, Duncan GS, Takimoto H, Mak TW. Abnormal development of intestinal intra-epithelial lymphocytes and peripheral natural killer cells in mice lacking the IL-2 receptor beta chain. J Exp Med. 1997;185:499–505.

55. Correa I, Bix M, Liao NS, Zijlstra M, Jaenisch R, Raulet D. Most gamma delta T cells develop normally in beta 2-microglobulin-deficient mice. Proc Natl Acad Sci USA. 1992;89:653–657.

56. Sydora BC, Brossay L, Hagenbaugh A, Kronenberg M, Cheroutre H. TAP-independent selection of CD8⁺ intestinal intraepithelial lymphocytes. J Immunol. 1996;156:4209–4216.

57. Schleussner C, Ceredig R. Analysis of intraepithelial lymphocytes from major histocompatibility complex (MHC)-deficient mice: no evidence for a role of MHC class II antigens in the positive selection of V delta 4[+] gamma delta T cells. Eur J Immunol. 1993;23:1615–1622.
58. Ohteki T, Yoshida H, Matsuyama T, Duncan GS, Mat TW, Ohashi PS. The transcription factor interferon regulatory factor 1 (IRF-1) is important during the maturation of natural killer 1.1[+] T cell receptor⁻ alpha/beta[+] (NK1[+] T) cells, natural killer cells, and intestinal intraepithelial T cells. J Exp Med. 1998;187:967–972.

8
Local proliferation and apoptosis of T cell subsets versus homing

J. WESTERMANN, M. KAISER and U. BODE

INTRODUCTION

Lymphocytes continuously migrate through the body to increase the chance of meeting the cognate antigen[1–5]. In the human body about 500×10^9 lymphocytes leave the blood each day to enter various organs and then return into the blood[6,7]. Many studies have attempted to clarify how these enormous migration streams are regulated. It is now well established that both lymphocyte subsets and the various types of vascular endothelium differ in the expression of adhesion molecules and ligands[8,9]. This heterogeneity was the basis for a widely accepted model proposing that migrating lymphocytes are guided to their target tissue via the interaction of site-specific adhesion molecule pathways, very much like a letter is delivered to the correct address via the postal code[10–12]. In accordance with this model, preferential accumulation of lymphocytes in a given tissue is most often associated with preferential entry. However, preferential accumulation of migrating lymphocytes can be due also to increased proliferation and reduced cell death within the tissue, and/or a reduced exit rate from the tissue[2,6,13,14].

To analyse the relative contribution of lymphocyte entry, proliferation, death and exit to their distribution *in vivo*, activated T lymphocytes will be taken as an example. This population is chosen because it shows preferential tissue accumulation in all species investigated so far (summarized in Ref. 15). In addition, it will be briefly outlined that even under non-pathological circumstances activated T cells preferentially accumulate in the lamina propria of ileum and colon, and not in that of jejunum.

MATERIAL AND METHODS

Preparation and injection of *in vitro* activated T cells

Cell suspensions were prepared as described in Ref 15. In brief, rat pLN (pooled axillary, brachial and cervical lymph nodes) and mLN (mesenteric lymph nodes[16]) were stimulated via the $\alpha\beta$ T cell receptor (antibody R73) and CD28 (antibody JJ319) as described[17,18], and cultured in the presence of 5 μM 5-bromo-2-deoxyuridine (BrdUrd) for 72 h. BrdUrd is incorporated into the DNA during the S-phase of the cell cycle and can be detected in cytological and histological preparations with specific antibodies (summarized in Ref. 19). Then $15-110 \times 10^6$ BrdUrd[+] T cells (mean 60×10^6) were injected over 2 min intravenously into unrestrained rats[20].

Identification of the activated T cells in various tissues

At various time points after injection the mesenteric lymph nodes, and the small and large intestine were removed, frozen in liquid nitrogen and stored at $-80°C$. Cryostat sections were prepared and the BrdUrd[+] cells were identified by immunohistology[19].

Identification of proliferating cells among the activated T cells in various tissues

Congenic (LEW.7B) pLN and mLN T cells were stimulated as described but without adding BrdUrd. Three days later the host animals received BrdUrd intravenously. By removing mLN and samples of the gut 1 h later it was guaranteed that BrdUrd[+] cells had incorporated BrdUrd within the respective organ[21]. After injection into LEW.7A recipients, the congenic cells were identified by a monoclonal antibody directed against LEW.7B cells[19].

Identification of apoptotic cells in macrophages

Cryostat sections were fixed with 4% paraformaldehyde (pH 7.4 in PBS) for 20 min. To localize macrophages in the paracortex, the sections were incubated with the monoclonal antibody ED1 and revealed in blue by the alkaline phosphatase anti-alkaline phosphatase technique as described[19]. To detect cells with DNA fragmentation, the TUNEL method was used as described[15].

RESULTS AND DISCUSSION

The preferential accumulation of activated T cells migrating through the body is due to increased proliferation and reduced cell death

T cells were activated via the T cell receptor and CD28, labelled, injected into rats, and their localization within mLNs was analysed. It was confirmed that activated mLN T cells were present in significantly higher numbers than activated pLN T cells in mLN (Fig. 1, upper panel). To study whether this localization is due to preferential immigration, the number of activated mLN and pLN T cells in the high endothelial venules (HEVs) was determined (Fig. 1). The HEVs are the main route of entry into lymph nodes, and preferential immigration of activated mLN T cells into mLN should be reflected by a higher number of these cells in the wall of the HEVs[20,22,23]. Surprisingly, both cell types were found in about comparable numbers in the HEVs, indicating a comparable entry rate[15].

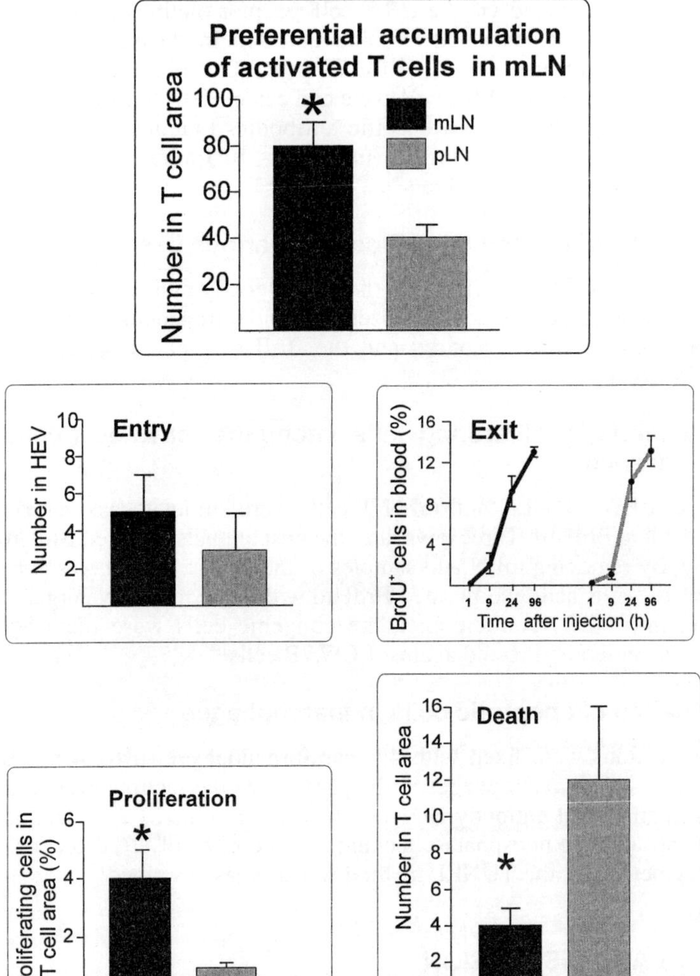

Figure 1 Increased proliferation and decreased apoptosis as causes for preferential accumulation of migrating activated T cells. Upper panel: One day after injection of activated T cells from either mesenteric lymph nodes (mLNs) or peripheral lymph nodes (pLNs), activated mLN T cells accumulate two times more in the T cell region of mLNs than activated pLN T cells. **Entry**: Both activated mLN and pLN T cells are found in comparable numbers in the high endothelial venules (HEV) of mLNs 1 h after injection, indicating a comparable entry rate for both populations. **Proliferation**: Three days after injection the percentage of activated mLN T cells proliferating in the lymph node is four times greater than that of activated pLN T cells. **Death**: The number of apoptotic cells contained by macrophages of mLNs is four times less 9 h after injection of activated mLN T cells compared with activated pLN T cells. **Exit**: The appearance rate of the progeny of the activated cells in the blood is comparable after injection of both activated mLN and pLN T cells, indicating that the exit rate of both populations is similar. Thus, preferential proliferation and reduced apoptosis rather than increased entry or reduced exit are responsible for the preferential accumulation of activated mLN T cells in mLNs (mean and standard deviations are indicated; asterisks indicate significant differences, $p < 0.05$; adapted from Ref. 15 and unpublished results)

The proportion of proliferating cells among the activated mLN and pLN T cells was then determined, showing that about three to four times as many activated mLN T cells were proliferating in mLNs as activated pLN T cells (Fig. 1). Since about 70% of activated lymphocytes migrating through the body die within 24 h[24,25], reducing the death rate of the migrating activated T cells could also lead to preferential accumulation. The death of the activated T cells was analysed using the TUNEL technique[26]. After injection of activated mLN T cells the total number of apoptotic cells contained by macrophages in the T cell region of mLNs was four times lower than after injection of activated pLN T cells (Fig. 1). This indicates that activated mLN T cells die at a lower rate in mLN, making the reduced death rate a likely cause of the preferential accumulation of activated mLN T cells in mLNs. In the rat the exit of lymphocyte subsets from different lymphoid organs is difficult to measure. Since activated T cells mainly proliferate within the tissue and not in the circulation, the appearance rate of the progeny of the activated T cells in the blood gives a rough indication of differences in the exit rate. Thus, activated mLN and pLN T cells were homogeneously labelled with BrdUrd and then injected intravenously. Since BrdUrd is distributed equally to both daughter cells during cell division, the progeny should contain less BrdUrd, leading to a decreased staining intensity. Indeed, BrdUrd^{low} cells (daughter cells) were identified in the blood from 24 h after injection onwards, the kinetics for activated mLN and pLN T cells being comparable. This indicates that preferential exit is not a likely cause of preferential accumulation of activated mLN T cells in mLNs.

Thus, in contrast to granulocytes, where it is possible to relate a high cell number in an inflamed tissue directly to an increased immigration rate[6,27], the explanation of changes in the numbers of migrating lymphocytes requires entry, proliferation, death and exit all to be considered[13,14,28].

The localization of activated mLN T cells in the lamina propria of the gut was then investigated. The injected cells could be clearly identified (Fig. 2), and the percentage of locally proliferating cells among them could be determined. About three to four times more activated mLN T cells were localized in the lamina propria of ileum and colon than in jejunum 72 h after injection (Table 1). However, there was no difference in the local proliferation rate among the activated T cells at the different sites (Table 1). Thus, at the moment it seems that differences in proliferation is not the reason for the preferential accumulation in ileum and colon. Whether preferential immigration, reduced cell death or local retention of activated T cells causes this phenomenon, remains to be studied.

CONCLUSION

Activated T cells produce cytokines and express co-stimulatory molecules and are, therefore, able to induce the proliferation of 'innocent' bystander lymphocytes[29]: the distribution of these potentially dangerous cells should be carefully regulated. Modifying the survival of activated T cells after random entry into the tissue represents an elegant way of making these cells available to the sites where they are needed, while retaining them in certain regions. Such a mechanism might explain how immune responses can spread from the jejunum to the ileum and colon but still remain confined to the small and large intestine.

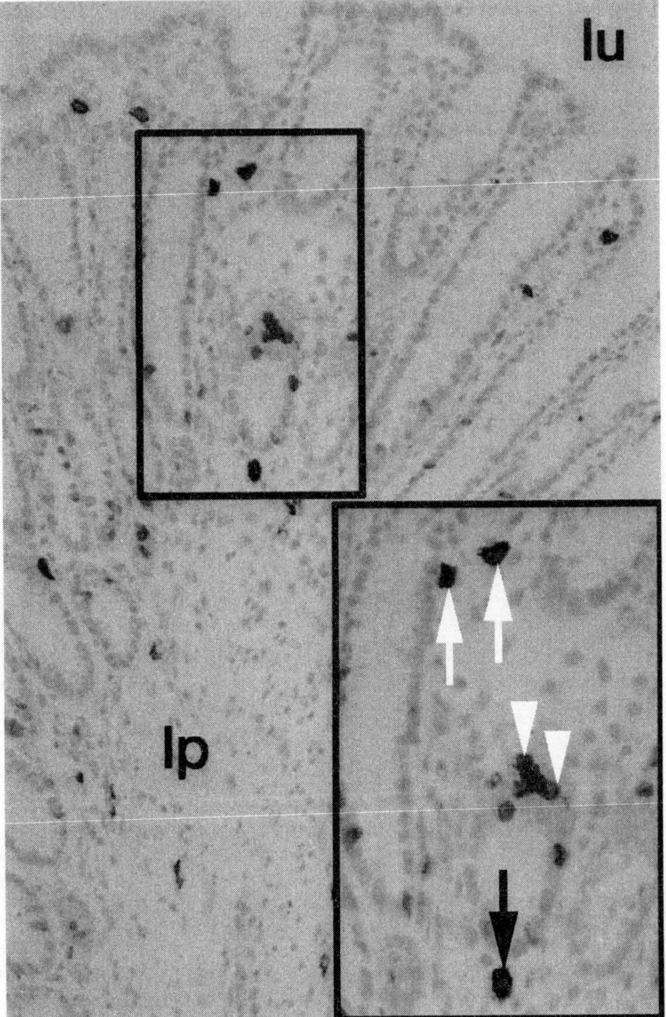

Figure 2 Local proliferation of activated mLN T cells in the lamina propria of the colon 72 h after injection. On cryostat sections of the rat colon activated mLN T cells are revealed shown by (white arrows. Those cells which were injected and incorporated BrdUrd while being in the lamina propria are shown by the (black arrow (inset represents a magnification of the encircled area). Proliferating cells of the recipient are shown by white arrowheads (lu: lumen; lp: lamina propria; irrelevant control antibodies showed no positive staining; alkaline phosphatase anti-alkaline phosphatase; counterstain, haematoxylin)

ACKNOWLEDGEMENTS

We thank K. Bankes, I. Dressendörfer, S. Lopez-Kostka and F. Weidner. The continuous support by R. Pabst (Department of Anatomy, Medical School of Hannover, Germany) and the help in preparing the figures by M. Peter are

Table 1 Number and local proliferation of activated mLN T cells in different regions of the gut[a]

	Jejunum (n = 6)	*Ileum* (n = 6)	*Colon* (n = 6)
Number[b]	1	3.3 ± 0.9[*]	4.2 ± 1.8[*]
Proliferation[c]	5.0 ± 1.5	6.2 ± 1.8	5.1 ± 1.9

[a] Activated mLN T cells were injected and 72 h later BrdUrd was given intravenously. One hour later the organs were removed and analysed.

[b] The number of cells per section is given. The area of lamina propria per section was comparable between jejunum, ileum and colon (data not shown), and is related to that in jejunum which is set at 1.

[c] Indicated is the percentage of BrdUrd[+] among the injected activated mLN T cells found at the different sites.

gratefully acknowledged. The authors' studies were supported by the Deutsche Forschungsgemeinschaft (SFB 244 A7 and We 1175/4-2).

References

1. Ford WL. Lymphocyte migration and immune responses. Prog Allergy. 1975;19:1–59.
2. Pabst R, Binns RM. Heterogeneity of lymphocyte homing physiology. Several mechanisms operate in the control of migration to lymphoid and non-lymphoid organs in vivo. Immunol Rev. 1989;108:83–109.
3. Abernethy NJ, Hay JB. The recirculation of lymphocytes from blood to lymph: Physiological considerations and molecular mechanisms. Lymphology. 1992;25:1–30.
4. Ager A. Lymphocyte recirculation and homing: roles of adhesion molecules and chemo-attractants. Trends Cell Biol. 1994;4:326–333.
5. Salmi M, Jalkanen S. How do lymphocytes know where to go: current concepts and enigmas of lymphocyte homing. Adv Immunol. 1997;64:139–217.
6. Westermann J, Pabst R. Lymphocyte subsets in the blood: A diagnostic window on the lymphoid system? Immunol Today. 1990;11:406–410.
7. Westermann J, Pabst R. How organ-specific is the migration of 'naive' and 'memory' T lympho-cytes? Immunol Today. 1996;17:278–282.
8. Springer TA. Adhesion receptors of the immune system. Nature. 1990;346:425–434.
9. Butcher EC, Picker LJ. Lymphocyte homing and homeostasis. Science. 1996;272:60–66.
10. Butcher EC. Leukocyte-endothelial cell recognition: three (or more) steps to specificity and diversity. Cell. 1991;67:1033–1036.
11. Adams DH, Shaw S. Leucocyte-endothelial interactions and regulation of leucocyte migration. Lancet. 1994;343:831–836.
12. Springer TA. Traffic signals for lymphocyte recirculation and leukocyte emigration: The multi-step paradigm. Cell. 1994;76:301–314.
13. Pabst R, Westermann J. Which steps of lymphocyte recirculation are regulated by interferon-gamma? Res Immunol. 1994;145:289–294.
14. Pabst R, Tschernig T. Lymphocyte dynamics: caution in interpreting BAL numbers. Thorax. 1997;52:1078–1080.
15. Bode U, Wonigeit K, Pabst K, Westermann J. The fate of activated T cells migrating through the body: rescue from apoptosis in the tissue of origin. Eur J Immunol. 1997;27:2087–2093.
16. Fritz FJ, Westermann J, Pabst R. The mucosa of the male genital tract – part of the common mucosal secretory immune system? Eur J Immunol. 1989;19:475–479.
17. Tacke M, Clark GJ, Dallmann MJ, Hünig T. Cellular distribution and costimulatory function of rat CD28. Regulated expression during thymocyte maturation and induction of cyclosporin A sensitivity of costimulated T cell responses by phorbol ester. J Immunol. 1995;154:5121–5127.
18. Tacke M, Hanke G, Hanke T, Hünig T. CD28-mediated induction of proliferation in resting T cells *in vitro* and *in vivo* without engagement of the T cell receptor: evidence for functionally distinct forms of CD28. Eur J Immunol. 1997;27:239–247.

19. Westermann J, Smith T, Peters U *et al.* Both activated and nonactivated leukocytes from the periphery continuously enter the thymic medulla of adult rats: phenotypes, sources and magnitude of traffic. Eur J Immunol. 1996;26:1866–1874.
20. Walter S, Micheel B, Pabst R, Westermann J. Interaction of B and T lymphocyte subsets with high endothelial venules in the rat: binding in vitro does not reflect homing in vivo. Eur J Immunol. 1995;25:1199–1205.
21. Westermann J, Ronneberg S, Fritz FJ, Pabst R. Proliferation of lymphocyte subsets in the adult rat: a comparison of different lymphoid organs. Eur J Immunol. 1989;19:1087–1093.
22. Westermann J, Blaschke V, Zimmermann G, Hirschfeld U, Pabst R. Random entry of circulating lymphocyte subsets into peripheral lymph nodes and Peyer's patches: No evidence in vivo of a tissue specific migration of B and T lymphocytes at the level of high endothelial venules. Eur J Immunol. 1992;22:2219–2223.
23. Westermann J, Nagahori Y, Walter S, Heerwagen C, Miyasaka M, Pabst R. B and T lymphocyte subsets enter peripheral lymph nodes and Peyer's patches without preference in vivo: No correlation occurs between their localization in different types of high endothelial venules and the expression of CD44, VLA-4, LFA-1, ICAM-1, CD2 or L-selectin. Eur J Immunol. 1994;24:2312–2316.
24. Smith ME, Martin AF, Ford WL. Migration of lymphoblasts in the rat. Monogr Allergy. 1980;16:203–232.
25. Binns RM, Licence ST, Pabst R. Homing of blood, splenic, and lung emigrant lymphoblasts: comparison with the behaviour of lymphocytes from these sources. Int Immunol. 1992;4:1011–1019.
26. Surh CD, Sprent J. T-cell apoptosis detected in situ during positive and negative selection. Nature. 1994;372:100–103.
27. Zimmermann GA, Prescott SM, McIntyre TM. Endothelial cell interactions with granulocytes: tethering and signaling molecules. Immunol Today. 1992;13:93–100.
28. Krug N, Tschernig T, Holgate S, Pabst R. How do lymphocytes get into the asthmatic airways? Lymphocyte traffic into and within the lung in asthma. Clin Exp Allergy. 1998;28:10–18:
29. Tough DF, Borrow P, Sprent J. Induction of bystander T cell proliferation by viruses and type 1 interferon in vivo. Science. 1996;272:1947–1950.

9
Mutant enterotoxins and cytokines for safe targeting of T_H1- and T_H2-type responses to mucosal vaccines

P. N. BOYAKA, J. W. LILLARD, Jr., S. YAMAMOTO and
J. R. MCGHEE

INTRODUCTION

Mucosal vaccines display the unique ability to promote both secretory IgA (S-IgA) and serum antibody (Ab) responses for mucosal and systemic immunity. In contrast to parenterally delivered vaccines which only promote immune responses in the systemic compartment, mucosal vaccines can potentially protect exposed mucosal surfaces against exogenous pathogens and toxins[1]. Previous studies have focused on the identification of adjuvants and delivery systems which promote mucosal and systemic immunity when administered by mucosal routes. In this regard, two bacterial enterotoxins (i.e., cholera toxin (CT) and heat labile (LT) toxin from *Escherichia coli,*) were identified as very effective mucosal adjuvants that are able to promote both mucosal and systemic immunity to co-administered protein antigens[2–4]. Unfortunately, these enterotoxins are quite toxic to humans and are therefore unsuitable for vaccine purposes. Attenuated live bacteria such as *Salmonella* and viruses (e.g. adenovirus) vectors have been used successfully for the delivery of immunogens by mucosal routes[5,6]; however, adverse side effects may be associated with use of these bacterial or viral recombinant vectors in humans.

Another important area of investigation for the development of vaccines is the nature of the immune response generated by mucosal adjuvants or delivery systems. Appropriate cell-mediated immunity (CMI) or humoral Ab responses are required for protection against intracellular or extracellular pathogens, respectively. Mouse studies have established that $CD4^+$ T helper (T_H) cells can be segregated into T_H1- and T_H2-types based on the patterns of cytokines secreted. Cytokines produced by $CD4^+$ T_H cells play a pivotal role in the development of CMI and Ab responses[7]. Thus, while T_H1-type cells secreting interferon-γ (IFN-γ) promote CMI as well as IgG2a Ab responses, T_H2-type cells which secrete interleukin (IL)-4, IL-5, IL-6, and IL-10 support IgE, IgG1 and IgG2b Ab responses in mice[8]. Recent studies have shown that the induction of dominant T_H1- or T_H2-type responses or mixed T_H1- and T_H2-type responses by mucosal vaccines can be achieved by selective use of mucosal adjuvants or delivery systems[3,4,6].

An alternative strategy for the preferential targeting of T_H1- or T_H2-type responses is the use of regulatory cytokines themselves as adjuvants. It is well known that IFN-γ and IL-4 are reciprocally regulated and give rise to T_H1- or T_H2-type CD4+ T cells. Further, some cytokines have been shown to enhance CMI and cytotoxicity (i.e., IFN-γ, IL-2, and IL-6)[9–11] or humoral Ab responses (IL-4, IL-5, IL-6, and transforming (TGF)-β) growth factor[12–14]. IL-12, a regulatory cytokine secreted by antigen presenting cells[15], is a potent inducer of IFN-γ synthesis[16] and thus stimulates the generation of T_H1-type responses[17]. However, large doses of parenterally administered cytokines are often required to achieve effective results *in vivo* and alternative methods for delivery of cytokines are needed to circumvent the toxicity often linked with high or frequent parenteral doses.

This chapter summarizes strategies currently being investigated to safely target T_H1- or T_H2-type immune responses to mucosal vaccines. The two major areas of investigation are the development of nontoxic mutants of bacterial enterotoxins and the mucosal delivery of regulatory cytokines (i.e., IL-12).

MUTANT ENTEROTOXINS AS SAFE MUCOSAL ADJUVANTS FOR INDUCTION OF PREDOMINANT T_H2-TYPE RESPONSES

Cholera toxin and related heat labile enterotoxin from *Escherichia coli*

CT and LT from *Escherichia coli* are very similar holotoxins which are highly immunogenic and strongly adjuvantogenic for mucosally co-administered protein antigens. Cholera toxin is a heterologous macromolecule made up of two structurally and functionally separate A and B subunits[18,19]. The B subunit of CT (CT-B) consists of five identical 11.6 kDa peptides that bind to GM1 gangliosides[20]. The binding of CT-B to GM1 ganglioside on mucosal epithelia allows the A subunit to reach the cytosol of target cells where it binds to nicotinamide adenosyl diphosphate (NADP) and catalyses the ADP ribosylation of Gsα[21]. The latter GTP-binding protein activates adenyl cyclase with subsequent elevation of cAMP in epithelial cells followed by secretion of water and chloride ions into the intestinal lumen[22]. The LT molecule is closely related to CT and the two enterotoxins share an approximate 80% amino acid sequence homology[23]. While both CT and LT bind GM1 gangliosides, LT also exhibits an affinity for GM2 and asialo-GM1[19].

Previous studies have shown that mucosally (i.e., orally or nasally) administered CT exerts its mucosal adjuvant effect by inducing Ag-specific CD4+ T_H2-type cells which support subsequent systemic development of IgG1 and IgG2b subclass, IgE and S-IgA Ab responses[2,3,24,25]. Further, IL-4 is required for the adjuvant effect of CT since the absence of IL-4 inhibits the CT mucosal adjuvant activity[3,26]. On the other hand, LT induces a mix of T$_H$1- and T$_H$2-type antigen-specific CD4$^+$ T cells and adjuvant activity occurs even in the absence of IL-4[4]. Despite their remarkable ability to promote both mucosal and systemic responses to nasally or orally administered vaccine antigens, the use of these enterotoxins as adjuvants in humans has been prevented by their toxicity[27]. Contrasting results were reported from earlier attempts to dissociate diarrhoeagenicity and adjuvanticity of CT by mucosal administration of the non-toxic B subunit. In this regard, the covalent linking of CT-B and the protein seems to be required for CT-B to exhibit mucosal adjuvant effects[28], although this point remains controversial.

Genetically engineered mutants of cholera toxin for induction of predominant T$_H$2-type responses

Our group has investigated the site-directed mutagenesis of CT as a strategy to circumvent the toxicity of this enterotoxin. For this purpose, two CT mutants were contructed by single amino acid substitution in the ADP-ribosyltransferase activity centre of the CT gene from *Vibrio cholerae* 01 strain GP14. The CT gene was cloned into phage M13mp19 followed by site directed mutagenesis

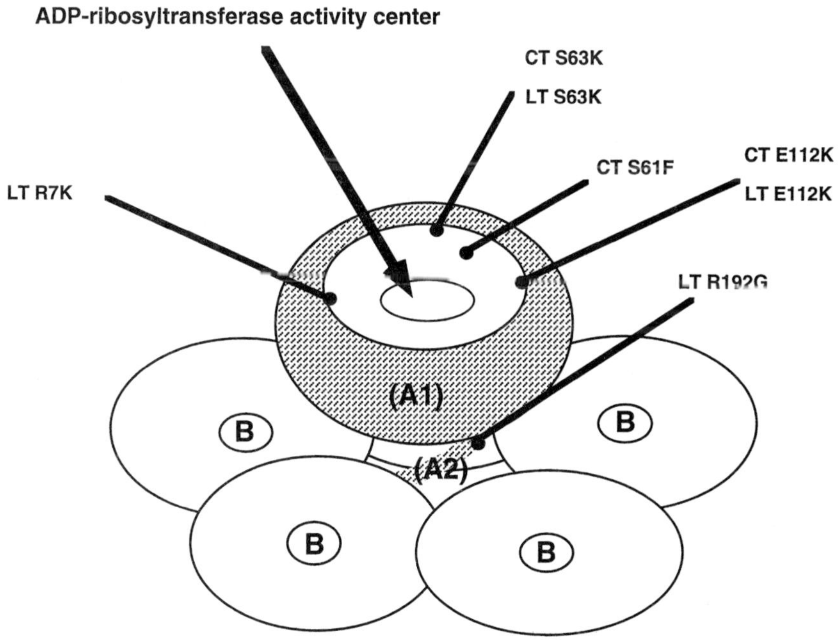

Figure 1 Sites of directed mutagenesis in the A subunit of cholera toxin (CT) and the related heat labile toxin (LT) from *Escherichia coli*. The main strategy used to obtain non-toxic mutants of CT and LT has consisted of single amino acid substitutions in the ADP-ribosyltransferase activity centre of the A1 subunit (i.e., R7K, S63K, S61F, and E112K mutants). Another strategy has involved single amino acid substitution outside the ADP-ribosyltransferase activity centre of the A2 subunit (LT R192G mutant)

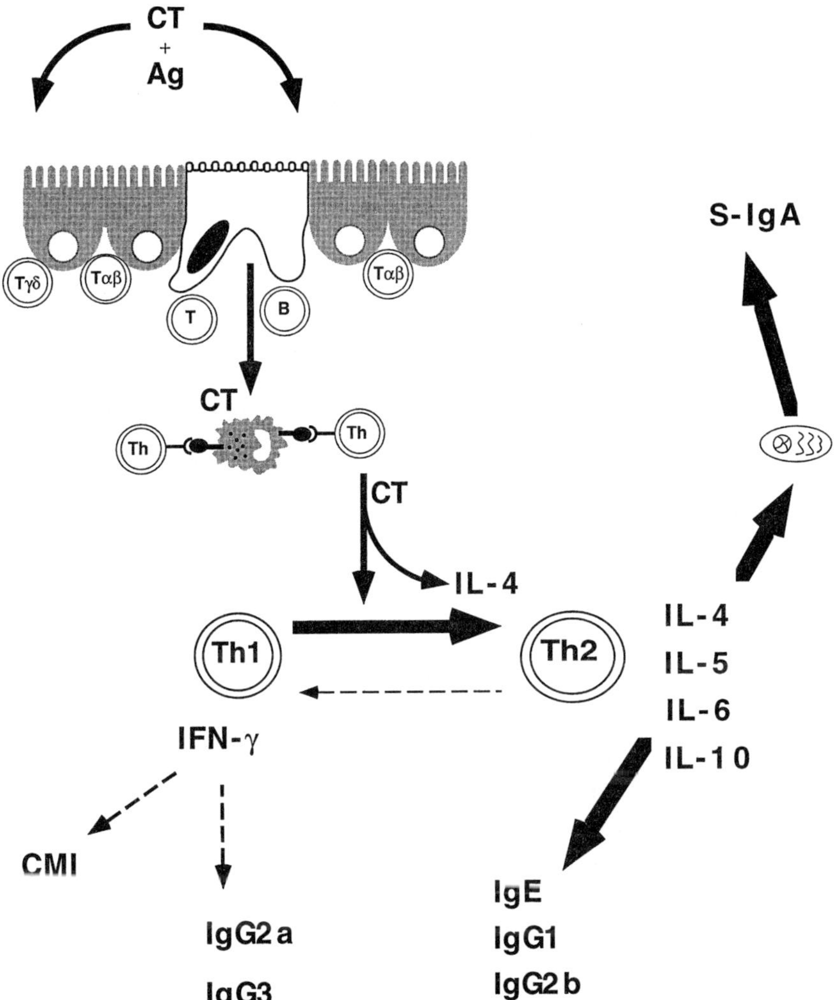

Figure 2 T helper cell-derived cytokines involved in the mucosal adjuvanticity of cholera toxin (CT). Mucosally administered CT as adjuvant promotes strong IL-4 responses which favour induction of antigen-specific T$_H$2-type cytokines with subsequent antigen-specific mucosal S-IgA Ab responses and serum IgE, IgG1 and IgG2b Ab responses

T$_H$2-type cells was involved in the adjuvant effect of these CT derivatives and native CT[39]. Taken together, these results show that directed mutagenesis in the ADP ribosyltransferase active centre of the A subunit of CT emphasizes the role of IL-4 and T$_H$2-type cytokines in the adjuvant effect of CT[3,26,40]. Most importantly, these studies provide evidence that these strategies allow a potent and safe way to induce dominant T$_H$2-type mucosal immune responses.

Mucosal and systemic immune responses to genetically engineered mutants of LT

Despite the structural and functional analogies between CT and LT, the latter binds to GM2 and asialo-GM1 gangliosides in addition to GM1 gangliosides[19]. Whether this tropism for a larger spectrum of cell surface carbohydrate influences the adjuvant effect of LT has not been established. Nevertheless, the adjuvanticity of mucosally administered LT results in serum Ab responses characterized by IgG1 and IgG2b Abs and, in contrast to CT, significant IgG2a Ab responses are also seen[4]. Further, LT induces a mixed CD4$^+$ T$_H$1- (i.e., IFN-γ) and T$_H$2-type (i.e., IL-4, IL-S, IL-6 and IL-10) response[4] and unlike nCT, the mucosal adjuvanticity of LT is not affected by the absence of IL-4[40].

Several groups have engineered mutants of LT by single amino acid substitution either inside or outside the ADP-ribosyltransferase cleft (Fig. 1). The mutant generated by amino acid substitution in position 112 (Glu for Lys) of the A subunit of LT lacked ADP-ribosylating activity but also lacked mucosal adjuvanticity when administered by the oral route[30,41]. The same strategy of single amino acid substitution has allowed the generation of other nontoxic mutants of LT, e.g., R7K[42], LTK63[39,42] and R192G[43]. The LTK63 and R192G mutants were also reported to retain the adjuvant effects of LT suggesting that the ADP-ribosylating activity and the related toxicity of LT can be dissociated from adjuvanticity. Thus, one might envision the use of mutants of LT when both T$_H$1- and T$_H$2-type responses are desired.

Mucosally administered IL-12 for targeting of T$_H$1- or T$_H$2-type responses to mucosal vaccines

The induction of T$_H$1- or T$_H$2-type responses by mucosal vaccination represents a major advance toward the preferential development of cell mediated immunity (CMI) or humoral Ab responses which would protect against intracellular or extracellular pathogens, respectively[7,8]. Since selected cytokines from T$_H$1- (i.e., IFN-γ) or T$_H$2-type (i.e., IL-4) cells can down-regulate the expression of the opposite T$_H$ cell phenotype[17,44], we have tested the effect that cytokines favouring T$_H$1-type responses would have on the immune response to mucosal vaccines containing nCT. IL-12, the product of macrophages and other APCs[45,46], is well known to be a strong inducer of IFN-γ secretion by NK and T cells[16,47]. Thus, IL-12 was used to test whether it could redirect the dominant T$_H$2-type responses induced by the mucosal adjuvant nCT.

Parenterally administered IL-12 shifts CT-induced T$_H$2-type responses and down-regulates secretory IgA (S-IgA) Ab responses to oral vaccines

IL-12 was parenterally administered to mice receiving an oral vaccine with nCT to test the potential of IL-12 to redirect T$_H$2-type responses induced by this regimen. Frequent intraperitoneal injections of recombinant IL-12 (100 ng/dose) down-regulated IgE Ab responses and significantly changed the pattern of antigen-specific serum IgG subclasses[34]. In fact, mice parenterally treated with IL-12 exhibited lower IgG1 and higher IgG2a and IgG3 Ab titres than mice that received the oral vaccine alone. The shift of CT-induced Ab subclass responses was shown to be due to T$_H$1-type cell responses. In this regard, antigen-specific CD4$^+$ T cells isolated from both systemic (i.e., spleen) and mucosal (i.e., Peyer's patches) compartments of mice parenterally treated with IL-12 displayed enhanced T$_H$1-type (i.e., IFN-γ and IL-2) cytokine secretion. Conversely, T$_H$2-type cytokine secretion was down-regulated when compared with groups given the oral vaccine only[34]. Mucosal IgA Ab responses were also altered by the parenteral treatment with IL-12, suggesting that parenteral IL-12 affects the mucosal adjuvanticity of CT. Antibody responses of all isotypes were abrogated when mice orally immunized with the combined vaccine were parenterally treated with 1 μg of IL-12. Furthermore, about 40% of mice treated with this dose (10–14 administrations) did not survive, confirming the potential toxicity associated with large and repeated parenteral doses of exogenous cytokines.

IL-12 delivered by the same mucosal route as mucosal vaccine with nCT shifts T$_H$2-type responses to T$_H$1-type but preserves S-IgA Ab responses

The mucosal delivery of IL-12 was investigated to circumvent the toxicity often linked to frequent or high parenteral doses of cytokines generally required to achieve effective results *in vivo*. In this regard, the effect of this regulatory cytokine on mucosal inductive sites has not been previously studied. For mucosal administration, IL-12 was complexed with preformed cationic liposomes (DOTAP) and the oral delivery of this cytokine did not result in significant serum IL-12[34]. In contrast, significant levels of serum IL-12 and subsequent IFN-γ secretion were achieved after nasal delivery of IL-12, confirming the uniqueness of nasal versus oral routes[48].

Mice that received oral IL-12 treatment exhibited reduced IgG1 and IgE Ab responses with enhanced antigen-specific IgG2a and IgG3 Abs, when compared with mice that received the oral vaccine alone[34]. Further, T$_H$2-type cytokine secretion (i.e, IL-4, IL-S, IL-6, and IL-10) by antigen-specific CD4$^+$ T cells from mice orally treated with IL-12 were significantly reduced when compared with the cytokine secretion pattern of cells from mice given the oral vaccine alone (Fig. 3). Conversely, T$_H$1-type cytokines (i.e., IFN-γ) were minimal in culture supernatants of cells from mice that received the oral vaccine with nCT alone but were enhanced by oral IL-12 treatment (Fig. 3). Similar results were obtained when IL-12 was co-nasally administered to mice receiving an intranasal vaccine[48]. Thus, IL-12 can be effectively administered by the oral or nasal routes to regulate immune responses to vaccines delivered by the same mucosal route. These results are consistent with the ability of IL-12 to promote T$_H$1-type cells and CMI responses.

An important result of our oral and nasal IL-12 studies was the inability of mucosally administered IL-12 to suppress S-IgA Ab responses. In fact, despite the shift induced for systemic Ab and T cell responses, mucosally administered IL-12 failed to down-regulate S-IgA Ab responses; however, this effect was achieved by parenteral administration of comparable IL-12 doses (1 μg)[34,48]. The fact that this regulatory effect could be observed in the absence of low or

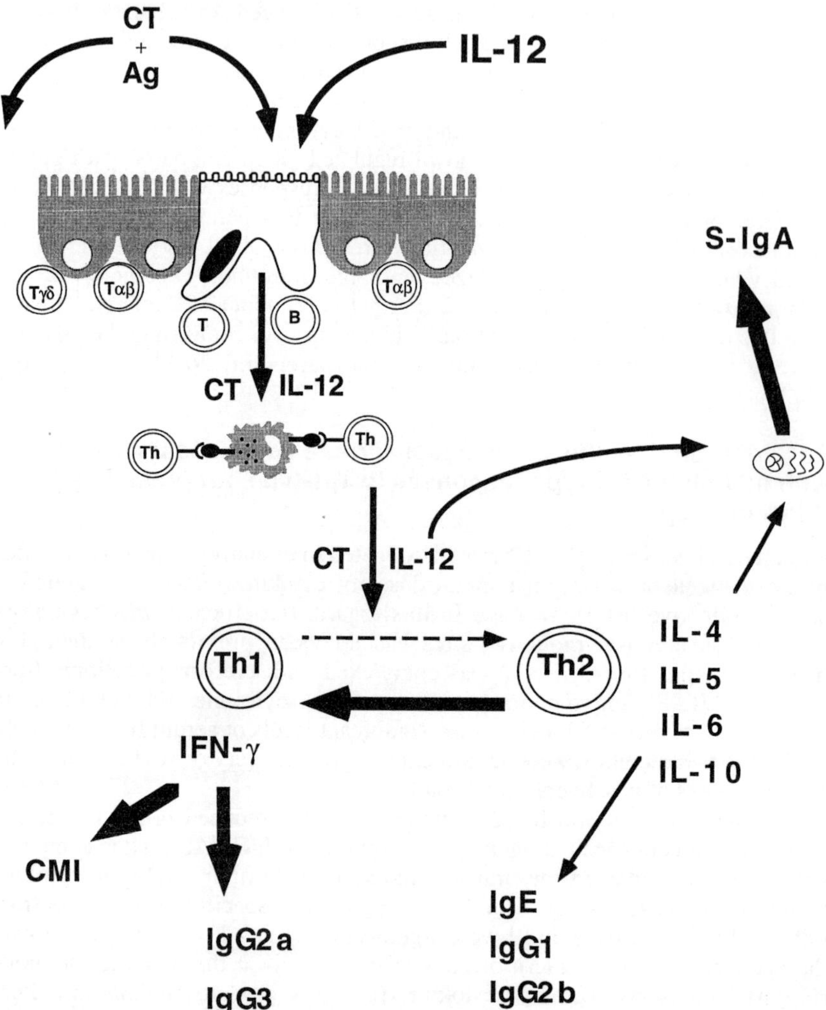

Figure 3 Effects of mucosal IL-12 delivered by the same mucosal route with a combined vaccine containing CT as adjuvant for CT-induced T_H2-type responses. When delivered by the same mucosal route as combined vaccine, IL-12 shifts CT-induced systemic T_H2-type responses toward a T_H1 type. This effect resulted in enhanced IFN-γ secretion and antigen-specific serum IgG2a and IgG3 Ab responses. Conversely, IL-4 and Th2-type responses were inhibited with a resultant abrogation of IgE Ab responses. Antigen-specific mucosal S-IgA Ab responses were not affected by this mucosal IL-12 treatment

negligible serum IL-12 levels prevented the adverse effects linked to large parenteral doses and suggested that IL-12 acted through direct effects on the inductive sites of the mucosa-associated lymphoreticular tissues (MALT).

IL-12 enhances both T_H1- and T_H2-type responses to mucosal vaccines given with nCT by a separate mucosal route

Since our results suggest that mucosally administered IL-12 acts directly on cells of the mucosal inductive site where the cytokine is introduced, we also addressed the effect of IL-12 when administered through a mucosal site different from where the vaccine containing nCT was given. For this purpose, IL-12 was delivered by the nasal route to mice which also received an oral vaccine with nCT as adjuvant. Interestingly, nasal IL-12 did not alter T_H2-type responses in the latter system. In fact, the nasal IL-12 treatment actually enhanced antigen-specific IgE Ab responses to the oral vaccine[48]. Nasal IL-12 also failed to down-regulate IgG1 and IgG2b Ab responses but actually enhanced IgG1 and IgG2b Abs and induced significant IgG2a and IgG3 Ab responses when compared with groups receiving the oral vaccine only[48]. Thus, as previously reported, IL-12 treatment can act as an adjuvant for humoral immunity[49] and enhance all IgG subclass responses[50].

The T helper cytokines responsible for the discrepancy between the effect of IL-12 on the immune response to vaccine delivered by the same or a separate mucosal route were determined by analysing cytokines secreted by antigen-specific CD4[+] T cells from the two groups. Nasal delivery of IL-12 induced IFN-γ and IL-2 (e.g., T_H1-type cytokine) secretion by *in vitro* restimulated antigen-specific CD4[+] T cells from mice receiving either the nasal or the oral vaccine, demonstrating that in both cases, IL-12 induced the development of T_H1-type subsets[48]. However, T_H2-type cytokines were differentially regulated by nasal IL-12 treatment: IL-4, IL-S, IL-6 and IL-10 secretion were inhibited by nasal IL-12 treatment of mice that received the nasal vaccine. Conversely, IL-4, IL-S and IL-6 were not affected and IL-10 was actually enhanced when nasal IL-12 was administered to mice orally immunized with nCT as adjuvant[48] (Fig. 4).

Our results clearly show that nasally administered IL-12 can either redirect T_H2-type responses toward T_H1-type or enhance both T_H1- and T_H2-type responses. This observation is consistent with previous reports that this cytokine could exacerbate ongoing T_H2-type responses[50,51] and act as adjuvant for humoral immunity through IFN-γ-dependent and -independent mechanisms[49]. To establish that the enhancing effect of nasal IL-12 on oral CT-induced T_H2-type responses was due to a delay of IL-12 to reach inductive sites in the GI tract, IL-12 was parenterally administered 24 h after oral immunization of mice. While parenteral administration of IL-12 on the day of oral immunization shifted the CT-induced T_H2-type responses toward a T_H1-type[34], a 24 h delay in the administration of this cytokine induced T_H1-type responses and enhanced CT-induced T_H2-type responses[48]. In fact, the pattern of serum and mucosal Ab responses as well as cytokine secretion by antigen-specific CD4[+] T cells were comparable to those observed in mice orally immunized with CT as adjuvant and nasally treated with IL-12[48].

CONCLUSION

The development of effective mucosal vaccines relies on safe mucosal adjuvants to promote CMI and/or Ab responses required to protect against intracellular pathogens or soluble antigens and toxins, respectively. Thus, future mucosal

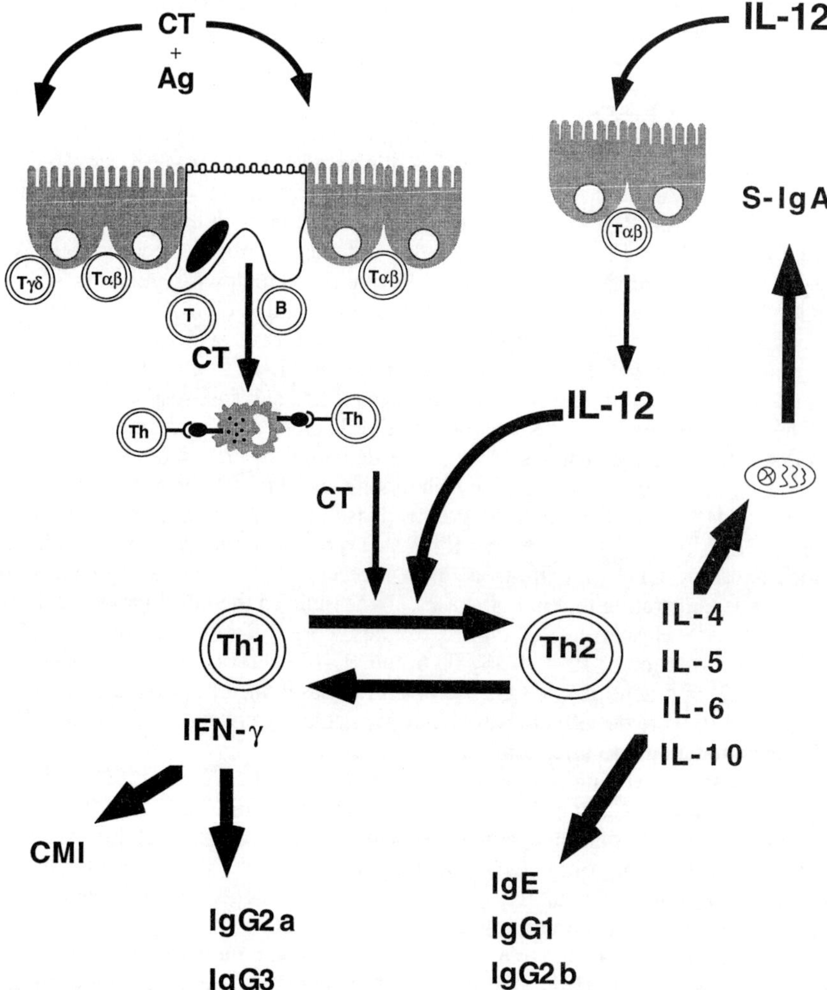

Figure 4 The enhancing effect of IL-12 on CT-induced T_H2-type responses when administered by separate mucosal routes as combined mucosal vaccine with CT as adjuvant. Both induction of antigen-specific T_H1-type responses and enhanced CT-induced T_H2-type responses occurred when IL-12 was administered by a separate mucosal route. Antigen-specific S-IgA Ab responses to the combined vaccine were not affected by mucosal IL-12 treatment

vaccines would benefit from strategies to safely trigger specific T_H cell subsets for T_H1, T_H2 or mixed T_H1/T_H2 responses in mucosal and systemic immune compartments. In this regard, site-directed mutagenesis of bacterial enterotoxins has provided mutants of CT and LT which may now be suitable for use in humans. This strategy will also allow the development of new tools for understanding the mechanisms responsible for the mucosal adjuvanticity of these enterotoxins. Specifically, single amino acid substitutions in the A subunit of

CT and LT have dissociated toxicity and ADP ribosyltransferase activity from adjuvanticity. Thus, two mutants of CT, E112K and S61F, can function as non-toxic mucosal adjuvants. However, the precise mechanisms involved in the regulatory effect of these mCT or other derivatives of nCT or nLT await elucidation.

The use of exogenous cytokines for the regulation of mucosal immune responses is a growing area of investigation. Cytokines represent a very attractive method to target desired immunity because of the large number of cytokines available and the multiple effects that each of these molecules exert on cells of the immune system. Thus, the mucosal administration of cytokines may provide a safe and effective way to regulate the immune response to mucosal vaccines by preventing potential toxicity associated with repetitive doses required for parenteral delivery. The differential effect of mucosal versus parenteral IL-12 on mucosal and systemic immune responses emphasizes the unique features of the mucosal and systemic immune compartments. In this regard, the failure of mucosally administered IL-12 to down-regulate secretory IgA responses in mucosal secretions might suggest a role of endogenous IL-12 in the control of these responses. We have also demonstrated that the timing and mucosal route of cytokine delivery influences the induction of targeted T$_H$1- and/or T$_H$2-type immune responses. These findings have important implications for the design of safe and effective future generations of mucosal adjuvants.

ACKNOWLEDGEMENTS

This work was supported by US PHS grants AI 18958, DK 44240, DE 04217, AI 35544, DE 09837, and NAID-DMID contracts NO1 AI 65298 and NO1 AI 65299.

References

1. Staats HF, Jackson RJ, Marinaro M, Takahashi I, Kiyono H, McGhee JR. Mucosal immunity to infection with implications for vaccine development. Curr Opin Immunol. 1994;6:572–583.
2. Xu Amano J, Kiyono H, Jackson RJ et al. Helper T cell subsets for immunoglobulin A responses: oral immunization with tetanus toxoid and cholera toxin as adjuvant selectively induces Th2 cells in mucosa associated tissues. J Exp Med. 1993;178:1309–1320.
3. Marinaro M, Staats HF, Hircoi T et al. Mucosal adjuvant effect of cholera toxin in mice results from induction of T helper 2 (Th2) cells and IL-4. J Immunol. 1995;155:4621–4629.
4. Takahashi I, Marinaro M, Kiyono H et al. Mechanisms for mucosal immunogenicity and adjuvancy of *Escherichia coli* labile enterotoxin. J Infect Dis. 1996;173:627–635.
5. Van Ginkel FW, Liu C, Simecka JW et al. Intratracheal gene delivery with adenoviral vector induces elevated systemic IgG and mucosal IgA antibodies to adenovirus and beta-galactosidase. Human Gene Ther. 1995;6:895–903.
6. VanCott JL, Staats HF, Pascual DW et al. Regulation of mucosal and systemic antibody responses by T helper cell subsets, macrophages, and derived cytokines following oral immunization with live recombinant *Salmonella*. J Immunol. 1996;156:1504–1514.
7. Mosmann TR, Coffman RL. T$_H$1 and T$_H$2 cells: different patterns of lymphokine secretion lead to different functional properties. Annu Rev Immunol. 1989;7:145–173.
8. Finkelman FD, Holmes J, Katona IM et al. Lymphokine control of *in vivo* immunoglobulin isotype selection. Annu Rev Immunol. 1990;8:303–333.
9. Luger TA, Krutmann J, Kirnbauer R et al. IFN-beta 2/IL-6 augments the activity of human natural killer cells. J Immunol. 1989;143:1206–1209.
10. Lorre K, Van DJ, Verwilghen J, Baroja ML, Ceuppens JL. IL-6 is an accessory signal in the alternative CD2-mediated pathway of T cell activation. J Immunol. 1990;144:4681–4687.

11. Mule JJ, Custer MC, Travis WD, Rosenberg SA. Cellular mechanisms of the antitumor activity of recombinant IL-6 in mice. J Immunol. 1992;148:2622–2629.

12. Beagley KW, Heldridge JH, Lee F et al. Interleukins and IgA synthesis: human and murine interleukin 6 induce high rate IgA secretion in IgA-commited B cells. J Exp Med. 1989;169:2133–2141.

13. McGhee JR, Mestecky J, Elson CO, Kiyono H. Regulation of IgA synthesis and immune response by T cells and interleukins. J Clin Immunol 1989;9:175–199.

14. Kim P-H, Eckmann L, Lee WJ, Han W, Kagnoff MF. Cholera toxin and cholera toxin B subunit induce IgA switching through the action of TGF-β1. J Immunol. 1998;160:1198-1203.

15. D'Andrea A, Rengaraju M, Valiante NM et al. Production of natural killer cell stimulatory factor (interleukin 12) by peripheral blood mononuclear cells. J Exp Med. 1992;176:1387–1398.

16. Chan SH, Perussia B, Gupta JW et al. Induction of interferon gamma production by natural killer cell stimulatory factor: characterization of the responder cells and synergy with other inducers. J Exp Med. 1991;173:869–879.

17. Coffman RL, Varkila K, Scott P, Chatelain R. Role of cytokines in the differentiation of CD4[+] T-cell subsets *in vivo*. Immunol Rev. 1991;123:189–207.

18. Gill DM. The arrangement of subunits in cholera toxin. Biochemistry. 1976;15:1242–1248.

19. Spangler BD. Structure and function of cholera toxin and the related *Escherichia coli* heat-labile enterotoxin. Microbiol Rev. 1992;56:622–647.

20. Heyningen SV. Cholera toxin: interaction of subunits with ganglioside GM1. Science. 1974;183:656–657.

21. Gill DM, King CA. The mechanism of action of cholera toxin in pigeon erythrocyte lysates. J Biol Chem. 1975;250:6424–6432.

22. Field M, Rao MC, Chang EB. Intestinal electrolyte transport and diarrheal disease. N Engl J Med. 1989;321:800–806.

23. Dallas WS, Falkow S. Amino acid sequence homology between cholera toxin and *Escherichia coli* heat-labile toxin. Nature. 1980;288:499–501.

24. Staats HF, Nichols WG, Palker TJ. Mucosal immunity to HIV-1: systemic and vaginal antibody responses after intranasal immunization with the HIV-1 C4/V3 peptide T1SP10 MN(A). J Immunol. 1996;157:462–472.

25. Staats HF, Montgomery SP, Palker TJ. Intranasal immunization is superior to vaginal, gastric, or rectal immunization for the induction of systemic and mucosal anti-HIV antibody responses. AIDS Res Hum Retroviruses. 1997;13:945–952.

26. Vajdy M, Kosco VM, Kopf M, Kohler G, Lycke N. Impaired mucosal immune responses in interleukin 4-targeted mice. J Exp Med. 1995;181:41–53.

27. Levine MM, Kaper JB, Black RE, Clements ML. New knowledge on pathogenesis of bacterial enteric infections as applied to vaccine development. Microbiol Rev. 1983;47:510–550.

28. Czerkinsky C, Russell MW, Lycke N, Lindblad M, Holmgren J. Oral administration of a streptococcal antigen coupled to cholera toxin B subunit evokes strong antibody responses in salivary glands and extramucosal tissues. Infect Immun. 1989;57:1072–1077.

29. Harford S, Dykes CW, Hobden AN, Read MJ, Halliday IJ. Inactivation of the *Escherichia coli* heat-labile enterotoxin by in vitro mutagenesis of the A-subunit gene. Eur J Biochem. 1989;183:311–316.

30. Tsuji T, Inoue T, Miyama A, Okamoto K, Honda T, Miwatani T. A single amino acid substitution in the A subunit of *Escherichia coli* enterotoxin results in a loss of its toxic activity. J Biol Chem. 1990;265:22520–22525.

31. Yamamoto S, Takeda Y, Yamamoto M et al. Mutants in the ADP-ribosyltransferase cleft of cholera toxin lack diarrheagenicity but retain adjuvanticity. J Exp Med. 1997;185:1203–1210.

32. Yamamoto S, Kiyono H, Yamamoto M et al. A nontoxic mutant of cholera toxin elicits Th2-type responses for enhanced mucosal immunity. Proc Natl Acad Sci USA. 1997;94:5267–5272.

33. Yamamoto S, Yamamoto M, Yamamoto M et al. Oral immunization with a nontoxic mutant of cholera toxin elicits mucosal adjuvanticity in mice. (submitted 1998).

34. Marinarco M, Boyaka PN, Finkelman FD et al. Oral but not parenteral interleukin (IL)-12 redirects T helper 2 (Th2)-type responses to an oral vaccine without altering mucosal IgA responses. J Exp Med. 1997;185:415–427.

35. Gill DM, Meren R. ADP-ribosylation of membrane proteins catalyzed by cholera toxin: basis of the activation of adenylate cyclase. Proc Natl Acad Sci USA. 1978;75:3050–3054.

36. Watkins PA, Moss J, Vaughan M. Effects of GTP on choleragen-catalyzed ADP ribosylation of membrane and soluble proteins. J Biol Chem. 1980;255:3959–3963.

37. Cong Y, Weaver CT, Elson CO. The mucosal adjuvanticity of cholera toxin involves enhancement of costimulatory activity by selective up-regulation of B7.2 expression. J Immunol. 1997;159:5301–5308.
38. Yamamoto M, Yamamoto S, Batanerco E, Fujihashi K, Kiyono H, Mcghee JR. Direct effects on antigen-presenting cells and T lymphocytes explain the adjuvanticity of a non toxic cholera toxin mutant. (Submitted 1998).
39. Douce G, Fontana M, Pizza M, Rappucoli R, Dougan G. Intranasal immuogenicity and adjuvanticity of site-directed mutant derivatives of cholera toxin. Infect Immun. 1997;65:2821–2828.
40. Okahashi N, Yamamoto M, Vanccott JL et al. Oral immunization of interleukin-4 (IL-4) knockout mice with a recombinant *Salmonella* strain or cholera toxin reveals that CD4$^+$ Th2 cells producing IL-6 and IL-10 are associated with mucosal immunoglobulin A responses. Infect Immun. 1996;64:1516–1525.
41. Lywaske N, Tsuji T, Holmgren J. The adjuvant effect of *Vibrio cholerae* and *Escherichia coli* heat-labile enterotoxins is linked to their ADP-ribosyltransferase activity. Eur J Immunol. 1992;22:2277–2281.
42. Douce G, Turcotte C, Cropley I et al. Mutants of *Escherichia coli* heat-labile toxin lacking ADP-ribosyltransferase activity act as nontoxic, mucosal adjuvants. Proc Natl Acad Sci USA. 1995;92:1644–1648.
43. Dickinson BL, Clements JD. Dissociation of *Escherichia coli* heat-labile enterotoxin adjuvanticity from ADP-ribosyltransferase activity. Infect Immun. 1995;63:1617–1623.
44. Seder RA, Paul WE. Acquisition of lymphokine-producing phenotype by CD4+ T cells. Annu Rev Immunol. 1994;12:635–673.
45. Kobayashi M, Fitz L, Ryan M et al. Identification and purification of natural killer cell stimulatory factor (NKSF), a cytokine with multiple biologic effects on human lymphocytes. J Exp Med. 1989;170:827–845.
46. Macatonia SE, Hosken NA, Litton M et al. Dendritic cells produce IL-12 and direct the development of Th1 cells from naive CD4+ T cells. J Immunol. 1995;154:5071–5079.
47. Seder RA, Gazzinelli R, Sher A, Paul WE. Interleukin 12 acts directly on CD4+ T cells to enhance priming for interferon gamma production and diminishes interleukin 4 inhibition of such priming. Proc Natl Acad Sci USA. 1993;90:10188–10192.
48. Marinaro M, Boyaka PN, Jackson RJ et al. Use of intranasal IL-12 to target predominantly Th1 responses to nasal and Th2 responses to oral vaccines given with cholera toxin. (Submitted 1998).
49. Metzger DW, McNutt RM, Collins JT, Buchanan JM, Van CV, Dunnick WA. Interleukin-12 acts as an adjuvant for humoral immunity through interferon-gamma-dependent and -independent mechanisms. Eur J Immunol. 1997;27:1958–1965.
50. Germann T, Guckes S, Bongartz M et al. Administration of IL-12 during ongoing immune responses fails to permanently suppress and can even enhance the synthesis of antigen specific IgE. Int Immunol. 1995;7:1649–1657.
51. Finkelman FD, Madden KB, Cheever AW et al. Effects of interleukin 12 on immune responses and host protection in mice infected with intestinal nematode parasites. J Exp Med. 1994;179:1563–1572.

Section III
Mechanisms of inflammatory disease 1: Abnormalities in IBD and related findings in animal models

10
Inflammatory bowel diseases: a breakdown of central and peripheral immunological homeostasis

W. STROBER, R. O. EHRHARDT AND B. R. LÚDVÍKSSON

INTRODUCTION: GENERALIZATIONS CONCERNING MOUSE MODELS OF MUCOSAL INFLAMMATION

Until recently, research into the immunopathogenesis of inflammatory bowel disease (IBD) was necessarily centred on the immunological responses of the patients themselves, rather than animal models of these diseases, either because the models then extant did not closely resemble the human disease and/or because knowledge of immune responses was not yet sufficiently advanced to allow models to be meaningfully analysed. The situation changed dramatically in the early 1990s with the appearance of reports of colitis occurring in SCID mice immunologically reconstituted by the transfer of naive, CD45RB[hi] T cells, followed by reports of colitis occurring in various knockout mice, the latter in the same issue of the journal, *Cell*[1–5]. These reports not only provided murine models of inflammation resembling Crohn's disease (reconstituted SCID mice as well as IL-2 and IL-10 knockout mice) and ulcerative colitis (TCR α chain knockout mice), they also provided an experimental universe within which the presence of colitis could be correlated with and understood by recourse to current notions of T cell differentiation, cytokine production and cell survival. In short, they revolutionized IBD research and, with other models that have appeared subsequently, are providing the first definitive insights into the cause and possible treatment of these diseases.

As illustrated in Table 1, a wide variety of murine models of intestinal inflammation, representing a wide variety of both induced and spontaneous colitides, have now been identified[1–19]. Several generalizations concerning these various models can now be put forward. The first is that in each instance they are characterized by various forms of immunological imbalance or dysregulation rather than gross immunological deficiency. This fact, plus the fact that mice with total lack of immune function, SCID mice or Rag-2-deficient mice, do not develop colitis, strongly suggests that mucosal inflammation in murine models is

Table 1 Rodent models of IBD

	Bowel pathology			Immune dysregulation		
	Histopathology	Peak time of onset	Microbial involvement	Peripheral	Central	Cytokine pattern
IL-2 –/–	Pancolitis, transmural, ulcerations, crypt abscesses, depending on the antigenic exposure	'Spontaneously' (12–15 weeks) or 7 days after immunization	+	CD4[+] LP T cells	Activated CD4[+]/CD69[+] SP T cells	IFN-γ and IL-12; TGF-β and IL-4
Gαi2 –/–	Pancolitis distal > proximal adenocarcinoma	8–13 weeks of age	?	CD4[+] LP T cells	Activated SP CD4[+] cells	IFN-γ, TNF-α, IL-1β, IL-6 and IL-12
IL-10 –/–	Focal colitis and ileitis, transmural	4–8 weeks of age	+	CD4[+] LP T cells	?	IFN-γ, IL-4
TGFβ –/–	Ileitis > colitis	3–5 weeks of age	SPF mice show delayed onset of inflammation	?	Thymocytes SPCD4[+]/DP ratio	IFN-γ
CD45RB[hi] Ø SCID	Transmural pancolitis, granuloma	5–8 weeks post-transfer	+	CD45Rb[hi] CD4[+] T cells	?	IFN-γ
TCRα –/–	Initial appendicitis, then pancolitis, microabscesses, UC-like lesions	4–6 months of age	+ (unpublished results)	Hyperproliferative CD4[+]/TCRβ[dim] T cells, IgG1/IgE autoantibodies	Aberrant thymocyte development	IL-4 and IL-1
C3H/HeJBir	Right-sided, distal colitis; mild submucosal inflammation	Onset 3–4 weeks of age; resolves after 10–12 weeks	+	CD4[+] LP T cell reactive to enteric bacterial antigens	?	?
TNBS	Pancolitis, transmural granulomatous	7 days after administration	+	CD4[+] LP T cells	–	IFN-γ, TNF-α and IL-12

not due to an infection with a known mucosal pathogen, if it is due to an infection at all. This conclusion is underscored by recent studies conducted by Kullberg and Sher, who have shown that, while IL-10 knockout mice rapidly develop colitis if exposed to the pathogen *Helicobactor hepaticus*, such infection is not more severe in the knockout mice than in their heterozygous control littermates (A. Sher, personal communication). The second generalization, one related to the first, is that in each of the models so far studied in the appropriate way, the presence of a germ-free or even a pathogen-free environment prevents or attenuates the expression of colitis. This striking fact strongly suggests that the normal mucosal microflora plays an essential role in the initiation and/or persistence of the mucosal inflammation[20]. Consistent with this is the observation that colitis can be induced in IL-2 knockout mice by the systemic administration of TNP-KLH (trinitrophenyl-substituted keyhole limpet haemocyanin), but not by KLH alone. We postulated that the TNP epitopes evoked an immune response that cross-reacts with self-epitopes associated with antigens in the mucosal microflora and it is the latter rather than the administered TNP that sustains the colitis. In addition, Duchmann *et al.* have shown that T cells from SJL/J mice with TNBS colitis can be stimulated *in vitro* by preparations of microflora whereas T cells from the same mice without colitis are not so stimulated[21]. That such responsiveness is related to the pathogenesis of the colitis is suggested by the fact that it disappears when the mice are successfully treated by anticytokine therapy. The obligate role of the normal microflora in the pathogenesis of colitis occurring in the various models revealed by the above studies provides an explanation for the fact that mice with very disparate immune defects all manifest a common disease manifestation, chronic colitis. Thus, if we assume that in each model the mucosal inflammation is an expression of an unregulated and excessive immune response to an antigenic challenge, the mucosal environment is the locus of the inflammation due to the heavy microbial load presented to the gut-associated lymphoid tissue (GALT). In effect, the mucosal immune system and its closely juxtaposed antigenic environment becomes the proverbial canary of the mine which is exposing the tendency of the entire system to manifest immune imbalanced immune responses. Finally, it is worth noting that the two generalizations about models of mucosal inflammation so far put forward may seem inherently contradictory in that on the one hand they suggest that a pathological organism is not responsible for the inflammation, but on the other hand they suggest that one or more non-pathological organisms are responsible for the inflammation. This contradiction is resolved if one recognizes that it is the response of the abnormal immune system to a mucosal organism or organisms in these murine models rather than intrinsic virulence factors associated with a particular pathogen that leads to and underlies the inflammation.

Yet another generalization relating to the murine models of mucosal inflammation concerns the rather remarkable fact that while the underlying defects in the various models are exceedingly diverse, the models resolve themselves into only one of two kinds of inflammatory process. The first and more common kind is exemplified by the inflammation found in SCID mice repleted by naive T cells, G_{i2} α, IL-2 and IL-10 knockout mice, and in the colitis induced by the instillation of TNBS per rectum to certain mouse strains. In each of these models the inflammation is histologically similar to Crohn's disease and is a

Th1 T cell-driven process characterized by the overproduction of IL-12 and IFN-γ[2,6,7,10,15,22–26]. The second kind is exemplified by the inflammation found in TCR α chain knockout mice or a newly described model of colitis induced by the instillation of oxazolone per rectum in which the inflammation is histologically reminiscent of ulcerative colitis and is a Th2 T cell-driven process characterized by the overproduction of IL-4[11,27]. Thus it appears that the diverse defects in the models have essentially two 'final common pathways' which in fact may well mimic the major immune processes present in the main forms of human IBD. One implication of the final common pathway in the models is that human IBD may itself be caused by several distinct immunological defects which nevertheless manifest themselves in a stereotypic fashion as one of the two forms of IBD. If this is indeed so, it could explain the fact that recent genetic studies of IBD are uncovering a large number of candidate disease genes. It should be noted, however, that the final common pathway concept predicts that treatment of the major forms of IBD will be successful if it addresses defects related to the final pathway regardless of the nature of the underlying immune defect.

A final generalization concerning the models concerns the fact that the distinction between induced and spontaneous colitides is more apparent than real. Thus, in those models in which colitis is induced in a presumably normal mouse by some immunological manipulation such as the administration of a contactant per rectum, the colitis induced also depends on a underlying genetic factor since it is now recognized that such colitis cannot be induced in all or even most mouse strains. Such mice are formally equivalent to knockout inasmuch as the latter also do not develop disease if maintained in a germ-free environment. Similarly, in the model of colitis represented by the SCID mouse reconstituted by naive T cells, the defect is equivalent to a genetic defect because, as we shall see, this mouse is lacking a counter-regulatory T cell population[28]. This aspect of the models points up the fact that even in murine models the occurrence of colitis requires both genetic and environmental factors, a fact increasingly evident in human IBD.

At this point we shall turn from the general to the particular with a discussion of one of the models of IBD, the IL-2 knockout mouse. We will use this discussion of a particular model to emphasize in a more immediate way the kinds of information that can be obtained from the models, and in doing so we will reiterate some of the generalizations concerning models already made above. Additionally, we will illustrate how the models illuminate human IBD.

THE IL-2 KNOCKOUT MOUSE MODEL OF COLITIS

Mice with the targeted deletion of the IL-2 gene, IL-2 knockout mice, were first developed by Sadlack and his colleagues who found, in initial studies, that such mice were surprisingly normal given the importance of IL-2 to the T cell responses[29]. This picture changed, however, when the animals were put in a more normal, and thus antigenically challenging, environment; at this point they were found consistently to develop a severe colitis as well as other pathological immune abnormalities. Initial studies of the colitis was complicated, however, by the fact that it occurred in a somewhat unpredictable fashion and thus could not be easily analysed for the critical immunological events immediately preceding the onset of colitis[3]. This problem was subsequently overcome by Ehrhardt and his colleagues, who found that administration of TNP-KLH (given with Freund's adjuvant by an intraperitoneal route) rapidly and reproducibly induced severe colitis in the knockout mice but not in heterozygous normal littermates[6]. Interestingly, while administration of TNP-ovalbumin also elicited colitis, unsubstituted KLH alone (or, indeed unsubstituted ovalbumin) were poor inducers of colitis. This strongly suggested, as already alluded to above, that only certain forms of immunization will induce colitis and that the TNP immunization is successful in this regard because it provides an antigenic epitope that may cross-react with epitopes in the mucosal microflora, thus greatly increasing the size of the T cell clonal population that ordinarily cause colitis.

Having devised a method for the controlled initiation of colitis in the IL-2 knockout mouse, the way was now open to study the cytokine responses accompanying and presumably causing the colitis. In initial studies it was found that administration of TNP-KLH to the mice led, within several days, to a massive and sustained infiltration of the lamina propria with activated T cells, whereas such administration to wild-type littermates led only to the transient appearance of activated cells at this site.

Further studies, in which TNP-KLH administration was accompanied by systemic administration of either anti-CD4 or anti-CD8 antibodies, led to the observation that anti-CD4, but not anti-CD8, prevented the cellular infiltration, and thus that the inflammation induced by TNP-KLH was a CD4$^+$ T cell-mediated process, as noted previously by others in the spontaneous colitis found in these mice[30]. In subsequent studies the cytokine profile of the infiltrating T cells was addressed. Here it was shown that extracted T cells stimulated *in vitro* (in the presence of exogenous IL-2) produced greatly increased amounts of IFN-γ, but reduced amounts of IL-4; similarly, studies of inflamed lamina propria with *in-situ* immunohistological techniques showed the presence of *in-vivo* secretion of large amounts of IFN-γ. These studies revealing the presence of Th1 cytokines in the inflamed tissue strongly suggested the presence of increased IL-12 secretion. This supposition was proven in two ways: first, *in-situ* immunohistological techniques were again used to show increased IL-12 production in tissues; second, and perhaps more importantly, anti-IL-12 was administered to mice either at the time of colitis induction with TNP-KLH or later when the inflammation was already well established and it was found that such antibody administration either prevented or abolished the pre-existing colitis. Taken together, these findings provided unequivocal evidence that the mechanism of colitis occurring in IL-2 knockout mice is a dysregulated IL-12-driven, Th1 T cell-mediated immune response. It is therefore very likely that the actual inflammation present is due to the stimulation of mucosal macrophages by Th1 cytokines (IFN-γ and TNF-α) and the subsequent release of the proximal causes of inflammation, the inflammatory cytokines IL-6, IL-1β and TNF-α itself.

The finding that IL-2 knockout manifested a dysregulated Th1 T cell response was by no means obvious given the central role of IL-2 in the proliferation of cells and thus its presumed essentiality to T cell differentiation of any type. Indeed, T cells extracted from the inflamed mucosa of IL-2 knockout mice did not proliferate in the absence of added IL-2. Nevertheless, these studies show quite definitively that, *in vivo*, vigorous T cell proliferation can occur in the absence of IL-2, perhaps under the proliferative drive of IL-12. This was further suggested by the observation described below that anti-IL-12 administration to mice with activated Th1 T cells is followed by the rapid loss of such cells.

The finding that the colitis of IL-2 knockout mice is a Th1 T cell-mediated inflammation places this model of colitis within a large group of murine models of colitis (as listed in Table 1) whose colitis is traceable to this same type of T cell response. This group includes mice with very different immune defects such as IL-10 knockout mice, Gi2α knockout mice, SCID mice reconstituted with naive T cells, CD3ε Tg mice, and SJL/J mice administered TNBS[16,25,31]. This observation recalls the discussion above concerning the 'final common pathway' concept of colitis and is only reiterated here to observe that a full understanding of the immunopathogenesis of any given model is to some extent incomplete if the mechanism of how this final common pathway is initiated is not fully clarified. In addition, it is germane to make this point again in the context of treatment of these various forms of Th1 T cell-mediated colitis. The fact is that not only IL-2 knockout mice can be successfully treated with anti-IL-12 administration, but all other Th1 models appropriately tested can also be so treated. Thus, again, treatment need only address the final common pathway, not the underlying immune defect, to be effective, temporarily at least.

Further studies of the colitis in IL-2 knockout mice were directed at addressing the question posed above, namely the cause of the excessive Th1 T cell response leading to colitis upon stimulation with TNP-KLH. One initial possibility considered was based on the knowledge that IL-2 is necessary for the induction of T cells producing IL-4. Thus, in the absence of IL-2 the powerful counter-regulatory influence of Th2 cytokines on the induction of Th1 T cells is weak or absent. Such counter-regulatory influence is exerted by IL-4 itself via its ability to down-regulate the expression of the β2 chain of the IL-12 receptor on developing Th1 T cells[32,33]. Another regulatory cytokine of Th1 response is IL-10, a cytokine produced by Th2 T cells, that alone or in concert with IL-4 will decrease the production of IL-12 by antigen-presenting cells[34-37]. However, while this explanation for the excessive Th1 response in IL-2 knockout mice is logical and compelling, it probably is not relevant in view of the fact that IL-4 knockout mice or IL-4 receptor knockout mice are not among the animal models of colitis. These knockout mice provide strong evidence that other, more immediate and cogent means of controlling excessive mucosal Th1 responses exist which act quite independently of IL-4.

Thus we come to a second and far more important explanation of the excessive Th1 response in IL-2 knockout mice leading to colitis, the fact that these mice do not produce appropriate levels of TGF-β under most circumstances[38]. The key to establishing this point was the serendipitous finding that the systemic administration of anti-CD3 antibody to IL-2 knockout mice, a manoeuvre that was initially expected to strongly stimulate T cells and thus to elicit colitis, did not elicit colitis and, in fact, prevented the immunization-induced colitis. Further examination of the response of IL-2 knockout mice to the administration of anti-CD3, disclosed that the latter was associated with induction of T cells producing

IL-4 as well as the suppressive cytokine, TGF-β. This last observation indicated that IL-2 knockout mice are able to produce IL-4 under some conditions and, in addition, suggested that the ability of anti-CD3 to prevent colitis might be due to its ability to elicit IL-4 production (which would prevent colitis by the mechanism discussed above) or to elicit TGF-β production. To test these possibilities IL-2 knockout mice were administered TNP-KLH and anti-CD3 as before, but this time these antibodies were given along with either anti-IL-4 or anti-TGF-β. The result was that the addition of anti-IL-4 had no effect, i.e. the mice still did not develop colitis; in contrast, the addition of anti-TGF-β had the dramatic effect of re-establishing the ability of TNP-KLH to induce colitis. These observations clearly indicated that the ability of TNP-KLH and not anti-CD3 to elicit colitis in the IL-2 knockout mouse is the former stimulates T cells without inducing a counter-regulatory TGF-β response; in addition, they show that the ability of anti-CD3 to inhibit colitis induction by TNP-KLH is due to its ability to stimulate a TGF-β response not its ability to stimulate an IL-4 response.

While the above studies satisfy the immediate question of why IL-2 knockout mice develop an excessive Th1 T cell response and colitis they raise additional questions concerning the effect of IL-2 on immune response that have yet to be answered. One question relates to why the administration of anti-CD3, but not TNP-KLH to IL-2 knockout mice elicits an IL-4/TGF-β response. One possible answer to this question is that IL-2 is necessary for the differentiation of IL-4-producing cells and TGF-β-producing T cells in the context of induction by conventional antigen presented by antigen-presenting cells (the TNP-based immunization). Here IL-2 would be an essential growth/proliferation factor without which Th2 lymphocyte differentiation cannot occur. However, at the same time IL-2 is not necessary for the cytokine production of such regulatory T cells when directly stimulated by anti-CD3 mAb. Proof of this possibility is difficult in that it involves studies of the ability of anti-CD3 to evoke IL-4/TGF-β responses in IL-2 knockout mice co-administered antibodies to various growth/proliferation factors. Another question relates to whether the inability of the IL-2 knockout mouse to produce TGF-β in response to TNP-KLH stimulation is in fact due to its inability to produce IL-4 in this situation. Here the question can be at least tentatively answered by the observation, already mentioned, that co-administration of anti-IL-4 to IL-2 knockout mice administered anti-CD3 and TNP-KLH neither reversed the protective effect of the anti-CD3 with respect to colitis nor affected TGF-β production. Thus, it appears that, at least in this situation, IL-4 was not necessary for the differentiation of T cells producing TGF-β despite the fact that in other situations it can be shown to be an enhancer of such differentiation[39]. As discussed below, a similar conclusion was also reached in a study of another model of colitis[40].

THE GENERAL REGULATION OF MUCOSAL RESPONSES: THE IFN-γ/TGF-β DICHOTOMY

The key role of TGF-β in the prevention of colitis in the IL-2 knockout mouse is not limited to this murine model of intestinal inflammation, but has been shown to play a similarly important role in TNBS-colitis and in the colitis developing in

SCID mice reconstituted with naive T cells[28,40]. TNBS-colitis is a colitis induced in SJL/J mice by the per-rectal administration of TNBS and is also a Th1 T cell-mediated colitis which in fact was the first murine model in which it was shown that administration of anti-IL-12 could treat the colitis. The counter-regulatory role of TGF-β in this model was demonstrated in studies in which it was shown that mice simultaneously fed TNP-lated colonic protein and given TNBS per rectum did not develop colitis because exposure to TNP by the oral route had induced lamina propria T cells producing TGF-β; in this case, as in the case of the IL-2 knockout mouse, the critical role of TGF-β as a counter-regulatory factor was shown by the ability of systemic anti-TGF-β to reverse the effect of feeding TNP-lated colonic protein. A similar situation obtained in studies of the colitis of SCID mice reconstituted with naive CD45RB[hi] T cells. In this case it was first shown that colitis could be prevented by the co-administration of mature CD45RB[lo] T cells, suggesting that the colitis was caused by the lack of counter-regulatory T cells in the naive T cell population and their presence in the mature T cell population. This possibility was proven true and the counter-regulatory cells were identified as TGF-β-producing T cells in studies showing that the administration of anti-TGF-β along with the mature T cell population neutralized the latter's effect and the mice now once again developed colitis. Parenthetically, in these studies, a mature T cell population obtained from IL-4 knockout mice also prevent colitis, indicating as in the IL-2 knock-out studies that IL-4 was not necessary for the induction of T cells producing TGF-β[28,38].

The counter-regulatory role of TGF-β and its ability to block the development of colitis in several very different models of Th1 T cell-mediated colitis, as detailed above, is not merely a phenomenon limited to colitis induction, but rather a general feature of the regulation of immune responses in the mucosal immune system. To understand this more fully, we need to digress for a moment to a discussion of certain aspects of the normal mucosal response to oral antigen administration.

The ingestion of antigen and its subsequent presentation to T cells in the mucosal follicles triggers a complex and inter-related immune response whose outcome depends on many factors. If the antigen is present at a relatively low concentration and is not accompanied by adjuvant, it evokes a bipartite response consisting on the one hand of Th1 T cells producing IFN-γ and on the other of T cells producing TGF-β[41]. These responses are mutually inhibitory, as shown by the fact that the administration of anti-IL-12 to mice at the time of oral antigen administration inhibits the Th1 response (as expected) and greatly enhances the TGF-β response[42]. In contrast, administration of anti-TGF-β to mice co-administered antigen that evokes a response that cross-reacts with normal microfloral antigens (TNP-KLH) results in colitis (presumably due to over-exuberant Th1 response). In the ordinary course of events, the TGF-β response is dominant and thus, in most instances, oral administration of a protein antigen results in oral tolerance. Thus, the organism is spared the necessity of mounting unnecessary and perhaps harmful responses to antigens that are unassociated with potential pathogens. Contrariwise, if oral administration of antigen is accompanied by a mucosal adjuvant, as it would if it were part of a pathological organism, an immunogenic pathway is brought into play and the individual mounts a successful Th1 (or Th2) T cell response that maintains host defence. Inherent in this description of the normal mucosal response is the exquisite balance between the Th1 T cell response and TGF-β-producing T cell response initially induced by mucosal antigen[43]. One factor that may be critical in maintaining this balance is IL-10, a potent inhibitor of IL-12 production and thus of Th1 T cell responses[35,44]. Thus, if oral antigen also has a propensity to elicit a vigorous early IL-10 response one would have an explanation for the initial dominance of the TGF-β response. This possibility suggests an explanation of adjuvant activity since adjuvant may act by shutting down early IL-10 production and thus give a nascent Th1 response an opportunity to take hold. This hypothesis finds some support in the observation that IL-10 knockout mice develop a Th1 colitis[22].

With this brief overview of the nature of the mucosal responses, particularly the Th1 T cell/TGF-β-producing T cell dichotomy, we can now understand that the multifaceted mucosal disease represented by the various models is best visualized as a disruption of the normal mucosal immune response balance and the emergence of an unregulated, unfettered Th1 (or Th2) response. Put more succinctly, chronic mucosal inflammation in the various animal models is best visualized as a failure of oral tolerance. Finally, it is important to mention that the tension between the Th1 T cell response and the TGF-β response that seems to govern mucosal homeostasis and inflammation, holds equally well with respect to normal and abnormal mucosal Th2 responses.

THE ROLE OF THE THYMUS IN THE DEVELOPMENT OF COLITIS IN THE IL-2 KNOCKOUT MOUSE

So far in our discussion of IL-2 knockout mice we have made the tacit assumption that all of the relevant pathological events leading to colitis following systemic TNP-KLH administration occur in the peripheral lymphoid tissues, rather than in the central thymic tissue. Theoretically, however, it is attractive to consider that intrathymic events constitute a critical part of the pathological loop, since negative selection of potentially self-reactive thymocytes is one of the most critically acclaimed functions of the thymus. Data consistent with this possibility were initially obtained by Krämer *et al.*, who showed using thymic (nu/nu) IL-2 knockout mice that the development of autoimmunity was dependent on the presence of an IL-2-deficient intrathymic microenvironment[45].

To more directly consider this possibility, the colitogenic potential of thymocytes in IL-2 knockout mice following TNP-KLH administration was determined. It was found that such systemic immunization caused a profound reduction in the number of double-positive (DP; CD4$^+$/CD8$^+$) thymocytes in the thymus accompanied by a proportional increase in the number of single-positive thymocytes in this organ[46]. In addition, the cytokine profile of the single-positive thymocytes was abnormal: these cells produced increased amounts of IFN-γ and decreased amounts of IL-4 in comparison to similar cells from normal thymuses. This constellation of findings could be explained if it were assumed that delicate balance of IL-12 and IL-2 was essential for maintaining homeostasis during the maturation and selection of naive thymocytes. In the absence of IL-2 this balance would therefore be lost, leading to maturation of potentially autoreactive dysregulated IL-12-driven Th1-like thymocytes. Powerful support for this scenario comes from two interrelated findings. First, administration of anti-IL-12 to IL-2 knockout mice restores the normal intrathymic microenvironment with 80% of thymocytes being DP, 15% SP and the rest being naive DN thymocytes. Second, the adaptive transfer of thymocytes from IL-2 knockout mice to naive normal mice led to the rapid development of severe colitis in the latter mice, thus indicating that the lack of IL-2 does indeed lead to the generation of autoreactive colitogenic thymocytes, in this case cells reacting with mucosal antigens. Overall, these studies lead to the conclusion that cells mediating colitis in the IL-2 knockout mouse initially develop in the thymus and then, upon trafficking to the mucosal tissues, are restimulated by mucosal antigens. Furthermore, these cells cause a colitis because in the IL-2 knockout they are unopposed by a normal complement of counter-regulatory, TGF-β-producing cells. In this way IL-2 deficiency causes a central dysregulation and a peripheral dysregulation that combine to produce disease. Similar conclusions have recently been drawn from other Th1-driven murine colitis models where either interference of the T cell receptor (CD3ε Tg mice) or intracellular signalling (Gαi2 knockout mice) has led to dysregulated intrathymic development of Th1-like thymocytes[9,10,16].

These studies of thymic function in IL-2 knockout mice raise the interesting question of the role of the thymus in other murine models of mucosal inflammation or indeed in human Crohn's disease. In some of the models it appears quite unlikely that the thymus is playing a significant role and the colitis appears to be an entirely peripheral lymphoid abnormality. However, further studies in which these mice are studied for the development of colitis following thymectomy will be necessary to resolve this question. As far as the human disease is concerned, the most conservative view is that it is possible, or even likely, that at least in some patients the disease is likely to have a central lymphoid component.

CONCLUDING REMARKS: THE RELATION BETWEEN MODELS OF COLITIS AND HUMAN IBD

The above analysis of the basis of the colitis occurring in murine models of mucosal inflammation, particularly IL-2 knockout mice, leads inevitably to the question of how these models help explain human IBD. The most cogent answer to this question is that the models provide a blueprint both for aforementioned 'final common pathways' of inflammation as well as the kinds of basic immunological abnormalities that lead to these pathways. The most frequent final common pathway seen in the various models is an IL-12-driven. Th1 T cell-mediated inflammation; characterized by the production of IL-12 by lesional antigen-presenting cells and increased IFN-γ production and decreased IL-4 and IL-5 production by lesional T cells. This pathway appears to be the one operative in Crohn's disease, since it produces a lesion very similar to that found in Crohn's disease, a mononuclear cellular infiltrate spanning the full thickness of the bowel wall. Perhaps more importantly, this pathway is relevant to Crohn's disease because the latter also exhibits a Th1 cytokine profile[47–52]. It has recently been demonstrated that in Crohn's disease one sees lamina propria macrophages that manifest greatly increased production of IL-12[53,54]. On this basis one can say that the pathogenesis of the granulomatous inflammation in Crohn's disease is the overproduction of IFN-γ which leads in turn to the production of the pro-inflammatory cytokines that are the immediate causes of inflammatory disease, TNF-α, IL-1β and IL-6. Also, on this basis, it seems likely that Crohn's disease would be highly responsive to treatment with anti-IL-12, just as such treatment is effective in the various models of colitis also driven by Th1 T cells.

A second 'final common pathway' occurring in the murine models is, as we have seen, the Th2 T cell-driven inflammation characteristic of the colitis occurring in TCR α chain knockout mice and in a newly developed model caused by the intra-rectal administration of oxazolone, oxazolone colitis. The inflammations associated with these models are very different from the Th1-type inflammations in that they are characterized by superficial and ulcerative inflammatory processes associated with a mixed lymphocyte/granulocyte infiltrate. In that this form of inflammation resembles that found in ulcerative colitis, the studies of the models of colitis suggest that a Th2-type response is the final common pathway of ulcerative colitis[8,27]. However, the parallelism between the models and ulcerative colitis is not as clear-cut as that between the models and Crohn's disease, because in ulcerative colitis the cytokine pattern of the lamina propria T cells is not completely typical of a skewed Th2 response. Thus, one cannot yet say that ulcerative colitis is definitely a Th2 T cell-driven disease despite the evidence from various animal models.

Implicit in the above formulation of Crohn's disease and ulcerative colitis as polar examples of Th1 and Th2-like final common pathway-related inflammations respectively, is that each of these diseases may arise from multiple 'primary' defects, some of which are represented by the various murine models. While these primary defects can in principle be quite varied, it seems likely that they fall into one of several rather limited categories that affect the final common pathway in one of several ways. One such category are factors that set the intrinsic activity of the Th1 T cell pathway, i.e. the tendency of a given individual to mount a Th1 T cell response via the production of IL-12 and IFN-γ. In this regard it is reasonable to postulate that certain individuals with Crohn's disease have a markedly increased ability to mount Th1 T cell responses, and while this may protect such individuals from certain kinds of infection, it may also make such individuals susceptible to the development of Crohn's disease. Another such category of factors are those that suppress or down-regulate Th1 responses. Into this category would fall defects relating to the production of cytokines that are known to inhibit Th1 responses such as the TGF-β response or the IL-10 response. On this basis, much of the focus in future studies of Crohn's disease may centre on delineating these categories of defects in the various patients and on the genetic factors underlying these defects.

As a final point relating to how the murine models elucidate the nature of IBD, we return to the point that the inflammations occurring in the models are almost undoubtedly immunological responses to the protein components of the endogenous microflora. This observation predicts that the antigenic driving force of either Crohn's disease or ulcerative colitis is not a long-sought-after mucosal pathogen, but rather one or more (probably more) of the commensal bacteria universally resident in the bowel. Already direct evidence for this hypothesis has been demonstrated by Duchmann and his co-workers, showing that while normal individuals cannot mount immunological responses to their own flora, patients with Crohn's disease are capable of such responses[55]. Does this insight imply that ultimately the IBD will be controlled by selective elimination of flora components that induce untoward responses? The answer to this question is far from clear, but it seems reasonable to say that such a therapeutic approach is not likely to be effective given the complexity and redundancy of the microflora and the fact that autoimmune responses in general are almost universally due to stimulation by a large number of separate epitopes, even in situations where the range of autoantigens seems far more restricted than in IBD.

Overall, a better and more feasible approach to the therapy of IBD involves the correction of the response to a given antigen universe rather than the correction of the universe.

References

1. Powrie F, Mason D. OX-22high CD4[+] T cells induce wasting disease with multiple organ pathology: prevention by the OX-22low subset [published erratum appears in J Exp Med. 1991;173:1037]. J Exp Med. 1990;172:1701- 8.
2. Powrie F, Leach MW, Mauze S, Menon S, Caddle LB, Coffman RL. Inhibition of Th1 responses prevents inflammatory bowel disease in SCID mice reconstituted with CD45RBhi CD4[+] T cells. Immunity. 1994;1:553–62.
3. Sadlack B, Merz H, Schorle H, Schimpl A, Feller AC, Horak I. Ulcerative colitis-like disease in mice with a disrupted interleukin-2 gene [see comments]. Cell. 1993;75:253–61.
4. Mombaerts P, Mizoguchi E, Grusby MJ, Glimcher LH, Bhan AK, Tonegara S. Spontaneous development of inflammatory bowel disease in T cell receptor mutant mice. Cell. 1993;75:275–82.
5. Kühn R, Löhler J, Rennick D, Rajewsky K, Müller W. Interleukin 10-deficient mice develop chronic enterocolitis. Cell. 1993;75:263–74.
6. Ehrhardt RO, Ludviksson BR, Gray B, Neurath M, Strober W. Induction and prevention of colonic inflammation in IL-2 deficient mice. J Immunol. 1997;158:566–73.
7. Elson CO, Beagley KW, Sharmonov AT *et al.* Hapten-induced model of murine inflammatory bowel disease: mucosa immune responses and protection of tolerance. J Immunol. 1996;157:2174–85.
8. Fuss IJ, Boirivant M, Chu AC, Strober W. Oxazolone-induced colitis: an animal model of ulcerative colitis treatable with antibodies to IL-4. Grastroenterology. 1998;114:64020 (abstract).
9. Hollander GA, Simpson SJ, Mizoguchi E *et al.* Severe colitis in mice with aberrant thymic selection. Immunity. 1995;3:27–38.
10. Hornquist CE, Lu X, Rogers-Fani PM *et al.* G(α)i2-deficient mice with colitis exhibit a local increase in memory CD4[+] T cells and proinflammatory Th1-type cytokines. J Immunol. 1997; 158:1068–77.
11. Kosiewicz MM, Krishnan A, Shah M *et al.* Characterization of a new spontaneous murine model of inflammatory bowel disease. Gastroenterology. 1998;114:64142 (abstract).
12. Kraft SC, Fitch FW, Kirsner JB. Histologic and immunohistochemical features of Auer 'colitis' in rabbits. Am J Pathol. 1963;43:913–23.
13. Leach, MW, Bean AG, Mauze S, Coffman RL, Powrie F. Inflammatory bowel disease in C.B-17 SCID mice reconstituted with the CD45RB[hi] subset of CD4[+] T cells. Am J Pathol. 1996;148: 1503-15.
14. Ludviksson BR, Gray B, Strober W, Ehrdhart RO. Dysregulated intrathymic development in the IL-2-deficient mouse leads to colitis-inducing thymocytes. J Immunol. 1997;158:104–11.
15. Neurath MF, Fuss I, Kelsall BL, Stuber E, Strober W. Antibodies to interleukin 12 abrogate established experimental colitis in mice. J Exp Med. 1995;182:1281–90.
16. Rudolph U, Finegold MJ, Rich SS *et al.* Gi2α protein deficiency: a model of inflammatory bowel disease. J Clin Immunol. 1995;15:101–55.

17. Spiegel AM, Elson CO, Sartor RB, Tennyson GS, Riddell RH. G protein gene knockout hits the gut: experimental models of inflammatory bowel disease. Nat Med. 1995;1:522–4.
18. Sundberg JP, Elson CO, Bedigian H, Birkenmeier EH. Spontaneous, heritable colitis in a new substrain of C3H/HeJ mice. Gastroenterology. 1994;107:1726–35.
19. Watanabe M, Ueno Y, Yajima T *et al.* Interleukin 7 transgenic mice develop chronic colitis with decreased interleukin 7 protein accumulation in the colonic mucosa. J Exp Med. 1998;187: 389–402.
20. Lúdvíksson BR, Ehrhardt RO, Fuss IJ, Strober W. Mucosal and thymic dysregulation. Role in human intestinal inflammation. Immunologist. 1997;5:202–9.
21. Duchmann R, Schmitt R, Knolle P, Meyer zum Buschenfelde KH, Neurath M. Tolerance towards resident intestinal flora in mice is abrogated in experimental colitis and restored by treatment with interleukin-10 or antibodies to interleukin-12. Eur J Immunol. 1996;26:934- 8.
22. Berg J, Davidson DJ, Kuhn R *et al.* Enterocolitis and colon cancer in interleukin-10-deficient mice are associated with aberrant cytokine production and CD4[+] Th1-like responses. J Clin Invest. 1996;98:1010–20.
23. Autenrieth IB, Bucheler N, Bohn E, Heinze G, Horak I. Cytokine mRNA expression in intestinal tissue of interleukin-2 deficient mice with bowel inflammation. Gut. 1997;41:793–800.
24. Aranda R, Sydora BC, McAllister PL *et al.* Analysis of intestinal lymphocytes in mouse colitis mediated by transfer of CD4[+], CD45RBhigh T cells to SCID recipients. J Immunol. 1997;158: 3464–73.
25. Bregenhold S, Claesson MH. Increased intracellular Th1 cytokines in SCID mice with inflammatory bowel disease. Eur J Immunol. 1998;28:379–89.
26. Davidson NJ, Leach MW, Fort MM *et al.* T helper cell 1-type CD4[+] T cells, but not B cells, mediate colitis in interleukin 10-deficient mice. J Exp Med. 1996;184:241–51.
27. Mizoguchi A, Mizoguchi E, Chiba C *et al.* Cytokine imbalance and autoantibody production in T cell receptor-alpha mutant mice with inflammatory bowel disease. J Exp Med. 1996;183:847–56.
28. Powrie F, Carlino F, Leach MW, Mauze S, Coffman RL. A critical role for transforming growth factor-beta but not interleukin 4 in the suppression of T helper type 1-mediated colitis by CD45RB(low) CD4[+] T cells. J Exp Med. 1996;183:2669–74.
29. Schorle H, Holtschke T, Hunig T, Schimp A, Horak I. Development and function of T cells in mice rendered interleukin-2 deficient by gene targeting. Nature. 1991;352:621–4.
30. Simpson SJ, Mizoguchi E, Allen D, Bhan AK, Terhorst C. Evidence that CD4[+], but not CD8[+] T cells are responsible for murine interleukin-2-deficient colitis. Eur J Immunol. 1995;25:2618–25.
31. Simpson SJ, Hollander GA, Mizoguchi E *et al.* Expression of pro-inflammatory cytokines by TCR alpha beta+ and TCR gamma delta+ T cells in an experimental model of colitis. Eur J Immunol. 1997;27:17–25.
32. Szabo SJ, Dighe AS, Gubler U, Murphy KM. Regulation of the interleukin (IL)-12R beta 2 subunit expression in developing T helper 1 (Th1) and Th2 cells. J Exp Med. 1997;185: 817–24.
33. Szabo S, Jacobson NG, Dighe AS, Gubler U, Murphy KM. Developmental commitment to the Th2 lineage by extinction of IL-12 signaling. Immunity. 1995;2:665–75.
34. Ria F, Penna G, Adorina L. Th1 cells induce and Th2 inhibit antigen-dependent IL-12 secretion by dendritic cells. Eur J Immunol. 1998;28:2003–16.
35. Aste-Amezaga M, Ma X, Sartori A, Trinchieri G. Molecular mechanisms of the induction of IL-12 and its inhibition by IL-10. J Immunol. 1998;160:5936–44.
36. Segal BM, Dwyer BK, Shevach EM. An interleukin (IL)-10/IL-12 immunoregulatory circuit controls susceptibility to autoimmune disease. J Exp Med. 1998;187:537–46.
37. Shnyra A, Brewington R, Alipio A, Amura C, Morrison DC. Reprogramming of lipo-polysaccharide-primed macrophages is controlled by a counterbalanced production of IL-10 and IL-12. J Immunol. 1998;160:3729–36.
38. Ludviksson BR, Ehrhardt RO, Strober W. TGF-beta production regulates the development of the 2,4,6-trinitrophenol-conjugated keyhole limpet hemocyanin-induced colonic inflammation in IL-2-deficient mice. J Immunol. 1997;159:3622–8.
39. Seder RA, Marth T, Sieve MC *et al.* Factors involved in the differentiation of TGF-beta-producing cells from naive CD4[+] cells: IL-4 and IFN-gamma have opposing effects, while TGF-beta positively regulates its own production. J Immunol. 1998;160: 5719–28.
40. Neurath MF, Fuss I, Kelsall BL, Presky DH, Waegell W, Strober W. Experimental granulo-matous colitis in mice is abrogated by induction of TGF-beta-mediated oral tolerance. J Exp Med. 1996;183: 2605–16.

41. Strober W, Kelsall B, Fuss I *et al.* Reciprocal IFN-gamma and TGF-beta responses regulate the occurrence of mucosal inflammation. Immunol Today. 1997;18:61–4.
42. Marth T, Strober W, Seder RA, Kelsall BL. Regulation of transforming growth factor-beta production by interleukin-12. Eur J Immunol. 1997;27:1213–20.
43. Weiner HL. Oral tolerance. Proc Natl Acad Sci USA. 1994;91:10762–5.
44. D'Orazio TJ, Niederkorn JY. A novel role for TGF-beta and IL-10 in the induction of immune privilege. J Immunol. 1998;160:2089–98.
45. Kramer S, Schimpl A, Hunig T. Immunopathology of interleukin (IL) 2-deficient mice: thymus dependence and suppression by thymus-dependent cells with an intact IL-2 gene. J Exp Med. 1995;182:1769–76.
46. Ludviksson BR, Gray B, Strober W, Ehrhardt RO. Dysregulated intrathymic development in the IL-2-deficient mouse leads to colitis-inducing thymocytes. J Immunol. 1997;158:104–11.
47. Fais S, Capobianchi MR, Pallone F *et al.* Spontaneous release of interferon gamma by intestinal lamina propria lymphocytes in Crohn's disease. Kinetics of *in vitro* response to interferon gamma inducers. Gut. 1991;32:403–7.
48. West GA, Matsuura T, Levine AD, Klein JS, Fiocchi C. Interleukin 4 in inflammatory bowel disease and mucosal immune reactivity. Gastroenterology. 1996;110:683–95.
49. Parronchi P, Romagnani P, Annunziato F *et al.* Type 1 T-helper cell predominance and interleukin-12 expression in the gut of patients with Crohn's disease. Am J Pathol. 1997;150:823–32.
50. Noguchi M, Hiwatashi N, Liu Z, Toyota T. Enhanced interferon-gamma production and B7-2 expression in isolated intestinal mononuclear cells from patients with Crohn's disease. J Gastroenterol. 1995;30(Suppl. 8):52–5.
51. Fuss IJ, Neurath M, Boirivant M *et al.* Disparate CD4+ lamina propria (LP) lymphokine secretion profiles in inflammatory bowel disease. Crohn's disease LP cells manifest increased secretion of IFN–gamma, whereas ulcerative colitis LP cells manifest increased secretion of IL-5. J Immunol. 1996;157:1261–70.
52. Breese E, Braegger CP, Corrigan CJ, Walker-Smith JA, MacDonald TT. Interleukin-2- and interferon-gamma-secreting T cells in normal and diseased human intestinal mucosa. Immunology. 1993;78:127–31.
53. Monteleone G, Biancone L, Marasco R *et al.* Interleukin 12 is expressed and actively released by Crohn's disease intestinal lamina propria mononuclear cells. Gastroenterology. 1997;112:1169–78.
54. Neurath MF, Fuss I, Schürmann G *et al.* Upregulation of the IL-12/STAT-4 signaling pathway distinguishes Crohn's disease from ulcerative colitis. Gastroenterology. 1998;114:64299 (abstract).
55. Duchmann R, Kaiser I, Hermann E, Mayet W, Ewe, K, Meyer zum Buschenfelde KH. Tolerance exists towards resident intestinal flora but is broken in active inflammatory bowel disease (IBD) [see comments]. Clin Exp Immunol. 1995;102:448–55.

11
Pathways of T cell pathology in models of experimental colitis

Y. P. DE JONG, S. J. SIMPSON, M. COMISKEY, S. VAN SCHAIK, D. ALLEN, B. WANG and C. TERHORST

INTRODUCTION

Ulcerative colitis (UC) and Crohn's disease (CD), collectively referred to as inflammatory bowel disease (IBD), are chronic, spontaneously relapsing disorders, which appear to be immunologically mediated and to have genetic and environmental components. The pathways that lead to these diseases can now in principle be dissected by using genetically well defined animal models. A distinct subset of immunodeficient mutant mice develop IBD-like diseases. As experimental IBD is dependent upon aberrant T lymphocytes and upon the presence of intestinal bacteria, a general model is being formulated in which specialized T lymphocytes initiate destructive cascades in the intestinal mucosa. This destruction is accelerated by the bacterial components infiltrating from the lumen of the intestine and by recruitment of neutrophils. Absence of disease in immunodeficient animals kept under gnotobiotic conditions strongly suggests that colonic bacteria are implicated in the initiation of the pathways leading to IBD. A majority of investigators in this field hold the view that ubiquitous (resident) anaerobic luminal bacteria and bacterial products initiate and exacerbate the disease in animals with a weakened immune system. Thus, intestinal homeostasis is a delicate balance between pro-inflammatory activities of luminal bacteria and host defences.

Early models for IBD were conceived from the observation that insult to the mucosal epithelium results in recruitment of cells to the intestine as a means of repairing the damage and/or dealing with the subsequent entry of infectious organisms; in essence local damage leading to local inflammation[1-3]. The application of agents such as dextran sodium sulphate or acetic acid to the colon mucosa has provided a simple means by which this could be achieved with some useful results. However there is little evidence to suggest that IBD is initiated by physical transgression of the mucosal/luminal barrier[1,4].

Recent years have seen the emergence of numerous genetic models for IBD which have resulted from either transgenic expression of proteins or from gene knockout techniques[2,3,5–9]. From the outset, the development of colitis in these modified animals highlighted the complex array of immunoregulatory pathways which operate to temper inflammatory responses within the colon. In most cases the modified immunological phenotypes in these animals are distinct and yet the outcome is often similar; namely the development of a wasting disease and inflammation of the colon. For example mice deficient in cytokine gene expression including interleukin (IL)-2, IL-10 and transforming growth factor β (TGFβ) each develop distinct forms of spontaneous chronic mucosal inflammation within the GI tract[10–13]. Similarly, alterations to the development of certain T cell subsets such as in TCR deficient mice has also been found to lead to the development of a colitis-like disease[14]. However, the observation that not all immunodeficiencies give rise to spontaneous colitis or the accompanying wasting disease and anaemia suggests a central defect in T cell function or regulation lies at the core of the pathology observed in each of these models.

A second group of genetically altered mice develop colitis as a result of mutations in development of the intestinal epithelial barrier[15,16]. In these cases it is possible that immunocompetent mice succumb to disease through inappropriate exposure of mucosal T cells to luminal antigens or bacterial products. Colitis has also been observed after disruption of a cell signalling G protein (Gαi2 in mice[17], although in this latter case it remains to be determined whether the disease is caused by a defect in epithelial cells or in immunocytes. The possibility that defects in mucosal barrier function can lead to IBD by enabling luminal bacteria or their products greater access to the intestinal mucosa is consistent with the early models of epithelial destruction and the observation that in many models of IBD, disease is significantly attenuated or absent when mice are kept under gnotobiotic conditions[5].

In this review we focus on a third, distinct group of IBD models, which result from transplant of bone marrow-derived precursor T cells or transfer of a specific subset of T cells into immunodeficient hosts.

THE BMT → TGε26 MODEL

We developed a model for IBD in our laboratory which involves reconstitution of T cell/NK cell-deficient mice termed Tgε26[18,19]. Despite the absence of T cells and NK cells, Tgε26 animals remain viable and healthy, although the thymuses of these mice are very small and lack normal stromal architecture, most prominently of the cortical epithelium[20]. Previously, it was demonstrated that this defect was due to the absence of thymocytes which are blocked in Tgε26 animals at a very early stage of development (CD25+ Thy-1−) through the high copy number expression of a human CD3ε transgene[18,21].

Bone marrow reconstitution experiments revealed that the thymuses of adult Tgε26 mice do not support normal ontogeny of donor-derived thymocytes[30], made evident by the observation that only small numbers of thymocytes could be detected in bone marrow cell (BMC)-reconstituted Tgε26 thymus (BM → Tgε26). In addition, these cells displayed a pattern of CD4 and CD8 expression inconsistent with normal thymocyte development seen in wild type animals. Most strikingly, thymocytes in reconstituted mice were predominantly

CD4⁻CD8⁻ (DN) and CD4⁺ or CD8⁺ (SP) with a paucity of CD8⁺CD4⁺ (DP) thymocytes. In contrast, BMC reconstitution in RAG[null] mice resulted in the appearance of larger numbers of thymocytes which displayed a relatively normal pattern of development[20]. Around 4 weeks after BMC transfer, BM → Tgε26 mice develop a wasting syndrome and severe inflammation in the colon mucosa which correlates with the expansion of activated peripheral and intestinal T cells[22]. Predominantly these cells are of the TCR$\alpha\beta^+$ CD4⁺ lineage (70–95%) although smaller numbers of TCR$\alpha\beta^+$ CD8⁺ and TCR$\gamma\delta^+$ T cells can be detected.

Several salient features of the BM → Tgε26 model make apparent that the disease in these mice is not the result of a classical graft-versus-host (GVH) response by donor derived T cells carried in the BM inoculum. First, the strain combinations used in these original studies were equivalent to an F1 → parent combination ((C57BL/6 × CBA/J)F1 into the mixed CD57BL/6 × CBA/J background of Tgε26 mice) and cause severe colitis. Second, although these animals develop severe cachexia, disease in the colons of Tgε26 mice bears little similarity to that seen in classical GVHD. Thirdly and most importantly, when the BM → Tgε26 animals are kept in a germ-free environment, no colitis or wasting disease develops (C. Veltkamp, Y. P. de Jong and R. B. Sartor, unpublished observations). Moreover, no disease is induced when RAG[null] animals are reconstituted with bone marrow from the same donor background, suggesting that a defect specific to Tgε26 mice is responsible for induction of colitis in these animals.

Unlike adult Tgε26 animals, the thymus of fetal and neonatal Tgε26 mice (1–8 days old) can be reconstituted with wild type stem cells. This correlates with a normal pattern of thymocyte development and restoration of thymic architecture delineated by the development of a normal cortico-medullary boundary. Furthermore, neonatal Tgε26 mice, like BM › RAG[null] mice, do not develop any signs of either cachexia or colitis. Engraftment of a fetal Tgε26 thymus under the kidney capsule of adult Tgε26 prior to BMC transplantation is sufficient to protect animals from disease, which we suggest highlights the point that the inability to normally reconstitute the Tgε26 thymi is central to the development of colitis in this model.

THE CD45RB[hi] TRANSFER MODEL OF COLITIS

Original studies by Powrie *et al.* and Morrisey *et al.* revealed important regulatory interactions between subsets of CD4⁺ T cells, the maintenance of which were required to prevent the development of chronic intestinal inflammation in mice[23,24]. Most significantly, the regulatory and potentially pathogenic T cells in this system could be identified by a single surface marker (CD45RB). In these original studies it was observed that reconstitution of CB.17*Scid* mice with wild-type (wt) co-isogenic (BALB/c) T cells separated according to the expression levels of CD45RB (either CD45RB[hi] or CD45RB[lo]) had very different consequences for the recipient animals[23–25]. Thus, animals reconstituted with CD4⁺ CD45RB[hi] T cells developed a wasting syndrome and severe transmural colitis 7–10 weeks after cell transfer. Conversely, *Scid* mice that received CD45RB[lo] CD4⁺ T cells remained healthy. Furthermore, co-transfer of the two populations was sufficient to protect against disease. These experiments have provided an important landmark in IBD research since they were the first evidence for the existence of a subset of T cells with the ability to regulate pathogenic T cells.

DIFFERENCES AND SIMILARITIES IN THE TWO MODELS

Colitis in BM → Tgε26 and CD45RB[hi] recipient mice can be distinguished by certain salient features. In the case of the CD45RB[hi] model, animals develop moderate wasting with significant cellular inflammation of the colon mucosa, which in its severest form is transmural and accompanies the development of granulomas[26]. Involvement of the distal small intestine has also been reported in this model. Collectively, these features have prompted comparisons of this model with CD, since this human form of IBD is distinguished from UC by regional transmural inflammation of the colon, granuloma formation and frequent involvement of the distal ileum[27]. Certain features of the CD45RB[hi] model are shared in BM → Tgε26 mice, although in these animals inflammation is limited to the colon and is not transmural. In BM → Tgε26 animals the mononuclear cell infiltration of the colon mucosa is predominated by T cells and neutrophils with evidence of macrophage and B cell presence[22]. As observed in the CD45RB[hi] model, crypt cell proliferation is markedly increased in BM → Tgε26 mice, leading to crypt elongation and thickening of the bowel wall. Crypt abscesses are also a common feature at later stages of disease.

Onset of colitis in the BM → Tgε26 and CD45RB[hi] models each correlates predominantly with the expansion of peripheral and intestinal CD4[+] T cells which display an activated/memory-like phenotype, as determined by their low expression of CD45RB and L-selectin and elevated CD69 and CD44 expression[28,29]. More strikingly, a very high frequency of colon-derived and peripheral CD4[+] T cells (30–60%) express IFNγ and TNFα, which suggests a polarized T_H1 phenotype[30–32].

Despite their less conspicuous representation, CD8[+] T cells in BM → Tgε26 mice display a phenotype similar to that observed in CD4[+] subsets, in that they express IFNγ and TNFα at a high frequency (20–30%). Potentially these cells represent previously described Tc1 type T cells, and may be involved in disease either through pro-inflammatory cytokine expression or cytotoxic activity.

A small number of T cells expressing the TCR$\gamma\delta$ chains are routinely detected in the colon intraepithelial (IE) and lamina propria (LP) compartments of BM → Tgε26 animals. Like the TCR$\alpha\beta^+$ T cells from the same animals, a high frequency of these cells are capable of IFNγ expression, a characteristic not observed in colon derived TCR$\gamma\delta^+$ T cells from healthy wt animals[33]. As discussed later, evidence exists to suggest that activated TCR$\gamma\delta^+$ T cells may play a role in the development of colitis in the BM → Tgε26 colitis model.

An additional feature of colon-derived T cells from both the Tgε26 and CD45RB[hi] models is that they display potent cytotoxic activity *ex vivo* when set up in antibody redirected cytotoxicity assays[22]. The significance of CTL activity in colitis will be discussed in more detail later.

APPROACHES TO STUDYING COLITIS

Since the appearance of donor-derived T cells in the BM $\rightarrow$ Tgε26 and CD45RB^{hi} colitis model is critical for the development of disease, each system is open to a novel experimental approach whereby genetically mutant donors can be used in substitution of wt donors as a means of repopulating the T cell repertoire. In cases where T cell-specific proteins are to be examined, this approach has distinct advantages over cross-breeding experiments, which are time consuming and costly. Using transplantation of genetic mutant BMC in the BM $\rightarrow$ Tgε26 model and CD4$^+$ CD45RB^{hi} T cells in the CD45RB^{hi} model, we have examined the role of a number of specific proteins produced by T cells in the development of colitis. We have observed that RAG^{null} mice, which like *Scid* mice are T cell and B cell deficient, also develop a chronic T$_H$1 induced colitis after transfer of CD45RB^{hi} T cells. Disease in these animals appears very similar to that originally described in the CD45RB^{hi} $\rightarrow$ *Scid* colitis model. This enables the transfer of T cells from a number of genetically deficient donors, since many of these share an identical or similar genetic background (129SvEv or 129SvEv $\times$ C57BL/6).

THE IL-12 PATHWAY

Under normal circumstances T$_H$1 type T cells mediate inflammatory effects predominantly through the production of cytokines such as IFNγ by which they incite other components of the non-adaptive immune system into action[30,34]. For the most part it is assumed that T$_H$1 cell cytokines induce the maturation of macrophage/monocyte function, facilitating the expression of cytokines such as IL-1, IL-6, IL-8 and TNFα as well as a host of other inflammatory mediators[30,34]. Collectively, these mediators induce profound effects within the local tissue environment, including changes to the endothelium leading to increased adhesion molecule expression, increased vascular permeability and attraction of polymorphonuclear cells such as neutrophils to the site of inflammation. In order for these events to happen, however, T cells must themselves differentiate under the influence of a defined stromal and cytokine environment. Thus, the nature of the cellular interactions between activated mucosal T cells and resident macrophages and the repertoire of cytokines they produce, collaborate to induce a differentiated T$_H$1 phenotype[30,31].

Of the cytokines known to promote T$_H$1 development, IL-12 is established as the most potent[35]. Produced by neutrophils, macrophages and in the earlier phase probably mostly by dendritic cells, IL-12 interacts with receptors expressed by naive T cells and NK cells[35–40]. Consequently antigen responsive T cells and NK cells are stimulated to produce IFNγ which correlates with the activation of specific cell signalling machinery within these cells[41]. In turn IL-12 expression is upregulated in monocytes and macrophages in response to IFNγ[42], indicating that the IL-12/IFNγ response pathway appears to be amplified by positive feedback.

Signal transducers and activators of transcription (Stat) proteins, as the name suggests, are responsible for mediating signals via cell surface receptors and associated JAK kinases and initiating transcription of cell specific genes[41,43,44]. The induction of IFNγ in T$_H$1 type cells by IL-12 has been closely correlated with the activity of Stat-4 proteins which are required for efficient expression of IFNγ[45–47]. Evidence that the IL-12/Stat-4 pathway is non-redundant in the development of IL-12 induced T_H1 type responses is corroborated by the observation that mice deficient in Stat-4 genes show an equivalent phenotype to IL-12[null] animals in which T_H1-type responses are severely impaired[47–49].

The expression of mediators such as IL-12 within the intestinal mucosa must profoundly influence the nature of T cell responses to different antigens and it is likely that in IBD IL-12 is one of the most prominent. We have provided evidence that IL-12 is responsible for much of the pathology in the BM $\rightarrow$ Tgε26 and CD45RB[hi] models[50]. After reconstitution of each model with Stat-4 deficient (Stat-4[null]) BMC or T cells, both the BM $\rightarrow$ Tgε26 and CD45RB[hi]-recipient mice developed significantly milder forms of wasting and colitis than in mice reconstituted with wt T cells. Analyses of T cell specific IFNγ production from Stat-4[null] reconstituted animals in both models further revealed a considerable reduction in the frequency of T cells capable of IFNγ expression. These data, which showed that T cells deficient in Stat-4 signalling are moderated in their pathogenic capacity, correlate well with the reduced responses to classical T_H1-inducing antigens observed in the original Stat-4[null] mice[47,49]. The link between the actions of IL-12 and Stat-4 signalling in generating colitis was further underscored by the observation that treatment of wt BM $\rightarrow$ Tgε26 mice with anti-IL-12 antibodies[51] had a very similar effect to that seen in Stat-4[null] BMC-reconstituted animals. A role for IL-12 in human IBD is supported by the observation that in CD, elevated levels of IL-12 are associated other proinflammatory cytokines such as IFNγ and TNFα within the intestinal mucosa[52–54].

The above experiments provide an interesting contrast with those from a study on a more acute T_H1 model of colitis, induced by rectal administration of the haptenizing agent 2,4,6-trinitrobenzene sulphonic acid (TNBS) and ethanol in mice[55]. In this study, anti-IL-12 administration almost completely prevented disease and correlated with a profound reduction in IFNγ expression by T cells. Furthermore, a continued presence of IL-12 was required for pathology in TNBS-treated mice, since neutralization of IL-12 up to 20 days after onset of disease, was sufficient to facilitate the recovery of mice from disease. Although in the BM $\rightarrow$ Tgε26 and CD45RB[hi] models both colitis and IFNγ expression by T cells was significantly reduced by inhibition of the IL-12/Stat-4 pathway, neither was completely prevented. In some cases moderate colitis was still evident by histological examination and a significant number of T cells capable of IFNγ expression was detected. Collectively, these comparisons between acute and more chronic T_H1 models of intestinal inflammation suggest a different emphasis on the T_H1-promoting pathways which might influence the course of disease in each case. Thus, under conditions such as those found in the BM $\rightarrow$ Tgε26 and CD45RB[hi] recipient mice, T_H1-type T cells may fall under the influence of additional pathways which determine their development towards a T_H1 phenotype.

IFNγ-DEPENDENT AND INDEPENDENT T CELL PATHOLOGY

The apparent correlation between the actions of IL-12 and expression of IFNγ in the CD45RB[hi] transfer, BM $\rightarrow$ Tgε26 and TNBS-induced models of colitis suggests that the pivotal actions of this cytokine are contingent on its ability to induce IFNγ expression in T lymphocytes. However, data from our laboratory suggest that the actions of IL-12 in colitis extend beyond this role[50]. Thus, in BM $\rightarrow$ Tgε26 and the CD45RB[hi] models, T cell reconstitution using IFNγ[null] donor animals resulted in a high incidence of colitis. Although in the BM $\rightarrow$ Tgε26 model many animals developed colitis of reduced severity compared with those that received wt BMC, both the wasting syndrome and colitis were for the most part more severe than in animals that had received anti-IL-12 treatment or Stat-4 deficient BMC. In the CD45RB[hi] model these differences were even more pronounced.

The above results reveal that induction of IFNγ gene expression in T cells is not the only defining step in the progression of T$_H$1-like pathology. However, in these experiments the influence of cytokines derived from recipient cells (resident non-T cells present within the adoptive host) cannot be excluded. Certainly, it has already been demonstrated that anti-IFNγ antibodies attenuated disease in the CD45RB[hi] transfer model suggesting, in this model at least, that T cell independent sources of IFNγ may be sufficient to drive disease[26]. *Scid* and RAG[null] mice both harbour large numbers of NK cells which are a potent source of IFNγ which can be induced by IL-12. Consequently, it is possible that IFNγ expression by resident NK cells in the adoptive host is sufficient to drive development of a pathogenic T$_H$1 phenotype after transfer of CD45RB[hi] T cells. In contrast to *Scid* and RAG[null] animals, Tgε26 mice are profoundly deficient in NK cells, and these cells appear only in very small numbers after BMC transfer in adult mice[56]. It seems very unlikely therefore that NK cells in this model offer a sufficient source of IFNγ in BM $\rightarrow$ Tgε26 animals. Indeed evidence exists to suggest that NK cells can to a limited extent protect against mucosal inflammation in the BM $\rightarrow$ Tgε26 colitis model (B. Wang, S. A. Shah and C. Terhorst, unpublished observations).

The above arguments notwithstanding, precedents for mucosal inflammation in the absence of IFNγ expression do exist in other T$_H$1-like models of colitis. For example, in IL-2[null] mice, which harbour moderate numbers of IFNγ-expressing cells, colitis has been observed after importation of the IFNγ[null] mutation[50]. Similarly Berg *et al.* recently reported that administration of anti-IFNγ antibodies was only sufficient to protect against colitis in IL-10[null] mice if administered up to 3 weeks of age[57]. Treatment after this time resulted in an incidence and severity of disease equivalent to that seen in animals left untreated. These latter data suggest distinct roles for IFNγ in early versus later stages of T$_H$1 induction in the development of colitis.

In many ways the data obtained from different models of colitis bear similarities to those observed in experimental autoimmune encephalomyelitis (EAE). Experiments in this T$_H$1 type autoimmune disease model have shown that induction of pathology in mice by proteolipid protein (PLP)-primed T cells could be inhibited by injection with anti-IL-12[58,59]. However, exacerbation of disease by pre-incubating PLP-primed T cells *in vitro* with IL-12 was heightened by co-incubation with anti-IFNγ. Equivalent results were also obtained in established EAE, whereby injection of anti-IFNγ antibodies into mice exacerbated disease[60]. One interpretation applied to these data was that through anti-proliferative effects, IFNγ might actually act so as to limit the expansion of pathogenic T cells during early stages of disease.

Collectively, the evidence so far discussed suggests that pathology normally associated with expression of IFNγ by T cells, can occur in the absence of this T_H1 'signature' cytokine. One interpretation for these findings is that T cells incapable of IFNγ production might undergo so-called 'immune deviation' whereby they start to express T_H2 rather than T_H1 associated cytokines, but maintain their ability to induce disease[61]. In recent experiments this was shown to occur in a second EAE model as well as in an autoimmune insulitis model previously characterized by T_H1 induced pathology[62,63]. In a similar fashion previous studies have shown that T cells from Stat-4^{null} mice express T_H2 type cytokines including IL-4 and IL-10, after stimulation using conditions normally shown to elicit T_H1 like responses in wt T cells[49]. In the context of experimental colitis, development of disease resulting from activity of T_H2 like T cells has been demonstrated in TCRα^{null} mice, which develop immuno-pathology similar to that in T_H1 colitis models, but which is characterized by elevated levels of IL-4[64,65].

In IFNγ^{null} recipient Tgε26 or *Scid* mice, we have been unable to detect significant production of either IL-10 or IL-4 by T cells, suggesting that if immune deviation does occur in these animals it is very limited. Additionally, the requirements for T cells to respond to IL-12 in both the CD45RB^{hi} transfer and BM $\rightarrow$ Tgε26 colitis models suggests that the T cells in each case retained characteristic responsiveness of T_H1 type T cells, even in the absence of IFNγ expression. Together, these observations argue against immune deviation as a principal mechanism of pathology in the absence of IFNγ expression. More accurately, in the context of these two colitis models, IFNγ^{null} T cells appear to possess a 'modified' T_H1 phenotype, by which they mediate pathology via other pathways associated with T_H1 cells. In light of this it is worth considering other mechanisms might which lead to pathological changes associated with colitis.

IL-18 and IL-1

Recently a cytokine capable of inducing IFNγ expression in T cells and NK cells was identified and termed 'interferon-γ inducing factor' or IL-18[66,67]. Like IL-12, IL-18 can be induced in macrophages by bacterial products such as LPS[68]. The precise role for IL-18 in cell mediated immunity has yet to be established although it has been postulated that it may be important in anti-tumour immunity and in inflammation[66]. IL-18 shares some structural homology with IL-1 and like IL-1 is converted to its active form by the enzyme caspase-1. Comparison of caspase-1^{null} and IL-1β^{null} mice has revealed a role for IL-18 in the expression of the pro-inflammatory mediators TNFα, IL-1α and IL-6. Furthermore, regulation of IL-18 receptor appears to be somewhat dependent on IL-12, suggesting that the pathways of these cytokines may to some extent overlap. Consistent with this, it has recently been demonstrated in mice that IL-18 is not able to drive T_H1 development on its own, but rather that it may synergize with IL-12 to promote IFNγ expression in T cells[69]. Interestingly, however, in mice this was dependent on the background strain: Balb/c mice (typically identified as generating predominantly T_H2 type responses) but not C57BL/6 mice (typically T_H1 responders) were responsive to IL-18 potentiation of IL-12 responses[69]. Unpublished findings by the same group revealed a similar role for IL-1α as a co-factor in T_H1 development. These observations suggest a potential role for co-factor cytokines such as IL-18 in colitis, a question which we are currently addressing in the BM $\rightarrow$ Tgε26 and CD45RB^{hi} models.

CD40

One of the critical pathways by which T cells activate macrophages and dendritic cells is the binding of CD40L (gp39, CD154) to CD40 on the APC. CD40L is up-regulated on T cells after stimulation through the TCR complex and after binding induces several signals in the APC, including up-regulation of CD80 and CD86, transcription of IL-12 and a number of pro-inflammatory cytokines. In the TNBS model, blocking CD40-CD40L interaction with antibody treatment at early time points, rescued the mice from colitis. When antibodies were given after colitis had developed, no effect on disease could be detected[70]. A similar situation has also been reported in experimental autoimmune diabetes.

Interleukin–15

Interleukin–15, an IL-2 like cytokine that shares the IL-2Rβ and common-γ receptor chains, is thought to be a potent activator of T cells and macrophages. The precise mechanisms are poorly understood but may involve autocrine and cell contact mediated activation. The observation that IL-15 has been suggested to play a major role in rheumatoid arthritis[71] and was reported to be transcribed by intestinal epithelial cells[72] is consistent with a potential role for this cytokine in IBD, although this remains to be investigated.

TNFα and TNFβ

TNFα and TNFβ (also called lymphotoxin α), are the most extensively characterized of the proinflammatory cytokines and are known to play pivotal roles in many aspects of local and systemic response to infectious pathogens, inducing significant events associated with inflammation[73]. The role of TNFα in immunopathological diseases such as rheumatoid arthritis and CD is now established and both TNFα and TNFβ have become key targets of potential immunotherapy for these conditions[73–75].

Elevated levels of circulating TNFα can be detected in colitic BM $\rightarrow$ Tgε26 mice, and, in these animals as well as in CD45RB^{hi} mice, a high proportion of both CD8$^+$ and CD4$^+$ T cells from the peripheral lymph nodes (10–20%) and the colon (20–40%) are capable of expressing this cytokine. *In vivo* neutralization of TNFα in both models, using anti-TNFα antibodies (V1q) effectively inhibited both cachexia and colitis (Mackay *et al.*, submitted for publication)[26] but required continued weekly treatment. In both BM $\rightarrow$ Tgε26 and CD45RB^{hi} models therefore, TNFα was revealed as a predominant inflammatory mediator both systemically, leading to cachexia, and at a local level within the colon. This was even more strongly emphasized by the finding that T cells from BM $\rightarrow$ Tgε26 and CD45RB^{hi}-recipient mice, transplanted with INFγ^{null} bone marrow or T cells (see above) were capable of equivalent TNFα production to those from animals transplanted with wt cells. These data suggest that TNFα may operate to an extent independently of IFNγ and may possibly be directly regulated through the IL-12 pathway. This would be consistent with the findings of other studies which have revealed that some IL-12 functions, including those associated with IL-12-dependent pathology, are mediated through TNFα[76]. At this point it is not clear whether T cell or monocyte/macrophage-specific TNFα production is predominantly responsible for colitis in either the BM $\rightarrow$ Tgε26 or CD45RB[hi] colitis models. One potential interpretation of the IFNγ[null] transfer experiments however, might be that in the absence of IFNγ expression by T cells, TNFα might take over as the principal effector cytokine produced by T_H1 cells.

Potentially TNFα could be involved at a number of levels in the development of colitis. At a direct level TNFα can induce profound changes to endothelium resulting in up-regulation of adhesion molecules and changes in permeability[73]. At a systemic level TNFα induces release of acute phase proteins from the liver and is responsible for weight loss in cachexic diseases resulting from systemic infections. TNFα also potentiates the cytokine induction by other cells including monocytes, macrophages and lymphocytes. These findings are consistent with the possibility that TNFα might be involved at an immunoregulatory level in the development of T_H1 type diseases such as colitis. This notion has recently been borne out by the observation in CD patients undergoing treatment with anti-TNFα antibodies, that TNFα is a co-factor in the development of T_H1 type responses in this disease[77].

Lymphotoxin $\alpha\beta$

Despite its close relationship with TNFα and TNFβ, the immunological significance of lymphotoxin $\alpha\beta$ (LT$\alpha\beta$) has only recently emerged and much about the biology of this system remains to be elucidated. LT$\alpha\beta$ comprises a hetero-trimeric complex of the unique LTβ chain associated with LTα chains[78] which, unlike TNF, remains membrane bound. The LT$\alpha\beta$ complex has been shown to bind to a receptor distinct from both the TNF receptors (TNFR60 and TNFR80) designated the LTβ-R.

Studies of LTα and LTβ deficient mice and the progeny of pregnant mice treated with soluble LTβ receptor have demonstrated an important and distinct role for LT$\alpha\beta$ in the development of secondary lymphoid organs[79–81]. To an extent the LT$\alpha\beta$ pathway shares requirements for lymph node organization with the TNF system; for example, both pathways are required for Peyer's patch development and splenic architecture. More recently, it was observed that this latter function for LT$\alpha\beta$ is required throughout life, since administration of soluble LTβ-R was sufficient to disrupt splenic architecture and alter certain T_H1 dependent humoral responses in adult mice[82]. Although LT$\alpha\beta$ does not appear to mediate the same potent inflammatory effects as TNFα, both molecules do share the ability to induce apoptosis in certain adenocarcinoma cell lines, which is synergistic with IFNγ[83,84]. These data suggest that a limited degree of redundancy does exist in the functions of these molecules.

Recently we have demonstrated that the LT$\alpha\beta$ system is involved in the development of IBD in both the CD45RB[hi] and BM $\rightarrow$ Tgε26 colitis models (Mackay *et al.*, submitted for publication). Animals in each system treated with a soluble

LTβ-R–Ig fusion protein showed markedly reduced weight loss and developed a significantly milder colitis, compared with those that received control protein. In the case of the BM $\rightarrow$ Tgε26 model, reduction in disease was comparable with that seen in TNFα-treated animals. The lack of previous data demonstrating a role for LT$\alpha\beta$ in downstream inflammatory functions such as associated with TNF corroborate the observations that anti-TNFα antibodies are sufficient to mediate a high degree of protection in both models of colitis (Mackay *et al.*, submitted for publication[26]). This would indicate that these systems are non-redundant in their points of action. It seems plausible therefore to suggest that LT$\alpha\beta$ operates at an earlier time point than TNFα in the development of disease, possibly acting during the initiation of T_H1 responses[50]. In light of the previous findings that LT$\alpha\beta$ affects follicular dendritic cell function, it would seem reasonable to speculate that the function of this pathway may centre on the developmental or functional maturation of cells of the dendritic or monocyte lineage which might subsequently affect progression of T_H1 responses. Whatever the mechanism of LT$\alpha\beta$ function, the evidence so far suggests a significant role in the development of at least some types of inflammatory T_H1 type responses and as such may represent a potential target for therapeutic intervention in disease.

CYTOTOXIC T CELLS IN IBD

Several studies have suggested that cytotoxic T cells (CTL) might be involved in the development of human IBD[85,86] and the observation that CTL activity is significantly elevated in T cells from diseased colon of both BM $\rightarrow$ Tgε26 and CD45RB[hi] recipient mice supports this contention[22,87]. Potential models for CTL involvement are principally based on the notion that aberrant CTL activity could lead to damage of the epithelial boundary thereby exposing the mucosal immune system to bacterial products and thus initiating inflammatory response. Although this is a somewhat simplistic view and the evidence circumstantial, the potential involvement of CTL in IBD is nevertheless worthy of consideration. This is emphasized by the fact that CTL play a significant role in other pathologies such as GVHD[88] and in some autoimmune conditions[89].

CTL capable of rapid induction of target cell death have been identified as utilizing either of two effector pathways[90,91]. The first, perforin, has been classically associated with CD8[+] CTL, although it is now recognized that some CD4[+] T cells also utilize this pathway[92,93]. Induction of apoptosis in target cells by perforin is induced by formation of perforin polymers in the target cell surface, which allows the subsequent entry of serine proteases (granzymes) into the cytoplasm. FAS-L also induces apoptosis in target cells, although this is achieved through the engagement of its receptor (FAS) on the target cell surface[94]. Originally FAS expression was detected on T cells and the FAS-L/FAS pathway has been identified as the means by which T cells regulate one another through programmed cell death. More recently the observation that FAS is expressed on cell types other than T cells has prompted speculation that FAS-L-expressing T cells might operate directly in host defence against infection and also possibly in certain types of autoimmune conditions[89].

To test the role of perforin and FAS-L in the development of colitis in BM $\rightarrow$ Tgε26 mice we reconstituted Tgε26 mice with bone marrow from mice genetically deficient in perforin (PFP[null] mice)[91,95], FAS-L (*gld/gld* mice)[96] or both molecules (PFP[null] $\times$ *gld*). Colitis still developed in each set of animals, although the incidence and severity was moderately reduced in the absence of perforin expression. These studies suggested that perforin participates to a limited extent in the development of pathology in BM $\rightarrow$ Tgε26 mice whilst FAS-L was not involved in disease. At this stage we have not attributed each CTL pathway with a particular subset of T cell. A likely scenario, however, is that CD8[+] T cells mediated perforin-dependent killing whilst CD4[+] T cells were responsible for FAS-dependent CTL activity. In the CD45RB[hi] transfer colitis model reconstitution with perforin-deficient CD45RB[hi] CD4[+] T cells had no effect on the development of colitis, which is consistent with the finding that colon-derived T cells from these animals predominantly utilize FAS-L in mediating cell death[87]. In light of these findings, it will be of interest to examine whether FAS-L deficient T cells are capable of inducing disease in this model.

The notion that colonic CD8[+] T cells are responsible for perforin-induced CTL activity in the BM $\rightarrow$ Tgε26 mice is consistent with the activated status of these cells made evident by their ability to produce IFNγ and TNFα. In IL-2[null] mice colon-derived CD8[+] T cells are capable of significant short-term CTL activity[97]. However, disruption of CD8[+] T cell development by crossing IL-2[null] mice with MHC class I deficient (β2m[null]) mice, did not inhibit the development of colitis[97]. Indeed, in the absence of CD8[+] T cell development many IL-2[null] mice developed colitis more rapidly. Furthermore, this correlated in older animals with a high incidence of colon adenocarcinoma[98], which does not develop (to our knowledge) in either β2m[null] or IL-2[null] animals. These data suggest that CD8[+] T cells at least in IL-2[null] mice play a protective rather than a pathogenic role. This would be consistent with the frequently postulated suggestion that mucosal CD8[+] T cells are important in the regulation of intestinal immunity. The appearance of adenocarcinoma in β2m[null] x IL-2[null] mice is further consistent with the notion that this T cell subset might be important in the immunosurveillance of the intestinal mucosa.

LYMPHOCYTE HOMING TO THE GUT AND COLITIS

The adhesion of leukocytes to other cells and extracellular matrix is fundamental to the process inflammation. In order to enter a site of inflammation lymphocytes need to cross the endothelial barrier, a process known as extravasation. This is initiated by rolling of lymphocytes over the endothelium, facilitated by interactions of selectins with their ligands. By mechanisms not completely understood, these rolling cells up-regulate a second type of adhesion receptor called integrins, which enable them to cease rolling and initiate diapedesis. Integrins are a family of transmembrane glycoproteins composed of α and β subunits. In many cases these chains associate in different heterodimeric forms to determine the specificity of an integrin and its tissue destination.

Lymphocytes which express distinct integrins preferentially recirculate to their tissue of origin, supposedly returning them to the site where they encountered their antigen. This specificity of 'homing' has been shown elegantly in the case of the intestinal LP and Peyer's patches (PP). Lymphocytes expressing $\alpha_4\beta_7$-integrin home to these two sites through binding of this integrin to the mucosal addressin cell adhesion molecule (MadCAM)-1, which is exclusively expressed on the high endothelial venules at these sites. More than 95% of IEL express a second distinct integrin, $\alpha_E\beta_7$.

The role of different integrins can be assessed using mutant mice. For example, mice whose T cells are deficient in α_4 have no CD3+ cells in the PP but show normal numbers of IEL, suggesting that either $\alpha_4\beta_1$ or $\alpha_4\beta_7$ is required for homing to the PP[99]. β_7-deficient mice show a 10 to 30-fold decrease in LP lymphocyte number and a 5-fold decrease in IEL[100]. These results confirm the notion that $\alpha_4\beta_7$-integrin is a crucial adhesion factor for lymphocytes to home to the PP and possibly the LP, with a lesser role for $\alpha_4\beta_1$ and $\alpha_E\beta_7$.

Levels of $\alpha_4\beta_7$-integrin expression on LP lymphocytes appear to be lower in CD, UC and in infectious colitis, than in healthy individuals. At the same time up-regulated MadCAM-1 expression on the LP endothelium has been reported[101]. Although other adhesion molecules, including ICAM-1 and a number of integrins, also seem to be up-regulated in CD, the specificity of this remains to be investigated.

Several studies have been published in which mAbs against either $\alpha_4\beta_7$ or MadCAM interfered with the onset of or prevented colitis in animal models. In the cotton top tamarin, antibodies to both α_4 and $\alpha_4\beta_7$ significantly attenuate the spontaneous colitis that occurs in these animals[102]. In the CD45RB^{hi} transfer model, antibodies directed against β_7 or to its ligand MadCAM-1 seem to severely disable lymphocytes in homing to the LP. Furthermore, when these colitic mice were treated with a combination of these antibodies, a significant decrease in colitis was observed[103].

We are currently studying the effect of the α_4^{null} mutation in T cells. Bone marrow from α_4^{null}/RAG^{null} chimeras was injected into Tgε26 recipients to see whether the T cells from these animals can home to the gut and whether they can cause colitis. So far none of the α_4^{null} BM → Tgε26 mice has developed colitis, although after many weeks these mice die from a wasting syndrome similar to the one that accompanies the colitis in wt BM → Tgε26 transplants (unpublished observations). By flow cytometry only small numbers of CD8α^+ α_E^+ cells were found in the intraepithelium (IE) and no CD4+ cells could be detected in either the LP or IE.

We can speculate on the dynamics of lymphocytes in experimental colitis. Apparently the CD4+ cells, that have been shown to cause the disease in this model, do not require activation within the LP since the α_4^{null} BM → Tgε26 mice still die of a wasting syndrome. This raises important questions as to the nature and site of T cell stimulation in models of IBD. Whether APC take up antigen in the LP, travel to the MLN and spleen and there present it to T cells, or whether T cell stimulation within the intestine can occur, and in the absence of recirculation cause a systemic disease, remains to be elucidated.

CONCLUDING REMARKS

The conceptual understanding of IBD is undergoing a rapid evolution, due largely to the study of animal models of intestinal inflammation. As discussed in this review, models in which colitis depends upon the transfer of cells into immunodeficient hosts provide highly versatile vehicles for exploring different aspects of T cell-mediated pathology and regulation. These studies, which are uncovering the multiplicity of pathways which contribute to IBD, will provide a sure foundation for specific immunotheraputic intervention in the future.

References

1. Sartor RB. Role of intestinal microflora in pathogenesis and complications. In: Scholmerich J, Goebel H, Ruis WD, Hohenberger W (eds) Inflammatory Bowel Diseases: Pathophysiology as Basis of treatment. Dordrecht: Kluwer Academic Publishers, 1992:175–187.
2. Bhan AK, Mizoguchi E, Mizoguchi A. New models for chronic intestinal inflammation. Curr Opin Gastroenterol. 1994;10:633–638.
3. Elson CO, Sartor RB, Tennyson GS, Riddel RH. Experimental models of inflammatory bowel disease. Gastroenterology. 1995;109:1344–1367.
4. Shanahan F. Pathogenesis of ulcerative colitis. Lancet 1993;342:407–411.
5. Sartor RB. Insights into the pathogenesis of inflammatory bowel diseases provided by new rodent models of spontaneous colitis. Inflamm Bowel Dis. 1995;1:64–75.
6. Simpson SJ, Hollander GA, Mizoguchi E, Bhan AK, Wang B, Terhorst C. Defects in T-cell regulation: lessons for inflammatory bowel disease. In: Kagnoff MF, Kiyono H (eds) Essentials of Mucosal Immunology. San Diego: Academic Press, 1996:291–304.
7. Taurog JD, Richardson JA, Croft JT et al. The germfree state prevents development of gut and joint inflammatory disease in HLA-B27 transgenic rats. J Exp Med. 1994;180:2359–2364.
8. Schorle H, Holkschke T, Hunig T, Schimple A, Horak I. Development and function of T cells in mice rendered interleukin-2 deficient by gene targeting. Nature. 1991;352:621–624.
9. Hammer RE, Maika SD, Richardson JA, Tang JP, Taurog JD. Spontaneous inflammatory disease in transgenic rats expressing HLA-B27 and human beta 2m: an animal model of HLA-B27-associated human disorders. Cell. 1990;63:1099–1112.
10. Sadlack B, Merz H, Schorle H, Schimpl A, Feller AC, Horak I. Ulcerative colitis-like disease in mice with a disrupted interleukin-2 gene. Cell. 1993;75:253–61.
11. Shull MM, Ormsby I, Kier AB et al. Targeted disruption of the mouse transforming growth factor-beta 1 gene results in multifocal inflammatory disease. Nature. 1992;359:693–699.
12. Diebold R, Eis MJ, Yin M et al. Early onset multifocal inflammation in the transforming growth factor b1-null mouse is lymphocyte mediated. Proc Natl Acad Sci USA. 1995;92:12215–12219.
13. Kuhn R, Lohler J, Rennick D et al. Interleukin-10-deficient mice develop chronic enterocolitis. Cell. 1993;75:263–274.
14. Mombaerts P, Mizoguchi E, Grusby MJ, Glimcher LH, Bhan AK, Tonegawa S. Spontaneous development of inflammatory bowel disease in T cell receptor mutant mice [see comments]. Cell. 1993;75:274–282.
15. Herminston ML, Gordon JI. Inflammatory bowel disease and adenomas in mice expressing a dominant negative N-cadherin. Science. 1995;270:1203–1207.
16. Mashimo H, Wu DC, Podolsky DK, Fishman MC. Impaired defense of intestinal mucosa in mice lacking intestinal trefoil factor. Science. 1996;274:262–265.
17. Rudolph U, Finegold MJ, Rich SS et al. Ulcerative colitis and adenocarcinoma of the colon in G alpha i2-deficient mice. Nature Genet. 1995;10:143–150.
18. Wang B, Biron C, She J et al. A block in both early T lymphocyte and natural killer cell development in transgenic mice with high-copy numbers of the human CD3E gene. Proc Natl Acad Sci USA. 1994;91:9402–9406.
19. Wang B, Simpson SJ, Hollander GA, Terhorst C. Development and function of T lymphocytes and natural killer cells after bone marrow transplantation of severely immunodeficient mice. Immunol Rev. 1997;157:53–60.
20. Hollander GA, Wang B, Nichogiannoploulou A et al. A developmental control point in the induction of thymic cortex regulated by a sub population of pro-thymocytes. Nature. 1995;373:350–353.
21. Wang B, Levelt C, Salio M et al. Abrogation of early T cell development by excessive signal transduction through CD3e. Int Immunol. 1995;7:435–448.

22. Hollander GA, Simpson SJ, Mizoguchi E et al. Severe colitis in mice with aberrant thymic selection. Immunity. 1995;3:27–38.

23. Morrissey PJ, Charrier K, Braddy S, Liggitt D, Watson JD. CD4+ T cells that express high levels of CD45RB induce wasting disease when transferred into congenic severe combined immunodeficient mice. Disease development is prevented by cotransfer of purified CD4+ T cells. J Exp Med. 1993;178:237–244.

24. Powrie F, Leach MW, Mauze S, Caddle LB, Coffman RL. Phenotypically distinct subsets of CD4+ T cells induce or protect from chronic intestinal inflammation in C. B-17 scid mice. Int Immunol. 1993;5:1461–1471.

25. Powrie F, Correa-Oliveira R, Mauze S, Coffman RL. Regulatory interactions between CD45RB^{high} and CD45RB^{low} CD4+ T cells are important for the balance between protective and pathogenic cell-mediated immunity. J Exp Med. 1994;179:589–600.

26. Powrie F, Leach MW, Mauze S. Inhibition of TH1 responses prevents IBD in SCID mice reconstituted with CD45RB^{high} CD4+ T cells. Immunity. 1994;1:553–562.

27. Podolsky DK. Inflammatory bowel disease. N Engl J Med. 1991;325:928–937, 1008–1016.

28. Bottomly K, Luqman M, Greenbaum L et al. A monoclonal antibody to CD45R distinguishes CD4+ T cell populations that produce different cytokines. Eur J Immunol. 1989;16:617–623.

29. Bradley LM, Atkins G, Swain SL. Long term CD4+ memory T cells from the spleen lack MEL-14, the lymph node homing receptor. J Immunol. 1992;148:324–331.

30. Abbas A, Murphy KM, Sher A. Functional diversity of helper T lymphocytes. Nature. 1996;383:787–793.

31. Seder RA, Paul WE. Acquisition of lymphokine-producing phenotype by CD4+ T cells. Annu Rev Immunol. 1994;12:635–673.

32. Mossmann TR, Coffman RL. Th-1 and Th-2 cells: different patterns of lymphokine secretion lead to different functional properties. Annu Rev Immunol. 1989;7:145–173.

33. Simpson SJ, Hollander GA, Mizoguchi E, Allen D, Wang BP, Terhorst C. Expression of pro-inflammatory cytokines by TCR$\alpha\beta^+$ and TCR$\gamma\delta^+$ T cells in an experimental model of colitis. Eur J Immunol. 1997;27:17–25.

34. Boehm U, Klamp T, Groot M, Howard JC. Cellular responses to interferon γ. Annu Rev Immunol. 1997;15:749–795.

35. Trinchieri G. Interleukin-12: a proinflammatory cytokine with immunoregulatory functions that bridge innate resistance and antigen specific immunity. Annu Rev Immunol. 1995;13:251–276.

36. Sutterwala FS, Noel GJ, Clynes R, Mosser DM. Selective suppression of interleukin-12 induction after macrophage receptor ligation. J Exp Med. 1997;185:1977–1985.

37. Heufler C, Koch F, Stanzl U et al. Interleukin-12 is produced by dendritic cells and mediates T helper 1 development as well as interferon-gamma production by T helper 1 cells. Eur J Immunol. 1996;26:659–668.

38. Gerosa F, Paganin C, Peritt D et al. Interleukin-12 primes human CD4 and CD8 T cell clones for high production of both interferon-gamma and interleukin-10. J Exp Med. 1996;183:2559–2569.

39. Schmitt E, Hoeh P, Huels C et al. T helper 1 development of naive CD4+ T cells requires the coordinate action of interleukin 12 and interferon gamma and is inhibited by transformig growth factor-beta. Eur J Immunol. 1994;24:793–798.

40. Kennedy MK, Picha KS, Shanebeck KD, Anderson DM, Grabstein KH. Interleukin-12 regulates the proliferation of Th1, but not Th2 or Th0, clones. Eur J Immunol. 1994;24:2271–2278.

41. Jacobson NG, Szabo SJ, Weber-Nordt RM et al. Interleukin 12 signaling in T helper type 1 (Th1) cells involves tyrosine phosphorylation of signal transducer and activator of transcription (Stat)3 and Stat4. J Exp Med. 1995;181:1755–1762.

42. Yoshida A, Koide Y, Uchijima M, Yoshida TO. IFNγ induces IL-12 mRNA expression by a murine macrophage cell line, J 774. Biochem Biophys Res Commun. 1994;198:857–861.

43. Ihle JN. STATs: Signal transducers and activators of transcription. Cell. 1996;84:331–334.

44. Zhong Z, Wen Z, Darnell JE, Jr. Stat3 and Stat4: members of the family of signal transducers and activators of transcription. Proc Natl Acad Sci USA. 1994;91:4806–4810.

45. Cho SS, Bacon CM, Sudarshan C et al. Activation of STAT4 by IL-12 and IFN-alpha: evidence for the involvement of ligand-induced tyrosine and serine phosphorylation. J Immunol. 1996;157:4781–4789.

46. Yamamoto K, Quelle FW, Thierfelder WE et al. Stat4, a novel gamma interferon activation site-binding protein expressed in early myeloid differentiation. Mol Cell Biol. 1994;14:4342–4349.

47. Thierfelder WE, van Deursen JM, Yamamoto K et al. Requirement for Stat4 in interleukin-12-mediated responses of natural killer and T cells. Nature. 1996;382:171–174.
48. Magram J, Connaughton SE, Warrier RR et al. IL-12-deficient mice are defective in IFN gamma production and type 1 cytokine responses. Immunity. 1996;4:471–481.
49. Kaplan MH, Sun YL, Hoey T, Grusby MJ. Impaired IL-12 responses and enhanced development of Th2 cells in Stat4-deficient mice. Nature. 1996;382:174–177.
50. Simpson S, Shah S, Comiskey M et al. T cell-mediated pathology in two models of experimental colitis depends predominantly on the interleukin-12/signal transducer and activator of transcription (Stat)-4 pathway, but is not conditional on interferon gamma expression by T cells. J Exp Med. 1998;187:1225–1234.
51. Ozmen L, Pericin M, Hakimi J, Chizzonite RA, Wysocka M, Trinchieri G. Interleukin 12, interferon gamma and tumour necrosis factor alpha are the key cytokines of the generalized Schwartzman reaction. J Exp Med. 1994;180:907–915.
52. Sartor RB. Cytokines in intestinal inflammation:pathological and clinical considerations. Gastroenterology. 1994;106:533–549.
53. Parronchi P, Romagnani P, Annunziato F et al. Type 1 T-helper cell predominance and interleukin-12 expression in the gut of patients with Crohn's disease. Am J Pathol. 1997;150: 823–832.
54. Murata Y, Ishiguro Y, Itoh J, Munakata A, Yoshida Y. The role of proinflammatory and immunoregulatory cytokines in the pathogenesis of ulcerative colitis. J Gastroenterol. 1995;30 (Suppl 8):56–60.
55. Neurath MF, Fuss I, Kelsall BL, Stuber E, Strober W. Antibodies to interleukin 12 abrogate established experimental colitis in mice. J Exp Med. 1995;182:1281–1290.
56. Wang B, Hollander GA, Nichogiannopoulou A et al. Natural killer cell development is blocked in the context of aberrant T lymphocyte ontogeny. Int Immunol. 1996;8:939–949.
57. Berg DJ, Davidson N, Kuhn R et al. Enterocolitis and colon cancer in interleukin 10-deficient mice are associated with aberrant cytokine production and CD4+ Th-1 like responses. J Clin Invest. 1996;98:1010–1020.
58. Leonard JP, Waldburger KE, Goldman SJ. Prevention of experimental autoimmune encephalomyelitis by antibodies against interleukin 12. J Exp Med. 1995;181:381–386.
59. Seder RA, Kelsall BL, Jankovic D. Differential role for IL-12 in the maintenance of immune responses in infectious versus autoimmune disease. J Immunol. 1996;157:2745–2748.
60. Duong TT, St Louis J, Gilbert JJ, Finkelman FD, Strejan GH. Effect of anti-interferon-gamma and anti-interleukin-2 monoclonal antibody treatment on the development of actively and passively induced experimental allergic encephalomyelitis in the SJL/J mouse. J Neuroimmunol. 1992;36:105–115.
61. Rocken M, Shevach EM. Immune deviation – the third dimension of nondeletional T cell tolerance. Immunol Rev. 1996;149:176–194.
62. Lafaille JJ, van de Keere AL, Hsu JL et al. Myelin basic protein-specific T helper (Th-2) T cells cause experimental autoimmune encephalomyelitis in immunodeficient hosts rather than protect them from disease. J Exp Med. 1997;186:307–312.
63. Pakela S, Kurrer MO, Katz JD. T helper cells (Th-2) T cells induce acute pancreatitis and diabetes in immune compromised nonobese diabetic (NOD) mice. J Exp Med. 1997;186: 299–306.
64. Mizoguchi E, Mizoguchi A, Bhan AK. Role of cytokines in the early stages of chronic colitis in TCRa mutant mice. Lab Invest. 1997;76:385–397.
65. Mizoguchi A, Mizoguch E, Chiba C et al. Cytokine inbalance and autoantibody production in T cell receptor α mutant mice with inflammatory bowel disease. J Exp Med. 1996;183:847–856.
66. Okamura H, Tsutsi H, Komatsu T et al. Cloning of a new cytokine that induces IFN-gamma production by T cells [see comments]. Nature. 1995;378:88–91.
67. Kohno K, Kataoka J, Ohtsuki T et al. IFN-gamma-inducing factor (IGIF) is a costimulatory factor on the activation of Th1 but not Th2 cells and exerts its effect independently of IL-12. J Immunol. 1997;158:1541–1550.
68. Micallef MJ, Ohtsuki T, Kohno K et al. Interferon-gamma-inducing factor enhances T helper 1 cytokine production by stimulated human T cells: synergism with interleukin-12 for interferon-gamma production. Eur J Immunol. 1996;26:1647–1651.
69. Robinson D, Shibuya K, Mui A et al. IGIF does not drive Th-1 development but synergises with IL-12 for Interferon g production and activates IRAK and NF kB. Immunity. 1997;7:571–581.

70. Stuber E, Strober W, Neurath M. Blocking the CD40L-CD40 interaction in vivo specifically prevents the priming of T helper 1 cells through the inhibition of interleukin 12 secretion. J Exp Med. 1996;183:693–698.
71. McInnes I, Leung B, Sturrock R, Field M, Liew F. Interleukin-15 mediates T cell-dependent regulation of tumor necrosis factor-alpha production in rheumatoid arthritis. Nature Med. 1997;3:189–195.
72. Reinecker H, MacDermott R, Mirau S, Dignass A, Podolsky D. Intestinal epithelial cells both express and respond to interleukin 15. Gastroenterology. 1996;111:1706–1713.
73. Eigler A, Sinha B, Hartmann G, Endres S. Taming TNF: strategies to restrain this pro-inflammatory cytokine. Immunol Today. 1997;18:487–491.
74. van Dulleman HM, Hommes DW, Meenan J et al. Complete remissions of steroid-refractory Crohn's disease after administration of monoclonal anti-TNF antibody cA2. Gastroenterology. 1994;106:A1054.
75. van Dulleman HJM, van Deventer SJH, Hommes DW et al. Treatment of Crohn's disease with anti-tumour necrosis factor chimeric monoclonal antibody (CA2). Gastroenterology. 1995;109: 129.
76. Orange J, Salazar-Mather TP, Opal SM et al. Mechanisms of interleukin 12-mediated toxicities during experimental viral infections: role of tumor necrosis factor and flucocorticoids. J Exp Med. 1995;181:901–914.
77. Plevey SE, Landers CJ, Prehn J et al. A role for TNF-alpha and mucosal T helper-1 cytokines in the pathogenesis of Crohn's disease. J Immunol. 1997;159:6276–6282.
78. Ware CF, VanArsdale TL, Crowe PD, Browning JL. The ligands and receptors of the lympho-toxin system. In: Griffiths GM, Tschopp J (eds) Pathways for cytolysis. Berlin-Heidelberg: Springer-Verlag, 1995:175–217.
79. Togni PD, Goellner J, Ruddle NH et al. Abnormal development of peripheral lymphoid organs in mice deficient in lymphotoxin. Science. 1994;264:703.
80. Rennert PD, Browning JL, Mebius R, Mackay F, Hochman PS. Surface lymphotoxin alpha/beta complex is required for the development of peripheral lymphoid organs. J Exp Med. 1996;184:1999–2006.
81. Koni PA, Sacca R, Lawton P, Browning JL, Ruddle NH, Flavell RA. Distinct roles in lymphoid organogenesis for lymphotoxins alpha and beta revealed in lymphotoxin beta-deficient mice. Immunity. 1996;6:491–500.
82. Mackay F, Majeau GR, Lawton P, Hochman PS, Browning JL. Lymphotoxin but not tumour necrosis factor functions to maintain splenic architecture and humoral responsiveness in adult mice. Eur J Immunol. 1997;27:2033–2042.
83. Browning JL, Miatkowski K, Sizing I et al. Signaling through the lymphotoxin beta receptor induces the death of some adenocarcinoma tumor lines. J Exp Med. 1996;183:867–878.
84. Abreu-Martin MT, Vidrich A, Lynch D, Targan SR. Divergent induction of apoptosis and IL-8 secretion in HT-29 cells in response to TNFα and ligation of Fas antigen. J Immunol. 1995;155:4147–4154.
85. James SP, Strober W. Cytotoxic lymphocytes and intestinal disease. Gastroenterology. 1986;90:235–240.
86. Ma A. Fas and the immunologically underprivileged intestine. Gastroenterology. 1997;113: 345–358.
87. Bonhagen K, Thoma S, Bland P et al. Cytotoxic reactivity of gut lamina propria CD4$^+$ $\alpha\beta$ T cells in SCID mice with colitis. Eur J Immunol. 1996;26:3074–3083.
88. Chu JL, Ramos PR, Rosendorff A et al. Massive upregulation of the Fas ligand in lpr and gld mice: implications for fas regulation and the graft versus host disease-like wasting sydrome. J Exp Med. 1995;181:393–398.
89. French LE, Tschopp J. Thyroiditis and hepatitis: Fas on the road to disease. Nature Med. 1997;3:387–388.
90. Berke G. The CTL's kiss of death. Immunol Today. 1995;81:9–12.
91. Lowin B, Hahne M, Mattmann C, Tschopp J. Cytolytic T cell cytotoxicity is mediated through perforin and Fas lytic pathways. Nature. 1994;370:650–652.
92. Williams NS, Engelhard VH. Identification of a population of CD4$^+$ CTL that utilize a perforin-rather than a Fas ligand-dependent cytotoxic mechanism. J Immunol. 1996;156:153–159.
93. Williams NS, Engelhard VH. Perforin-dependent cytotoxic activity and lymphokine secretion by CD4$^+$ T cells are regulated by CD8$^+$ T cells. J Immunol. 1997;159:2091–2099.
94. Nagata S, Goldstein P. The Fas death factor. Science. 1995;267:1449–1456.

95. Kagi D, Ledermann B, Burki K et al. Cytotoxicity mediated by T cells and natural killer cells is greatly impaired in perforin deficient mice. Nature. 1994;369:31–37.
96. Ettinger R, Wang JK, Bossu P et al. Functional distinctions between MRL-lpr and MRL-gld lymphocytes. Normal cells reverse the gld but not the lpr immunoregulatory defect. J Immunol. 1994;152:1557–1568.
97. Simpson SJ, Mizoguchi E, Allen D, Bhan AK, Terhorst C. Evidence that CD4[+], but not CD8[+] T cells are responsible for murine interleukin-2-deficient colitis. Eur J Immunol. 1995;25:2618–2625.
98. Shah SA, Simpson SJ, Brown LF et al. Development of colonic adenocarcinoma in a mouse model of ulcerative colitis. Inflammatory Bowel Diseases 1998;4:196–202.
99. Arroyo AG, Yang JT, Rayburn H, Hynes RO. Differential requirements for alpha4 integrins during fetal and adult hematopoiesis. Cell. 1996;85:997–1008.
100. Wagner N, Loehler J, Kunkel EJ et al. Critical role for beta7 integrins in formation of the gut-associated lymphoid tissue. Nature. 1996;382:366–370.
101. Briskin M, Winsor-Hines D, Shyjan A et al. Human mucosal adressin cell adhesion molecule-1 is preferentially expressed in the intestinal tract and associated lymphoid tissue. Am J Pathol. 1997;151:97–110.
102. Podolsky DK, Lobb R, King N et al. Attenuation of colitis in the cotton-top tamarin by anti-alpha 4 integrin monoclonal antibody. J Clin Invest. 1993;92:372–380.
103. Picarella D, Hurlbut P, Rottman J, Shi X, Butcher E, Ringler DJ. Monoclonal antibodies specific for beta 7 integrin and mucosal addressin cell adhesion molecule-1 (MadCAM-1) reduce inflammation in the colon of scid mice reconstituted with CD45RBhigh CD4[+] T cells. J Immunol. 1997;158:2099–2106.

12
Murine colitis induced by adoptive transfer of immunocompetent CD4$^+$ T cells into immunodeficient hosts

J. REIMANN

INTRODUCTION

Ulcerative colitis (UC) and Crohn's disease (CD) are human inflammatory bowel diseases (IBD) of unknown aetiology and pathogenesis. It is generally assumed that inappropriate regulation of mucosal immune responses to gut-derived antigens plays a role in eliciting or maintaining intestinal inflammatory reactions in these diseases. As many molecular details of mucosal immunity are currently elucidated in man and experimental animals by extensive research efforts, the available new information has the potential to reveal key events in the pathogenesis of these diseases (reviewed in Ref. 1). Experimental animal models that reproduce features of human IBD are of major interest to study the immuno-pathogenesis of IBD and to allow the design of novel therapeutic approaches. Recently, many animal models for the study of IBD have emerged, either through purposeful design of experimental protocols, or as unexpected 'byproducts' of genetically engineered mouse lines (reviewed in Refs 2–12). These models can be grouped into four classes.

- Models of 'spontaneous' heritable colitis in mice and monkeys (assumed to result from mutations in unknown genes).
- Induction of IBD by local challenge with chemical irritants (e.g. acetic acid, ethanol, trinitrobenzene sulfonic acid, dextran sulphate, indomethacin), immunostimulants (e.g. immune complexes), or bacterial antigens (e.g. peptidoglycans).
- Genetically engineered mice and rats that either express a transgene-encoded MHC-I molecule (B27), or display a gene-targeted 'knock-out' (KO) phenotype for genes encoding cytokines (IL-2, IL-10), TCR $\alpha\beta$ chains, T cell homing/adhesion receptors (N/E-cadherin) or signal transduction molecules (Giα2).
- Adoptive transfer of immunocompetent, non-fractionated or fractionated CD45RB^{hi} CD4$^+$ T cells into murine congenic/syngeneic, severely immuno-deficient hosts.

Our interest is focused on the induction of IBD in adoptive transfer models of the latter category.

THE EXPERIMENTAL SYSTEM

Immunodeficient mice homozygous for the autosomal recessive mutation severe combined immunodeficiency *scid* (SCID mice)[13] were used. Histocompatible, nonfractionated CD4$^+$ T cells were adoptively transferred into young SCID mice of different genetic backgrounds: i.e. transfer of 10^5–10^6 CD4$^+$ T cells from congenic C.B-17$^{+/+}$ or histocompatible BALB/c or BALB/c^{dm2} (dm2) mice into H-2^d C.B-17 *scid/scid* mice, or of C57BL/6 CD4$^+$ T cells into H-2^b C57BL/6 *scid/scid* mice reconstituted the hosts with gut-seeking CD49d^{hi} CD4$^+$ T cells of the memory CD44^{hi} CD45RB^{lo} CD62L^{lo} phenotype (reviewed in Refs 10, 14, 15).

The basic features of the system are outlined in Table 1. CD4$^+$ T cell repopulation of the SCID host was observed either after cell transfer[16–24], or after heterotopic transplantation of gut wall from an immunocompetent, histocompatible donor into the skin of the SCID host[25]. The SCID host animals were kept either under standard pathogen-free (SPF), or under germ-free (GF) conditions. Transplanted SPF but not GF SCID mice developed clinical and histological signs of chronic, progressive IBD in 3–6 months. Histopathology indicated that CD4$^+$ T cell-repopulated SPF SCID mice developed inflammatory changes confined to the colonic mucosa. The small intestine down to the terminal ileum was usually devoid of inflammation. The degree of colitis along the large intestine in individual animals was variable, and there was interindividual variability. Histopathologically, this murine colitis resembles human ulcerative colitis.

This experimental system allowed us to address a number of questions about the immunopathogenesis of IBD. The following themes were of particular interest to us.

● Which CD4$^+$ T cell subsets induce IBD in the course of repopulating the immunodeficient, histocompatible host?

Table 1 Adoptive transfer systems used to construct a model of murine colitis

	Immunocompetent donor	*Immunodeficient host*	
	H-2 haplotype	*Strain*	*Status*
Cell transfer	H-2^d BALB/c; BALB/c^{dm2}; C.B-17^{++}	C.B-17 *scid/scid*	SPF GF
	H-2^b C57BL/6	C57BL/6 *scid/scid*	SPF
Heterotopic transplant	H-2^d C.B-17^{++}; BALB/c	C.B-17 *scid/scid*	SPF

SPF, specific pathogen-free; GF, germ-free; scid, severe combined immunodeficiency; cell transfer, injection of purified CD4$^+$ T cells; heterotopic transplant, transplantation of gut wall from an immunocompetent donor into the skin of a histocompatible SCID host

- Why is there a preferential repopulation of gut-associated lymphoid tissues of the immunodeficient host with immunocompetent CD4+ T cells?
- What drives the polyclonal activation, *in situ* expansion, and differentiation into a T_H1 phenotype of CD4+ T lymphocytes in the colonic lamina propria of the histocompatible, immunodeficient host?
- Which CD4+ T cell-mediated immune effector mechanisms prevalent in mucosal tissues may contribute to the tissue damage characteristic of IBD?

In the following, we will discuss these issues. None of the questions has a definite answer yet. We will try to relate our findings to those obtained in other murine IBD models. Finally, we will ask which new therapeutic approaches are suggested by the available data.

CD4+ T CELL SUBSETS INDUCING IBD AFTER TRANSFER INTO SEVERELY IMMUNODEFICIENT HOSTS

Immunocompetent $CD3^+$ $CD4^+$ $CD8\alpha^-$ $TCR\alpha\beta$ T cells derived from many different sources induced IBD in our system (Table 2). This was observed irrespective of the route of cell transfer, i.e. intravenous and intraperitoneal cell injections were equally effective. CD4+ T cells prepared from primary lymphoid organs (thymus), secondary lymphoid tissues (spleen; inguinal, popliteal or mesenteric lymph nodes) or peripheral tissues (lamina propria of the small or large intestine) displayed comparable IBD-inducing potential. Following transfer into histocompatible SPF SCID mice, all tested CD4+ T cells repopulated the adoptive host and induced IBD[21,22,24] (and unpublished data). Only CD4+ T cells recovered from the gut epithelial layer of transplanted SCID mice showed a poor repopulation efficiency after transfer into a 'second generation' SCID mouse group[21]. CD4+ T cells selectively migrated out of a heterotopic gut wall

Table 2 CD4+ T cell subsets that induce IBD after adoptive transfer into a histocompatible SCID host

Tissue origin	Thymic medulla
	Spleen, lymph nodes
	Gut lamina propria
Developmental origin	Thymic
	Extrathymic
CD45RB surface phenotype	High
	Low
TCR $\alpha\beta$ repertoire	Monoclonal populations
	Oligoclonal populations
	Polyclonal populations
Activation status	Resting lymphocytes
	Activated lymphoblasts

transplant from an immunocompetent, histocompatible donor into gut-associated tissues of the immunodeficient host[25].

Gut lamina propria CD4$^+$ T cells from euthymic and athymic donor mice induced an IBD in the SCID host; manifestation of colitis was delayed for 2–4 weeks after transfer of CD3$^+$ CD4$^+$ CD8$^-$ TCR$\alpha\beta$ T cells from nude donor mice compared with the transfer of CD4$^+$ T cells from congenic, euthymic donor mice[26].

CD4$^+$ T cells expressing the CD45RB^{high} phenotype are assumed to be naïve while CD45RB^{low} (CD45RO) CD4$^+$ T cells seem to be primed. CD45RB^{hi} CD4$^+$ T cells from normal rats have the potential to induce autoimmune diseases in congenic, immunodeficient hosts[27–29]. CD45RB^{hi} CD4$^+$ T cells from healthy animals thus seem to express an autoaggressive potential that can be revealed *in vivo*. This concept has been applied to the study of murine inflammatory bowel disease (IBD): CD45RB^{hi} CD4$^+$ T cells from immunocompetent mice induced clinical and histopathological signs of colitis after transfer into a histocompatible, immunodeficient host. In this system, peripheral CD45RB^{hi} CD4$^+$ T cells from BALB/c donor mice induced colitis after adoptive transfer into C. B-17 *scid/scid* hosts, while non-fractionated CD4$^+$ T cells or CD45RB^{lo} CD44^{hi} CD4$^+$ T cells did not[9,30–38]. We could not reproduce these findings in the SPF SCID mice of our colony. CD45RB^{high} CD4$^+$ T cells as well as CD45RB^{low} CD4$^+$ T cells from spleen or lymph nodes of immunocompetent donor mice induced colitis after transfer into SCID mice although the IBD tended to run a more rapid course after transfer of the former subset (K. Bonhagen and J. Reimann, unpublished).

We transferred polyclonal, oligoclonal or monoclonal CD4$^+$ TCR$\alpha\beta$ T cell populations into SPF SCID mice. Polyclonal CD4$^+$ T cell populations were obtained from normal BALB/c, C.B-17$^{+/+}$, dm2 or C57BL/6 mice. Oligoclonal CD4$^+$ T cell populations were isolated from aged, leaky SCID donor mice that expressed a rearranged, MHC-I-restricted TCR$\alpha\beta$ receptor; these mice develop an oligoclonal CD4$^+$ T cell population composed of 8–20 individual clones that express a transgene-encoded TCRβ-chain and an endogenous ('leaky') TCRα-chain[22]. Monoclonal CD4$^+$ T cells were derived from D011.10 transgenic BALB/c mice that express a rearranged TCR$\alpha\beta$ receptor specific for the A^d/OVA323-339 epitope; the T cell system of these animals is composed of a monoclonal population of CD4$^+$ T cells. Transfer of all three types of CD4$^+$ T cell populations induced an IBD in histocompatible SPF SCID hosts.

The state of activation of the transferred CD4$^+$ T cells is relevant to their IBD-inducing potential: mitogen- or antigen-stimulated CD4$^+$ T lymphoblasts are more efficient in inducing IBD than are the respective resting CD4$^+$ T lymphocytes (K. Bonhagen and J. Reimann, unpublished). After transfer of blasts, IBD developed 3–5 weeks earlier than after transfer of an equal number of resting lymphocytes.

Taken together, these data reveal that most tested CD4$^+$ T cell subsets could induce an IBD after adoptive transfer into histocompatible SPF SCID mice. There is little evidence that a particular CD4$^+$ T cell subset is involved but the relative efficiency with which different CD4$^+$ T cell subsets induced the disease varied.

PREFERENTIAL REPOPULATION OF GUT-ASSOCIATED TISSUES OF THE IMMUNODEFICIENT HOST WITH IMMUNOCOMPETENT CD4+ T CELLS

Transferred CD4+ T cells repopulated the lamina propria and epithelial layer of the small and large intestine, the mesenteric lymph nodes, the peritoneal cavity and the spleen of the SPF-raised SCID host. Very few (or no) CD3+ T cells were detectable in other peripheral lymph nodes or in other peripheral tissues of the adoptive host. This reconstitution pattern was seen with all CD4+ T cell populations tested, irrespective of their origin. CD4+ T cells recovered from the blood, spleen, peritoneal cavity, mesenteric lymph nodes or the gut lamina propria of a transplanted SCID mouse could reconstitute a naïve SCID host and showed a similar repopulation pattern. Transfer of even high numbers of CD4+ T lymphocytes or T lymphoblasts into GF SCID mice did not lead to stable repopulation and did not induce IBD. Activation of macrophages pre- or post-transplantation (by repeated intraperitoneal injections of LPS or bacterial plasmid DNA) did not support CD4+ T cell engraftment into GF SCID mice (K. Bonhagen and J. Reimann, unpublished).

The selective reconstitution of the immunodeficient host with gut-seeking CD4+ T cells was confirmed by the surface phenotype of repopulating T cells. Almost all T cells repopulating the SCID host express the $\alpha_4\beta_7$ integrin, a homing receptor for mucosa-seeking leucocytes[24,25]. The cells exchange the α_4-chain with the α_E-chain when migrating from the gut lamina propria into the epithelial layer[21]. Murine IBD induced by CD4+ T cell transfer is suppressed by treatment with a monoclonal antibody to the β_7-integrin chain[38]. This integrin is overexpressed on peripheral blood leucocytes from patients with IBD[39]. CD4+ T cells repopulating the SCID host express high levels of the P-selectin-binding ligand PSGL-1[40] which is involved in leucocyte–endothelial cell interactions during intestinal inflammation[41]. The surface phenotype profile of CD4+ T cells repopulating the SCID host thus confirms the selective engraftment of mucosa-seeking T cells in this model. It is unclear whether the mucosa-seeking T cell subset is selectively expanded in the SCID host, or if repopulating T cells are 'imprinted' with the mucosa-seeking phenotype during repopulation. The data indicate that a microbial gut flora is an essential prerequisite for successfully repopulating the SCID host with T lymphocytes.

IN SITU ACTIVATION AND EXPANSION OF T_H1 CD4+ T LYMPHOCYTES IN THE COLONIC LAMINA PROPRIA OF THE HISTOCOMPATIBLE, IMMUNODEFICIENT HOST

Donor-derived, $\alpha\beta$ lineage CD3+ CD4+ CD8− T cells isolated from different tissues of transplanted SCID mice are mucosa-seeking memory/effector cells expressing high levels of CD44 and the CD2 and CD28 co-stimulator molecules, but low levels of CD45RB and CD62L (Table 3). Most of these T cells are CD95+ and hence susceptible to apoptosis or 'activation-induced cell death' (AICD). A large fraction of these cells shows evidence of *in vivo* activation, i.e. are CD25+ and CD69+[18,22–25]. Most CD25+/CD69+ CD4+ T cells are found in the

Table 3   Surface phenotype of CD4$^+$ T cells repopulating the adoptive SCID host

Marker	Indicates
L^{d-}	Donor (dm2)-derived[a]
CD3^{hi} CD4^{hi} CD8$^-$	Mature peripheral T cell
TCR$\alpha\beta^+$	$\alpha\beta$ lineage
CD62L(LECAM-1)^{lo} CD45RB^{lo}	Not naive
CD44^{hi} CD2^{hi} CD28^{hi}	Memory T cells
CD49d^{hi} (α_4-chain of $\alpha_4\beta_7$ integrin)	Mucosa-seeking
CD103^{hi} (α_{IEL}-chain of $\alpha_{IEL}\beta_7$ integrin)	Stimulated by TGFβ, homing to epithelial layer
CD25^{hi} CD69^{hi}	*In situ* activated
CD95^{hi}	Receptive to apoptotic signal
CD95L$^{hi\ b}$	Triggers apoptotic death of recognized cell

[a] in the dm2→SCID system; [b] by about 30% of colonic lamina propria CD4$^+$ T cells

colonic lamina propria of transplanted SCID mice, and the fraction of *in situ* activated CD4$^+$ T cells increases strikingly with the progression of the disease. The gut lamina propria seems to be the major (and possibly exclusive) site of CD4$^+$ T cell proliferation[24]. *In vitro*, these lamina proria CD4$^+$ T cells require both IL-2 and IL-7 to support their proliferation[24].

When polyclonal populations of CD4$^+$ T cells are transferred into SPF SCID mice, the TCR$\alpha\beta$ repertoire of repopulating T cell populations remains polyclonal[24], i.e., there is no evidence for preferential expansion of an oligoclonal population in the immunodeficient, histocompatible host. Even when CD4$^+$ T cell populations are repeatedly 'passaged' through SCID mice, and only 10^5 cells are transferred to initiate each new passage, T cell expansion during the 3–5 month period in the SCID host is extensive but apparently does not introduce a reproducible bias into the TCR β-chain repertoire. Furthermore, we have not been able to select *in vivo* by repeated passage through different SCID hosts a CD4$^+$ T cell line with an enhanced IBD-inducing phenotype and a restricted TCR β-chain repertoire. Oligoclonal and monoclonal CD4$^+$ T cell lines are as efficient as polyclonal CD4$^+$ T cell lines in repopulating the SCID host and in inducing IBD[22] (and data not shown). It is surprising that monoclonal CD4$^+$ T cell lines can repopulate the SCID host in the absence of the relevant antigen; we have observed this with OVA-specific CD4$^+$ T cell lines cloned *in vitro*[19], and with monoclonal CD4$^+$ T cells from D011.10 transgenic mice (K. Bonhagen and J. Reimann, unpublished). These data suggest that a TCR-independent (mitogen-like) stimulus drives T cell activation and expansion in the colonic lamina propria of transplanted SCID mice although stimulation by 'cross-reactive' antigens or expression of additional TCR specificities by 'monoclonal' CD4$^+$ T cell populations from transgenic mice (resulting from co-expression of rearranged endogenous TCRα-chains) cannot be formally excluded. The stimulus that drives T cell expansion in the adoptive host is (directly or indirectly) dependent on the microbial flora of the gut because repopulation of GF SCID mice with mono- or polyclonal CD4$^+$ T cell populations was repeatedly unsuccessful (J. Reimann, unpublished).

A T$_H$1 cytokine expression profile is inducible in CD4$^+$ T cells repopulating the adoptive SCID host[20,23,40]. CD4$^+$ T cells freshly isolated from different tissues of the SCID host release only low levels of IFNγ and TNFα during a 12–24 h incubation period. In contrast, following a 5 h stimulation of these T cells with phorbol ester/ionomycin *in vitro*, these CD4+ T cells release abundant amounts of these two cytokines (but no IL-4) detectable by ELISA (at the population level) and in intracellular staining and FCM analyses (at the single cell level). These analyses revealed that > 60% of the CD4+ T cells produce large amounts of IFNγ and TNFα but very few (or no) IL-4-producing T cells are detectable. ELISA showed that inducible IL-12 levels in a mononuclear cell population from repopulated tissues of the adoptive SCID host were high, but IL-10 levels were low or undetectable. Hence, the cytokine profile detectable in diseased, transplanted SCID mice displayed the characteristics of a T_H1 phenotype. This observation is in line with findings in many other murine IBD models[36,42–50]. Unexpected was the observation that CD4+ T cells recovered from diseased tissue (colonic lamina propria) as well as from non-diseased tissues (mesenteric lymph nodes, spleen, peritoneal cavity) of transplanted SCID mice expressed equally high levels of inducible T_H1-type cytokines. Hence, the complete CD4+ T cell population in the reconstituted SCID host and not only CD4+ T cells residing in the inflamed colonic tissues has the potential to produce abundant amounts of proinflammatory cytokines. The *in situ* levels of cytokines released from CD4+ T cells and antigen-presenting cells (APC) in inflamed and non-inflamed tissues of the transplanted SCID mice *in vivo* are unknown. This question will have to be approached by immunohistological studies. When the cytokine expression profile of cells in the murine IBD is compared to that reported for lamina propria cells from UC or CD patients, the cytokine expression profile is similar to CD but not UC (Table 4). This is puzzling because the localization and histopathology of the murine IBD resembles human UC.

The critical question of which immunoregulatory mechanism drives CD4+ T cell differentiation into the T_H1 phenotype remains unresolved. Conceivably, the mode of antigen/mitogen-induced cell activation has a decisive effect on the functional differentiation of CD4+ T cell populations. Alternatively, a critical regulatory cell type that prevents T_H1 differentiation or promotes T_H2 differentiation may be deficient in this system. Different APC, i.e. CD11b+ macrophages and CD11c+ dendritic cells (DC), accumulate in the colonic lamina propria during the development of IBD. These have not been functionally characterized up to now. These APC may bias the T cell response towards a T_H1 pathway of

Table 4 Cytokine expression by lamina propria cells in human and murine IBD

Cytokine	Human IBD		Murine IBD
	CD	*UC*	
IL-12	↑↑	N	↑↑
IFNγ	↑↑	N (↑)	↑↑
TNFα	↑↑↑	↑	↑↑↑
IL-4	↓↓	↓↓	↓↓
IL-10	↓↓	(↓)	↓↓

N, normal; UC, ulcerative colitis; CD, Crohn's disease;
murine IBD: adoptive CD4+ T cell system in SCID mice.

differentiation. Alternatively, evidence has emerged for the presence of IL-10-producing immunoregulatory CD4[+] T cells (Tr1) that prevent T_H1 differentiation and may be an important physiological control for preferential T_H2 type differentiation in mucosal immune responses[51,52]. An effect of such regulatory cells on the differentiation-inducing phenotype of APC is likely; hence, these potential regulatory effects on CD4[+] T cell differentiation may not be alternative pathways but sequential events in a common pathway. Further experimental data are needed to clarify this issue.

CD4[+] T CELL-MEDIATED PATHOGENESIS OF IBD

CD4[+] T cell-mediated immune effector mechanisms in mucosal tissues apparently contribute to the tissue damage characteristic of IBD. Although a number of different candidate mechanisms have been proposed, formal evidence for the decisive role of any one of these mechanisms is not available in animal models or in human IBD.

T_H1 CD4[+] T cells isolated from the colonic lamina propria of transplanted SCID mice are cytolytic[23,26,53,54]. The TCR-mediated cytolytic effect operates through the CD95(Fas)/CD95L(FasL) pathway. CD95-expressing targets of this cytolytic attack relevant in the pathogenesis of IBD are intestinal epithelial cells (IEC), APC and the CD4[+] T cells themselves. A central role of epithelial damage in the pathogenesis of IBD as a result of the immune attack by T cells has been postulated[55–60]. IFNγ-up-regulated MHC-II expression by IEC and the extensive migration of CD4[+] T cells into the colonic epithelium would support this hypothesis. Some types of APC express CD95 and are susceptible to attack by CD4[+] T cells that recognize the antigen presented by these cells[61]. This may effect a selection of APC that bias the response towards the T_H1 direction. In different assay systems, we detected massive AICD in 50–70% of the colonic lamina propria CD4[+] T cells from transplanted SCID mice *in situ,* in gut-derived CD4[+] T cells explanted *in vitro,* and in gut-derived CD4[+] T cell populations after TCR-dependent stimulation. AICD is a well established homeostatic control mechanism of T cell responses[62,63]. It is possible that a relative inefficiency of this process in the colonic lamina propria allows the accumulation of numbers of functional CD4[+] T cells in this tissue that are deleterious. Drugs that facilitate the ongoing apoptotic response of T cells may, therefore, be of benefit.

Cytotoxic damage caused by IEC or APC is certainly not the only tissue-damaging mechanism in IBD that should be considered. Proinflammatory mediators may directly or indirectly introduce lesions into the stroma, the integrity of the mucosal barrier or the tissue matrix. These questions are at the status nascendi of being approached experimentally, and animal models may be of help to solve some of these questions.

DESIGN OF NOVEL THERAPEUTIC APPROACHES FOR IBD

If a T cell response underlies the pathogenesis of IBD, options to treat the disease could include the following approaches (Table 5):

Table 5 Therapeutic approaches to experimental IBD

Target	Approach	Procedure
Eliminate stimulus of the response	??	
Suppress or attenuate stimulated response	Block T cell homing into the gut	Anti-β_7 integrin antibody antagonize endothelial selectins
	Block T cell activation	Cyclosporine A, sulphasalazine, NF-κB anti-sense
	Suppress development of T_H1 phenotype	Neutralizing antibodies to IL-12, IFNγ, TNFα; cytokine receptor antagonists inhibit cytokine-triggered signalling, block cytokine gene transcription
	Prevent release of proinflammatory cytokines	Caspase inhibitors
Promote early termination of the response	Facilitate AICD	
Change polarization of the response	Cytokine therapy (IL-10, TGFβ)	

- elimination of the stimulus that drives the response;
- suppression or attenuation of the response;
- promotion of the early termination of the response;
- changing the polarization of the response (i.e., converting a pathogenic into a non-pathogenic response).

The stimulus that drives the T cell response in IBD is unknown in all experimental systems characterized so far. Substantial evidence indicates that the bacterial flora of the gut plays a major role in stimulating the response[64]. Murine IBD (elicited by adoptive CD4+ T cell transfer) has been interpreted as an immunity-mediated condition triggered by infection with *Helicobacter hepaticus*[65]. The growing number of newly identified *Helicobacter* species raises the possibility that bacteria of this genus play a role in the disease. Identifying a bacterial species that can induce colitis would certainly represent a major breakthrough in the field, and would allow the most specific and rational therapeutic approach.

Because the immune response can usually not be prevented, suppression or attenuation of the ongoing response seems the appropriate choice. T cell homing into the gut could be blocked by treatment with anti-$\beta7$ integrin antibody[38] or inhibitors to endothelial selectins. The T cell response activated in the gut lamina propria could be suppressed by cyclosporine[66–68], sulphasalazine or NF-κB antisense oligonucleotide treatment[69]. The differentiation of T_H1 effector CD4+ T cells could be inhibited by treatment with neutralizing antibodies to IL-12, IFNγ or TNFα[43,44,49,69–72], by cytokine receptor antagonists, or by drugs that inhibit cytokine signalling or cytokine gene transcription. Thalidomide is an interesting candidate mediating the latter effect[73]. Release of the proinflammatory cytokines IL-1 and IL-18 could be inhibited by caspase inhibitors.

The deleterious effects of an ongoing T cell response could possibly be limited by facilitating apoptosis (activation-induced cell death) that can be considered a negative regulator of T cell activation. An established polarization of a CD4[+] T cell response towards the T_H1 phenotype can be changed into a T_H2 response by administration of IL-10 or TGFβ[36,44,50,52,74]. Animal models will be helpful to screen for new ways to treat IBD.

CONCLUSION

Many new animal models for the study of the immunopathogenesis of IBD have emerged durung the last years. It is uncertain how faithfully these systems reproduce the forms of IBD prevalent in patients. Despite the diversity of the experimental approaches used to construct these models, almost all murine and rat systems point to immunocompetent, mucosal T_H1 CD4[+] T cells as central agents in the disease process. The origin of these CD4[+] T cells, their activation and differentiation in the gut mucosa and the molecular details of the IBD-inducing phenotype are under intense study by many groups. It is hoped that this will yield new successful therapeutic approaches for these diseases.

ACKNOWLEDGEMENTS

The contributions of Kerstin Bonhagen, Dr Stefan Thoma and Stefan Rütten are greatly appreciated. The study was supported by grants from the Deutsche Forschungsgemeinschaft (SFB322/B12), the Fritz-Thyssen-Stiftung and the EC Biomed 2 contract PL 950612 to J.R.

References

1. Kagnoff MF, Kiyono H (eds) Mucosal Immunology. San Diego: Academic Press, 1997.
2. Podolsky DK. Inflammatory bowel disease. N Engl J Med. 1991;325:928–937.
3. Grisham M. Animal models of inflammatory bowel disease. Curr Opin Gastroenterol. 1993;9:524–533.
4. MacDonald TT. Aetiology of Crohn's disease. Arch Dis Child. 1993;68:623–625.
5. Strober W, Ehrhardt RO. Chronic intestinal inflammation: an unexpected outcome in cytokine or T cell receptor mutant mice. Cell. 1993;75:203–205.
6. Conner EM, Aiko S, Grisham M. Genetically engineered models of inflammatory bowel disease. Curr Opin Gastroenterol. 1994;10:358–364.
7. Herfarth HH, Sartor RB. Cytokine regulation of experimental intestinal inflammation. Curr Opin Gastroenterol. 1994;10:625–632.
8. Sartor RB. Cytokines in intestinal inflammation: pathophysiological and clinical considerations. Gastroenterology. 1994;106:533–539.
9. Powrie F. T cells in inflammatory bowel disease: protective and pathogenic roles. Immunity. 1995;3:171–174.
10. Reimann J, Rudolphi A, Claesson MH. Novel experimental approaches in the study of the immunopathology in inflammatory bowel disease. J Mol Med. 1995;73:133–140.
11. Neurath MF, Meyer zum Büschenfelde KH. Protective and pathogenic roles of cytokines in inflammatory bowel diseases. J Investig Med. 1996;44:516–521.
12. Bhan AK, Mizoguchi E, Mizoguchi A. New models of chronic intestinal inflammation. Curr Opin Gastroenterol. 1994;10:633–638.
13. Bosma MJ, Carroll AM. The SCID mouse mutant: definition, characterization, and potential uses. Annu Rev Immunol. 1991;9:323–350.

14. Reimann J, Rudolphi A, Claesson MH. Selective reconstitution of T lymphocyte subsets in scid mice. Immunol Rev. 1991;124:75–95.

15. Reimann J, Rudolphi A, Claesson MH. Reconstitution of SCID mice with low numbers of CD4+ TCR$\alpha\beta$+ T cells. Res Immunol. 1994;145:332–336.

16. Rudolphi A, Spiess S, Conradt P, Claesson MH, Reimann J. CD3+ T-cells in scid mice. I. Transferred purified CD4+, but not CD8+ T-cells are engrafted in the spleen of congenic scid mice. Eur J Immunol. 1991;21:523–533.

17. Rudolphi A, Claesson MH, Reimann J. CD3+ T cells in severe combined immunodeficiency (scid) mice. VI. Intravenous injection of CD4+ CD8- T cells from spleen, lymph node or thymus of adult dm2 donor mice into young scid mice rescues host-derived, IgM-producing B cells. Immunology. 1992;77:157–164.

18. Reimann J, Rudolphi A, Tscherning T, Claesson MH. Selective engraftment of memory CD4+ T cells with an unusual recirculation pattern and a diverse T cell receptor-Vb repertoire into scid mice. Eur J Immunol. 1993;23:350–356.

19. Rudolphi A, Reimann J. Transplantation of CD4+ T cell clones into SCID mice. J Immunol Methods. 1993;158:27–36.

20. Rudolphi A, Enssle K-H, Claesson MH, Reimann J. Adoptive transfer of low numbers of CD4+ T cells into SCID mice chronically treated with soluble IL-4 receptor does not prevent engraftment of IL-4-producing T cells. Scand J Immunol. 1993;38:57–64.

21. Reimann J, Rudolphi A. Coexpression of CD8α in peripheral CD4+ TCR$\alpha\beta$+ T cells migrating into the murine small intestine epithelial layer. Eur J Immunol. 1995;25:1580–1588.

22. Reimann J, Rudolphi A, Spiess S, Claesson MH. A gut-homing, oligoclonal CD4+ T cell population in severe-combined immunodeficient mice expressing a rearranged, transgenic class I-restricted $\alpha\beta$ T cell receptor. Eur J Immunol. 1995;25:1643–1653.

23. Bonhagen K, Thoma S, Bland PW et al. Cytotoxic reactivity of gut lamina propria CD4+ $\alpha\beta$ T cells in SCID mice with colitis. Eur J Immunol. 1996;26:3074–3083.

24. Rudolphi A, Bonhagen K, Reimann J. Polyclonal expansion of adoptively transferred CD4+ $\alpha\beta$ T cells in the colonic lamina propria of scid mice with colitis. Eur J Immunol. 1996;26: 1156–1163.

25. Rudolphi A, Boll G, Poulsen SS, Claesson MH, Reimann J. Gut-homing CD4+ TCR$\alpha\beta$+ T cells in the pathogenesis of murine inflammatory bowel disease. Eur J Immunol. 1994;24: 2803–2812.

26. Bonhagen K, Thoma S, Leithäuser F, Möller P, Reimann J. A pancolitis resembling human ulcerative colitis is induced by oligoclonal, extrathymic CD4+ TCR$\alpha\beta$ T cells in histocompatible SCID mice.Clin Exp Immunol. 1998;112:443–452.

27. Powrie F, Mason DW. OX22high CD4+ T cells induce wasting disease with multiple organ pathology: prevention by the OX22low subset. J Exp Med. 1990;172:1701–1712.

28. Fowell D, McKnight AJ, Powrie F, Dyke R, Mason DW. Subsets of CD4+ T cells and their roles in the induction and prevention of autoimmunity. Immunol Rev. 1991;123:37–63.

29. Fowell D, Mason DW. Evidence that the T cell repertoire of normal rats contains cells with the potential to cause diabetes. Characterization of the CD4+ T cell subset that inhibits this autoimmune potential. J Exp Med. 1993;177:627–636.

30. Morrissey PJ, Charrier K, Braddy S, Liggitt D, Watson JD. CD4+ T cells that express high levels of CD45RB induce wasting disease when transferred into congenic severe combined immuno-deficient mice. Disease development is prevented by cotransfer of purified CD4+ T cells. J Exp Med. 1993;178:237–244.

31. Powrie F, Leach MW, Mauze S, Caddle LB, Coffman RL. Phenotypically distinct subsets of CD4+ T cells induce or protect from chronic intestinal inflammation in C. B-17 scid mice. Int Immunol. 1993;5:1461–1471.

32. Morrissey PJ, Charrier K. Induction of wasting disease in SCID mice by the transfer of normal CD4+/CD45RBhi T cells and the regulation of this autoreactivity by CD4+/CD45RBlo T cells. Res Immunol. 1994;145:357–362.

33. Powrie F, Correa Oliveira R, Mauze S, Coffman RL. Regulatory interactions between CD45RBhigh and CD45RBlow CD4+ T cells are important for the balance between protective and pathogenic cell-mediated immunity. J Exp Med. 1994;179:589–600.

34. Powrie F, Leach MW, Mauze S, Menon S, Barcomb-Caddle L, Coffman RL. Inhibition of Th1 responses prevents inflammatory bowel disease in scid mice reconstituted with CD45RBhi T cells. Immunity. 1994;1:553–562.

35. Leach MW, Bean AG, Mauze S, Coffman RL, Powrie F. Inflammatory bowel disease in C.B-17 scid mice reconstituted with the CD45RB^{high} subset of CD4$^+$ T cells. Am J Pathol. 1996;148: 1503–1515.
36. Powrie F, Carlino J, Leach MW, Mauze S, Coffman RL. A critical role for transforming growth factor-β but not interleukin 4 in the suppression of T helper type 1-mediated colitis by CD45RB^{low} CD4$^+$ T cells. J Exp Med. 1996;183:2669–2674.
37. Aranda R, Sydora BC, McAllister PL et al. Analysis of intestinal lymphocytes in mouse colitis mediated by transfer of CD4$^+$ CD45RB^{hi} T cells to SCID recipients. J Immunol. 1997;158:3464–3473.
38. Picarella D, Hurlbut P, Rottman J, Shi X, Butcher E, Ringler DJ. Monoclonal antibodies specific for β7 integrin and mucosal addressin cell adhesion molecule-1 (MAdCAM-1) reduce inflammation in the colon of scid mice reconstituted with CD45RB^{hi} CD4$^+$ T cells. J Immunol. 1997;158:2099–2106.
39. Meenan J, Spaans J, Grool TA, Pals ST, Tytgat GNJ, van Deventer SJH. Altered expression of a4b7, a gut-homing integrin, by circulating and mucosal T cells in colonic mucosal inflammation. Gut. 1997;40:241–246.
40. Thoma S, Bonhagen K, Vestweber D, Hamann A, Reimann J. Expression of the P-selectin-binding epitope and cytokines by CD4$^+$ T cells repopulating SCID mice with colitis. Eur J Immunol. 1998;28:1785–1797.
41. Arndt H, Palitzsch KD, Anderson DC, Rusche J, Grisham MB, Granger DN. Leucocyte-endothelial cell adhesion in a model of intestinal inflammation. Gut. 1995;37:374–379.
42. Simpson SJ, Hollander GA, Mizoguchi E et al. Expression of pro-inflammatory cytokines by TCR $\alpha\beta^+$ and TCR $\gamma\delta^+$ T cells in an experimental model of colitis. Eur J Immunol. 1997;27: 17–25.
43. Neurath MF, Fuss I, Kelsall BL, Meyer zum Büschenfelde KH, Strober W. Effect of IL-12 and antibodies to IL-12 on established granulomatous colitis in mice. Ann NY Acad Sci. 1996;795:368–370.
44. Strober W, Kelsall BL, Fuss I et al. Reciprocal IFN-γ and TGF-β responses regulate the occurrence of mucosal inflammation. Immunol Today. 1997;18:61–64.
45. Berg DJ, Davidson N, Kuhn R et al. Enterocolitis and colon cancer in interleukin-10-deficient mice are associated with aberrant cytokine production and CD4$^+$ TH1-like responses. J Clin Invest. 1996;98:1010–1020.
46. Ludviksson BR, Gray B, Strober W, Ehrhardt RO. Dysregulated intrathymic development in the IL-2-deficient mouse leads to colitis-inducing thymocytes. J Immunol. 1997;158:104–111.
47. Ehrhardt RO, Ludviksson BR, Gray B, Neurath MF, Strober W. Induction and prevention of colonic inflammation in IL-2-deficient mice. J Immunol. 1997;58:566–573.
48. Hörnqvist E, Lu X, Rogers-Fani PM et al. Gαi2-deficient mice with colitis exhibit a local increase in memory CD4$^+$ T cells and proinflammatory Th1-type cytokines. J Immunol. 1997;158:1068–1077.
49. Stuber E, Strober W, Neurath MF. Blocking the CD40L-CD40 interaction *in vivo* specifically prevents the priming of T helper 1 cells through the inhibition of interleukin 12 secretion. J Exp Med. 1996;183:693–698.
50. Neurath MF, Fuss I, Kelsall BL, Presky DH, Waegell W, Strober W. Experimental granulomatous colitis in mice is abrogated by induction of TGF-β-mediated oral tolerance. J Exp Med. 1996;183:2605–2616.
51. Hagenbaugh A, Sharma S, Dubinett SM et al. Altered immune responses in interleukin 10 transgenic mice. J Exp Med. 1997;185:2101–2110.
52. Groux H, O'Garra A, Bigler M et al. A CD4$^+$ T-cell subset inhibits antigen-specific T-cell responses and prevents colitis. Nature. 1997;389:737–742.
53. De Maria R, Boirivant M, Cifone MG et al. Functional expression of Fas and Fas ligand on human gut lamina propria T lymphocytes. A potential role for the acidic sphingomyelinase pathway in normal immunoregulation. J Clin Invest. 1996;97:316–322.
54. Boirivant M, Pica R, DeMaria R, Testi R, Pallone F, Strober W. Stimulated human lamina propria T cells manifest enhanced Fas-mediated apoptosis. J Clin Invest. 1996;98: 2616–2622.
55. Möller P, Koretz K, Leithäuser F et al. Expression of APO-1 (CD95), a member of the NGF/TNF receptor superfamily, in normal and neoplastic colon epithelium. Int J Cancer 1994;57:371–377.
56. Iwamoto M, Koji T, Makiyama K, Kobayashi N, Nakane PK. Apoptosis of crypt epithelial cells in ulcerative colitis. J Pathol. 1996;180:152–159.

57. Sträter J, Walczak H, Wellisch I et al. Normal colon epithelium is highly sensitive to CD95-induced apoptosis. Indication for a role of cell death-induced CD95/CL95L systems under inflammatory conditions? Verh Dtsch Ges Pathol. 1996;80:217–267.

58. Sträter J, Wedding U, Barth TF, Koretz K, Elsing C, Möller P. Rapid onset of apoptosis *in vitro* follows disruption of β1-integrin/matrix interactions in human colonic crypt cells. Gastroenterology. 1996;110:1776–1784.

59. Sträter J, Wellisch I, Riedl S et al. CD95 (APO-1/Fas)-mediated apoptosis in colon epithelial cells: a possible role in ulcerative colitis. Gastroenterology. 1997;113:160–167.

60. Sakai T, Kimura Y, Inagaki OK, Kusugami K, Lynch DH, Yoshikai Y. Fas-mediated cytotoxicity by intestinal intraepithelial lymphocytes during acute graft-versus-host disease in mice. Gastroenterology. 1997;113:168–174.

61. Ashany D, Song X, Lacy E, Nikolic Zugic J, Friedman SM, Elkon KB. Th1 CD4+ lymphocytes delete activated macrophages through the Fas/APO-1 antigen pathway. Proc Natl Acad Sci USA. 1995;92:11225–11229.

62. Zhang X, Brunner T, Carter L et al. Unequal death in T helper cell (Th)1 and Th2 effectors: Th1, but not Th2, effectors undergo rapid Fas/FasL-mediated apoptosis. J Exp Med. 1997;85:1837–1849.

63. Golstein P. Fas-based T cell-mediated cytotoxicity. Curr Top Microbiol Immunol. 1995;198:25–37.

64. Sartor RB. The role of endogenous luminal bacteria and bacterial products in the pathogenesis of experimental enterocolitis and systemic inflammation. In: Kagnoff MF, Kiyono H (eds) Mucosal Immunology. San Diego: Academic Press, 1997;307–320.

65. Cahill RJ, Foltz CJ, Fox JG, Dangler CA, Powrie F, Schauer DB. Inflammatory bowel disease: an immunity-mediated condition triggered by bacterial infection with *Helicobacter hepaticus*. Infect Immun. 1997;65:3126–3131.

66. Murthy SN, Cooper HS, Shim H, Shah RS, Ibrahim SA, Sedergran DJ. Treatment of dextran sulfate sodium-induced murine colitis by intracolonic cyclosporin. Dig Dis Sci. 1993;38:1722–1734.

67. Sartor RB. Cyclosporine therapy for inflammatory bowel disease. N Engl J Med. 1994;330:1897–1898.

68. Breese EJ, Michie CA, Nicholls SW et al. The effect of treatment on lymphokine-secreting cells in the intestinal mucosa of children with Crohn's disease. Aliment Pharmacol Ther. 1995;9:547–552.

69. Neurath MF, Pettersson S, Meyer zum Büschenfelde KH, Strober W. Local administration of antisense phosphorothioate oligonucleotides to the p65 subunit of NF-κB abrogates established experimental colitis in mice. Nature Med. 1996;2:998–1004.

70. Neurath MF, Fuss I, Pasparakis M et al. Predominant pathogenic role of tumor necrosis factor in experimental colitis in mice. Eur J Immunol. 1997;27.1743 1750.

71. Duchmann R, Schmitt E, Knolle P, Meyer zum Büschenfelde KH, Neurath M. Tolerance towards resident intestinal flora in mice is abrogated in experimental colitis and restored by treatment with interleukin-10 or antibodies to interleukin-12. Eur J Immunol. 1996;26:934–938.

72. Neurath MF, Fuss I, Kelsall BL, Stuber E, Strober W. Antibodies to interleukin 12 abrogate established experimental colitis in mice. J Exp Med. 1995;182:1281–1290.

73. Wettstein AR, Meagher AP. Thalidomide in Crohn's disease. Lancet 1997;350:1445–1446.

74. Powrie F, Menon S, Coffman RL. Interleukin-4 and interleukin-10 synergize to inhibit cell- mediated immunity *in vivo*. Eur J Immunol. 1993;23:3043–3049.

13
Biochemical characterization of CD4[+], $\alpha^-\beta^+$ T cells in TCR-α mutant mice with inflammatory bowel disease

I. TAKAHASHI, H. IIJIMA, D. KISHI, S. HAMADA, R. KATASHIMA, M. ITAKURA and H. KIYONO

A number of murine models of inflammatory bowel disease (IBD have been developed in the last 5 years[1,2]. These IBD mice exhibited the common feature of disrupting a T cell-dependent regulatory system which includes the alterations in T cell subpopulations and T cell selection[3–15] as well as those with targeted disruption of cytokine genes[16–19] and cytokine receptor genes[20–22]. Results obtained from these experimental IBD models indicate that either destruction of homeostasis in regulatory T cells or emergence of forbidden T cells plays a crucial role in the development of intestinal immune disorders. It has also been shown that ubiquitous non-pathogenic microorganisms in the gut flora worsen IBD, while symptoms are much milder and slower in progress, or even completely absent, in germ-free mice[13,17].

Accumulated results from a number of these different experimental models of IBD indicated that a subpopulation of CD4[+] T cells and their cytokines play a critical role for the induction of IBD. For example, either T-helper type 1 (T_H1) or T_H2 subset supports the development of IBD. T_H2 cells and their cytokines, particularly interleukin-4 (IL-4), have been suggested to enhance the development of IBD[6,10,11,22]. IL-2 gene disrupted mice that harbour abnormal B cell responses, including production of autoantibodies and antibodies directed against gut constituents, developed IBD[17]. On the other hand, the CD4[+]/CD45RB[high] T cell-transfer model of colitis in SCID mice resembles a dysregulated T_H1 response[3,14,23].

TCR-$\alpha^{-/-}$ mice develop inflammatory bowel disease characterized by diarrhoea and wasting syndrome by 3–4 months of age[4,6,10,13]. Necropsy of the diseased mice revealed bowel inflammation, while histological examination of the colon showed hyperplasia and distortion of epithelial crypts with infiltration of inflammatory lymphocytes within the lamina propria of the colon[4,6,10]. A

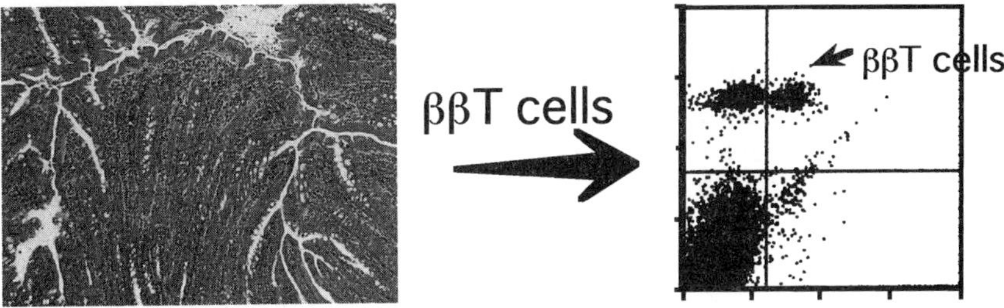

- Clonal accumulation

- Helper function (IgE responses to food/self-Ag)

- Production of Th 2 -type cytokine

Figure 1 General characteristics of infiltrated CD4+,$\alpha^-\beta^+$ T cells for the development of inflammatory bowel disease (IBD) in TCR α-chain deficient mice. Increase in T_H2-biased CD4+, $\alpha^-\beta^+$ T cells was associated with the IBD

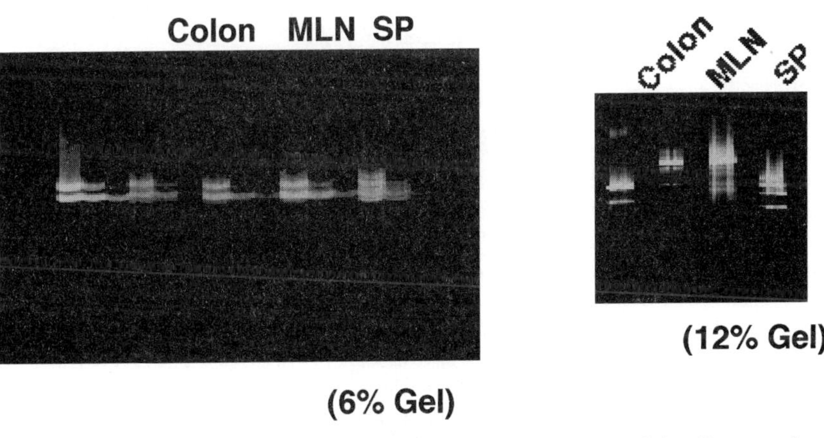

Figure 2 PCR-single strand conformation polymorphism (SSCP) analysis of clonally accumulated TCR Vβ 8-subsets of CD4+, $\alpha^-\beta^+$ T cells. PCR-amplified TCR Vβ 8-transcripts of CD4+, $\alpha^-\beta^+$ T cells isolated from the colon gave clonal mobility on the SSCP slab gel. On the other hand, those isolated from spleen gave multiple band pattern. SSCP slab gel containing 12% acrylamide shows the difference of clonality more clearly

unique subset of T cells expressing CD4 and TCR β-chain without the TCR α-chain is increased in TCR-$\alpha^{-/-}$ mice with IBD[5,6,8,10] (Figure 1). TCR-$\alpha^{-/-}$ mice showing signs of IBD developed massive enlargement of peripheral lymphoid tissues associated with polyclonal B cell activation[5,6,10,12]. There was also a prominent increase in the levels of faecal and serum antibodies, especially IgA followed by IgG, in the diseased mice[6,10]. Infiltration of CD4[+] TCR-$\alpha^-\beta^+$ T cells in Peyer's patches, lamina propria of the intestine and mesenteric lymph nodes was also associated with the hyperplasia of epithelial crypts[6,10]. Purified CD4[+] TCR-$\alpha^-\beta^+$ T cells from the lamina propria of the intestine of IBD mice were found to produce prominently IL-4 and were massively proliferated upon stimulation with staphylococcal enterotoxin B and luminal bacterial antigens[10]. Addition of the CD4[+] TCR-$\alpha^-\beta^+$ T cells to Peyer's patch B cell cultures markedly enhanced IgA, IgG, and IgM antibody responses of the B cells[10]. Furthermore, IgE antibodies were elevated in sera of the diseased mice, which reacted with milk casein and myelin basic protein[10]. These findings suggest dysregulation of systemic and oral tolerance in TCR-$\alpha^{-/-}$ mice with IBD[4,6,10]. In addition, depletion of the CD4[+], TCR-$\alpha^-\beta^+$ cells by the treatment of TCR-$\alpha^{-/-}$ mice with mAb against TCR β (clone # H57-597) suppressed the onset of IBD[10]. Thus, the CD4[+] TCR-$\alpha^-\beta^+$ T cells from the TCR-$\alpha^{-/-}$ mice mediate development of IBD and production of antibodies specific for self and food antigens.

In order to investigate whether recognition of gut antigens by a subset of monoclonal CD4[+] T cells leading to the intestinal inflammation, the clonotype of the T cell subset was assessed by PCR-single strand conformation polymorphism (SSCP) analysis[24]. The PCR-SSCP analysis used in this study has been shown to be so sensitive that a corresponding band can be detected when a T cell clone exists at a frequency of < 1 in 1000[25]. Therefore, this method has been effectively used to compare accumulating T cell clones among individual animals and different organs of an animal[25–27].

SSCP analyses of PCR-amplified TCR Vβ chain transcripts indicated that the TCR Vβ repertoire in CD4[+], TCR $\alpha^-\beta^+$ cells in the diseased mice was relatively monoclonal to oligoclonal (invariant): TCR Vβ 8 was most frequently used followed by TCR Vβ 6 and TCR Vβ 14, and clonality of the respective TCR Vβ in the diseased colon exhibited nearly identical mobility among the individual IBD mice (Figure 2)[28]. However, the clonality of the cDNA products of TCR Vβ in peripheral lymphoid tissues such as spleen and mesenteric lymph nodes was more divergent than that of the colon.

To verify that these common bands with identical mobility on the SSCP gels represent the same TCR Vβ chain sequences, PCR products corresponding to CDR3 regions of TCR Vβ8 of several diseased mice were extracted from the SSCP slab gels, and were cloned into a TA cloning vector. DNA sequences of 15 independent clones were determined for each band extracted[28]. Most of segments encoding the CDR3 of TCR Vβ8 used TCR Vβ 8.2, Dβ2, and Jβ2.4 structural genes.

Random addition and subtraction of nucleotides at the sites of recombination (i.e. VDJ junction) were also observed. The VDJ junctional sequence, which mostly appeared at a frequency of 75%, was identical among the PCR products from the respective mice, confirming that cDNA products with the identical mobility in the diseased mice were derived from the same T cell clones[28]. These results strongly suggest that the T_H2-biased CD4[+], TCR $\alpha^-\beta^+$ cells might be clonally expanded upon the stimulation with gut antigens. Thus, an oligoclonal population of the aberrant CD4[+], TCR $\alpha^-\beta^+$ cells is positively selected and prominently proliferated upon stimulation with gut-derived antigens in the intestinal inflammatory lesion.

References

1. Powrie F. T cells in inflammatory bowel disease: protective and pathogenic roles. Immunity. 1995;3:171–174.
2. Strober W, Ehrhardt RO. Chronic intestinal inflammation: an expected outcome in cytokine or T cell receptor mutant mice. Cell. 1993;75:203–205.
3. Powrie F, Leach MW, Mauze S, Caddle LB, Coffman RL. Phenotypically distinct subsets of CD4+ T cells induce or protect from chronic intestinal inflammation in C. B-17 scid mice. Int Immunol. 1993;5:1461–1471.
4. Mombaerts P, Mizoguchi E, Grusby MJ, Glimcher LH, Bhan AK, Tonegawa S. Spontaneous development of inflammatory bowel disease in T cell receptor mutant mice. Cell. 1993;75:275–282.
5. Mombaerts P, Mizoguchi E, Ljunggren HG et al. Peripheral lymphoid development and function in TCR mutant mice. Int Immunol. 1994;6:1061–1070.
6. Mizoguchi A, Mizoguchi E, Chiba C et al. Cytokine imbalance and autoantibody production in T cell receptor-α mutant mice with inflammatory bowel disease. J Exp Med. 1996;183:847–856.
7. Mizoguchi A, Mizoguchi E, Tonegawa S, Bhan AK. Alteration of a polyclonal to an oligoclonal immune response to cecal aerobic bacterial antigens in TCRα mutant mice with inflammatory bowel disease. Int Immunol. 1996;8:1387–1394.
8. Mizoguchi A, Mizoguchi E, Chiba C, Bhan AK. Role of appendix in the development of inflammatory bowel disease in TCR-α mutant mice. J Exp Med. 1996;184:707–715.
9. Mizoguchi A, Mizoguchi E, Smith RN, Preffer Fl, Bhan AK. Suppressive role of B cells in chronic colitis of T cell receptor α mutant mice. J Exp Med. 1997;186:1749–1756.
10. Takahashi I, Kiyono H, Hamada S. CD4+ T-cell population mediates development of inflammatory bowel disease in T-cell receptor α chain-deficient mice. Gastroenterology. 1997;112: 1876–1886.
11. Wen L, Roberts SJ, Viney JL et al. Immunoglobulin synthesis and generalized autoimmunity in mice congenitally deficient in $\alpha\beta$ (+) T cells. Nature. 1994;369:654–658.
12. Wen L, Pao W, Wong FS et al. Germinal center formation, immunoglobulin class switching, and autoantibody production driven by non α/β T cells. J Exp Med. 1996;183:2271–2282.
13. Dianda L, Hanby AM, Wright NA, Sebesteny A, Hayday AC, Owen MJ. T cell receptor-$\alpha\beta$-deficient mice fail to develop colitis in the absence of a microbial environment. Am J Pathol. 1997;150:91–97.
14. Morrissey PJ, Charrier K, Braddy S, Liggitt D, Watson JD. CD4+ T cells that express high levels of CD45RB induce wasting disease when transferred into congenic severe combined immunodeficient mice. Disease development is prevented by cotransfer of purified CD4+ T cells. J Exp Med 1993;178:237–244.
15. Holländer GA, Simpson SJ, Mizoguchi E et al. Severe colitis in mice with aberrant thymic selection. Immunity. 1995;3:27–38.
16. Kühn R, Löhler J, Rennick D, Rajewsky K, Müller W. Interleukin-10-deficient mice develop chronic enterocolitis. Cell. 1993;75:263–274.
17. Sadlack B, Merz H, Schorle H, Schimpl A, Feller AC, Horak I. Ulcerative colitis-like disease in mice with a disrupted interleukin-2 gene. Cell. 1993;75:253–261.
18. Sadlack B, Loller J, Schorle H et al. Generalized autoimmune disease in interleukin-2-deficient mice is triggered by an uncontrolled activation and proliferation of CD4+ T cells. Eur J Immunol. 1995;25:3053–3059.
19. Krämer S, Schimpl A, Hünig T. Immunopathology of interleukin (IL) 2-deficient mice: thymus dependence and suppression by thymus-dependent cells with an intact IL-2 gene. J Exp Med. 1995;182:1769–1776.
20. Willerford DM, Chen J, Ferry JA, Davidson L, Ma A, Alt FW. Interleukin-2 receptor α chain regulates the size and content of the peripheral lymphoid compartment. Immunity. 1995;3:521–530.
21. Suzuki H, Kündig TM, Furlonger C et al. Deregulated T cell activation and autoimmunity in mice lacking interleukin-2 receptor β. Science. 1995;268:1472–1475.
22. Cao X, Shores EW, Hu-Li J et al. Defective lymphoid development in mice lacking expression of the common cytokine receptor γ chain. Immunity. 1995;2:223–238.
23. Powrie F, Leach MW, Mauze S, Caddle LB, Coffman RL. Inhibition of Th1 responses prevents inflammatory bowel disease in scid mice reconstituted with CD45RB^{hi} CD4+ T cells. Immunity. 1994;1:553–562.

24. Iwahana H, Fujimura M, Takahashi Y, Iwabuchi T, Yoshimoto K, Itakura M. Multiple fluorescence-based PCR-SSCP analysis using internal fluorescent labeling of PCR products. BioTechniques. 1996;21:510–519.
25. Komagata Y, Masuko K, Tashiro F et al. Clonal prevalence of T cells infiltrating into the pancreas of prediabetic non-obese diabetic mice. Int Immunol. 1996;8:807–814.
26. Nakajima A, Kodama T, Yazaki Y et al. Specific clonal T cell accumulation in intestinal lesions of Crohn's disease. J Immunol. 1996;157:5683–5688.
27. Probert CS, Chott A, Turner JR et al. Persistent clonal expansions of peripheral blood CD4[+] lymphocytes in chronic inflammatory bowel disease. J Immunol. 1996;157:3183–3191.
28. Takahashi I, Iijima H, Katashima R, Itakura M, Kiyono H. Clonal expansion of CD4[+] $\beta\beta^+$ T cells in T-cell receptor α-chain deficient mice by gut-derived antigens. J Immunol., in revision.

14
The inhibition of the CD40L–CD40 interaction prevents the intestinal manifestations of acute murine graft-versus-host disease

E. STÜBER, A. von FREIER and U. R. FÖLSCH

INTRODUCTION

T cell-mediated diseases of the intestine manifest in different clinical and histological patterns, including severe epithelial damage in inflammatory bowel disease (Crohn's disease and ulcerative colitis), villous atrophy and crypt hyperplasia (coeliac disease) and mainly lymphocytic infiltrates in the colonic mucosa (microscopic colitis). So far, the exact mechanisms by which activated T cells lead to these different intestinal lesions are not fully understood. For this reason, we began to study the mechanisms of T cell activation in T cell-mediated murine acute graft-versus host (GvH) disease, which manifest as lymphocytic inflitrates, crypt hyperplasia and villous atrophy[1].

The activation and the differentiation of naive T cells is a process involving more than the one signal delivered by MHC-bound peptides presented by antigen-presenting cells (APC). In order to elicit T cell activation (and not T cell anergy) certain co-stimulatory molecules on the T cell surface have to be cross-linked. These molecules consist of CD28[2] as well as numerous other receptors of various families[3]. Members of the TNF-R/NGF-R family of receptors and their ligands are implicated in T cell co-stimulation (CD40L, OX40, 4-1BB, CD30) and also in T cell apoptosis (Fas, TNF-R, TRAIL, TRAMP)[4].

CD40 is primarily expressed by resting B cells, but also by macrophages and dendritic cells, whereas its ligand is found on activated T cells[5]. The CD40L–CD40 interaction was first shown to be of critical importance in T cell-dependent B cell activation[6]. A few years later, it was discovered that co-stimulation of T cells is incomplete without a functional CD40L–CD40 interaction[7]. Several mechanisms for this latter effect have been proposed, including a down-regulation of B7-1, B7-2 on B cells[8] and, probably more important, down-regulation of IL-12 production by macrophages and dendritic cells[9,10].

In order to begin to understand the complex activation cascade in T cell-mediated diseases that lead to villous atrophy and crypt hyperplasia of the small bowel mucosa, we first studied the relevance of the CD40L–CD40 interaction *in vivo* for the induction of villous atrophy and crypt hyperplasia during acute murine GvH disease.

MATERIALS AND METHODS

Animals, cell preparations and induction of acute semi-allogenic GvH disease

C57/BL6, DBA2 and the F_1 generation of these two mouse strains (B6D2F1) were raised and kept under standard conditions in the animal facility of the University Hospital of Kiel, Germany.

To induce semi-allogenic GvH disease a slight modification of the procedure described by Guy-Grand and Vassalli[1] was performed. To prepare donor lymphocytes, spleen and mesenterial lymph nodes of C57/BL6 mice were removed and pressed through a cell filter (40 μm pore size). Red blood cells were subsequently lysed by a hypotonic lysing buffer (ACK-buffer, Böhringer Ingelheim, Germany). The resulting lymphocytes (80×10^6 cells/animal) were transferred to 8 to 14-week-old irradiated (7.5 Gy) B6D2F1 mice of the same sex by i.p. injection. At various time points after the induction of semi-allogenic GvH disease (1–6 days) recipient animals were given 5 mg/kg bodyweight 5-bromo-2-deoxy-uridine (BrdUr) (Sigma Chemicals, St. Louis, Mo, USA) by i.p. injection and were sacrificed 60 min later. Spleens, inguinal and mesenteric lymph nodes as well as the small bowel were removed and frozen in liquid nitrogen or fixed in 10% phosphate buffered (pH 7.4) formalin for further analysis. Control animals consisted of irradiated B6D2F1 mice, which were transferred with the same amount of syngenic (B6D2F1) cells.

Treatment regimens of recipient animals

After induction of GvH disease one group of recipient B6D2F1 mice was treated with the monoclonal anti-gp39 (MR-1) antibody[11] (Parmingen, San Diego, CA, USA) or hamster IgG as control. The antibody (200 μg) was injected i.p. daily on days 0–4 after the induction of GvH disease. The animals were sacrificed and organs were removed as described above.

Detection of mucosal atrophy and epithelial proliferation

Formalin-fixed jejunal specimens were embedded in paraffin and cut in 6–8 μm sections. To detect mucosal atrophy some slides were stained with haematoxylin and eosin and the villous height and crypt depth were measured using a graded ocular. Furthermore, to visualize proliferating cells which had incorporated BrdUr *in vivo*, the BrdUr Detection Kit was used according to the manufacturer's instructions (Calbiochem, San Diego, CA, USA). Slides were counterstained with haematoxylin and mounted in Eukit mounting medium (Merck, Darmstadt, Germany).

Detection of apoptotic cells

In order to determine the rate of apoptosis in the during acute GvH disease, treated and untreated recipient animals were sacrificed at various times (1–6 days) after the induction of GvH disease, and the jejunum was removed and snap frozen in liquid nitrogen. Apoptotic cells were detached by the TUNEL technique, using the ApopTag *in situ* apoptosis detection kit (Oncor, Gaithersburg, PA, USA) according to the manufacturer's instructions.

RESULTS

The effect of anti-gp39 treatment on the histological changes in the jejunum after the induction of acute GvH disease

Figure 1A and B depicts the profound effect of semi-allogenic lymphocyte transfer on the histological architecture of the jejunum 6 days after the beginning of the experiment. In addition to the increased numbers of lymphocytes, the villi in the animals with GvH disease appeared much thicker and shorter than those in syngeneic controls. In contrast, the crypts were significantly elongated. Figure 1C shows the dramatic effect of the anti-gp39 treatment on these changes in the intestinal architecture. Inhibition of the CD40L–CD40 interaction totally prevented the intestinal manifestations of acute GvH disease. Table 1 gives the exact measurements of villous length, crypt depth and crypt/villus ratio, indicating a complete restitution of the mucosal architecture by anti-gp39.

Effect of gp39 on the rate of epithelial cell apoptosis

It has previously been shown by our group that apoptosis of crypt epithelium plays a major role in the pathogenesis of the intestinal transformation in GvH (Stüber *et al.*, manuscript submitted). As shown in Figure 2A and B, there are roughly five times more apoptotic cells in the animals with GvH disease than in the controls. Treatment with anti-gp39 completely prevented the induction of apoptosis in this animal model (Figure 2C).

Effect of anti-gp39 on epithelial cell proliferation

We estimated the number of proliferating cells by *in vivo* labelling with BrdUr, which is incorporated by cells during the S-phase of the cell cycle. As shown in

Table 1 Animals were treated as described in the text. Villus length and crypt depth were measured after 6 days by a graded ocular in at least 15–20 complete, straight crypt–villus axes per slide of syngenic, semi-allogenic and of semi-allogenic + MR-1 treated animals. The depicted data represent the average (± SD) of these measurements.

	Villus length (µm)	Crypt depth (µm)	Crypt/villus ratio
Syngenic control	310 ± 29	94 ± 9	0.31
GvH	198 ± 21	176 ± 11	0.88
GvH + MR-1	337 ± 8.85	79.3 ± 7	0.24

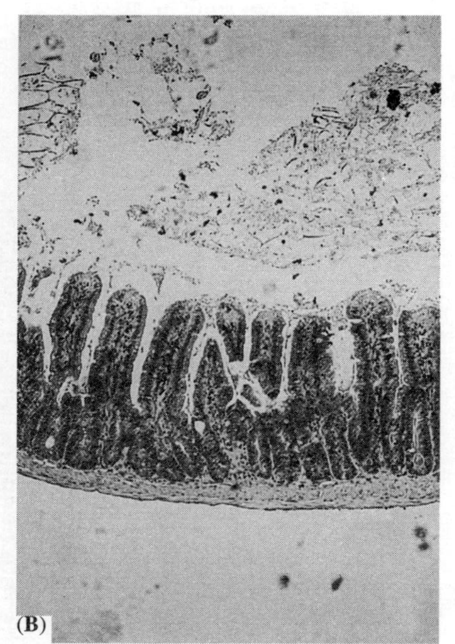

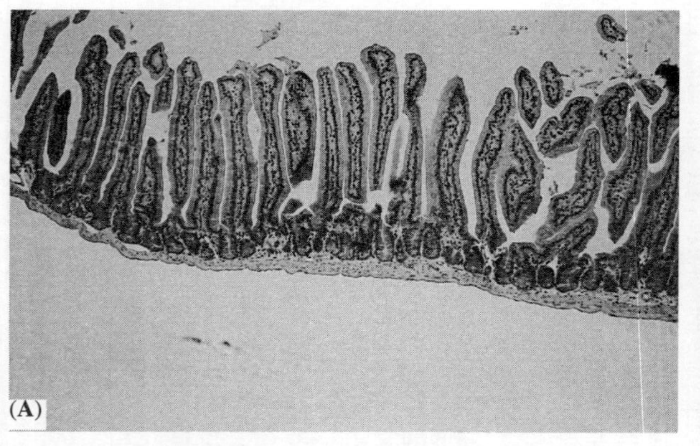

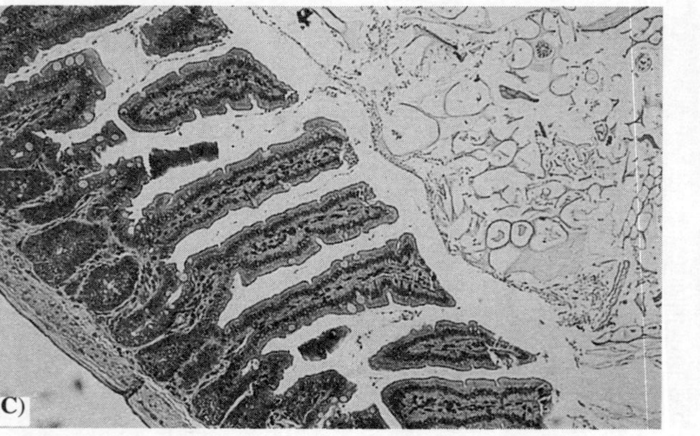

Figure 1 Irradiated B6D2F1 mice received either 80×10^6 B6D2F1 lymphocytes (syngenic control) (**A**) or 80×10^6 C57/BL6 lymphocytes (semi-allogenic) (**B**) without or with 200 μg MR-1 (**C**) each day by i.p. injection. Animals were sacrificed at day 6, the jejunum was removed and formalin fixed. After paraffin-embedding 6–8 μm sections were made and the slides were stained with haematoxylin and eosin according to standard procedures. Treatment with control hamster IgG did not change the intestinal morphology compared to GvH animals (data not shown)

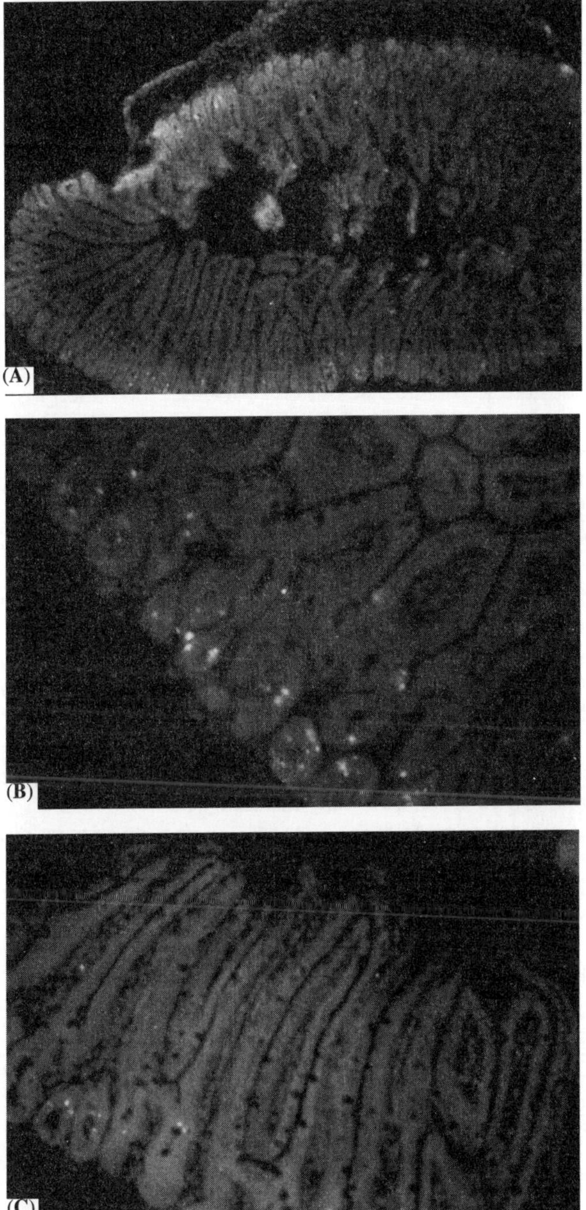

Figure 2 Irradiated B6D2F1 mice either received 80×10^6 B6D2F1 lymphocytes (syngenic control) (**A**) or 80×10^6 C57/BL6 lymphocytes (semi-allogenic) (**B**) without or with 200 μg MR-1 (**C**) each day by i.p. injection. Animals were sacrificed at day 3, the jejunum was removed and snap-frozen. Cryosections were cut at 6–8 μm, slides were stained with the ApopTag Direct Apoptosis *in situ* detection kit (Oncor, Gaithersburg, USA) and counterstained with propidium-iodide. Bright fluorescent nuclei indicate TUNEL-positive cells undergoing apoptosis

Figure 3A and B, we found approximately twice as many BrdUr-positive epithelial cells in the crypts of animals with GvH disease than in syngeneic controls, indicating a doubling of the proliferating cell pool. The treatment with anti-gp39 reversed this change completely (Figure 3C).

DISCUSSION

Murine acute GvH disease has been proposed to be mediated by activated CD4[+] donor-T cells[1], with CD8[+] T cells being important regulatory cells[12]. The resulting intestinal lesions are characterized by lymphocytic infiltrates, crypt hyperplasia and villous atrophy. Thus, this experimental animal model has been used to study the pathogenesis of similar human transformation processes of the intestinal mucosa (e.g. coeliac disease, GvH disease, food allergies).

The superfamily of TNF-R/NGF-R and their ligands (TNF-R, CD40, OX40, CD27, Fas, CD30, TRAIL, 4-1BB, TRAMP) is involved in multiple steps during the activation of lymphocytes and in apoptosis[4]. Furthermore, not only the receptor molecules of this family but also their respective ligands seem to be involved in cell signalling. This kind of cross-talk between the interacting cells thus blurs the distinction between receptor and ligand[4,13,14].

CD40 and its ligand CD40L is one of the receptor/ligand pairs belonging to this superfamily. The interaction of activated T cells expressing CD40L with B cells and with dendritic cells which are positive for CD40 is important for the differentiation of these cells[9,14–16]. This interaction is also crucial for T cell co-stimulation by different mechanisms: cross-linking of CD40L directly stimulates activated T cells[14], and the CD40L–CD40 interaction up-regulates B7-1 and B7-2 on B cells and dendritic cells, which co-stimulate T cells[8]. The interaction of CD40L and CD40 is also a main inducer of interleukin-12 secretion by macrophages and dendritic cells *in vivo* and *in vitro*[9,17,18], thus guiding the T cell differentiation into a T_H1 direction.

We demonstrated that the CD40L–CD40 interaction is crucial for the development of mucosal transformation in the acute murine GvH disease. Treatment with the anti-gp39 antibody (MR-1) totally prevented lymphocytic infiltrates, apoptosis, compensatory hyperregeneration and crypt hyperplasia. This study is corroborated by earlier findings of Durie and co-workers[19], who demonstrated the systemic effect of anti-gp39 in this animal model. How this inhibition is mediated is not clear at the moment. We are currently investigating whether IL-12 is down-regulated by anti-gp39 in this animal model, thereby preventing a T_H1 type of differentiation, as occurs in T_H1-mediated murine TNBS colitis[9]. Mowat and co-workers have shown that the manifestation of GvH disease is mainly mediated by T_H1 T cells[20,21]. Thus, anti-gp39 might interfere with the stimulation of macrophages and dendritic cells to produce IL-12 and thereby preventing a T_H1 type of T cell differentiation.

Inhibition of the OX40–OX40L interaction (another member of the TNF-R/NGF-R superfamily) by the administration of the fusion protein OX40–Ig also totally prevents the development of the mucosal transformation in the acute GvH disease. However, the occurrence of apoptosis and hyper-regeneration is not prevented by this treatment, indicating that while the CD40–CD40L interaction is

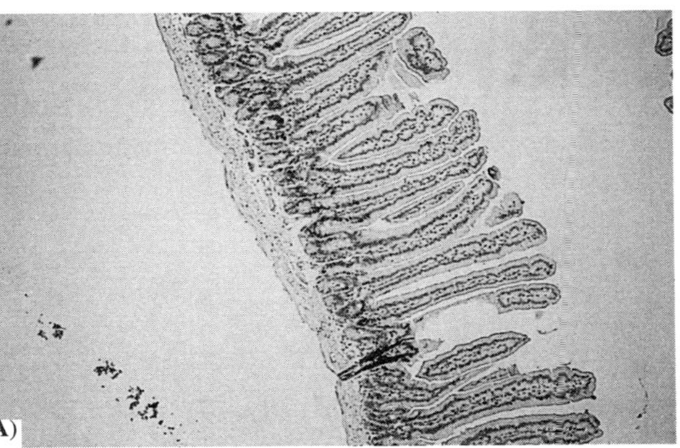

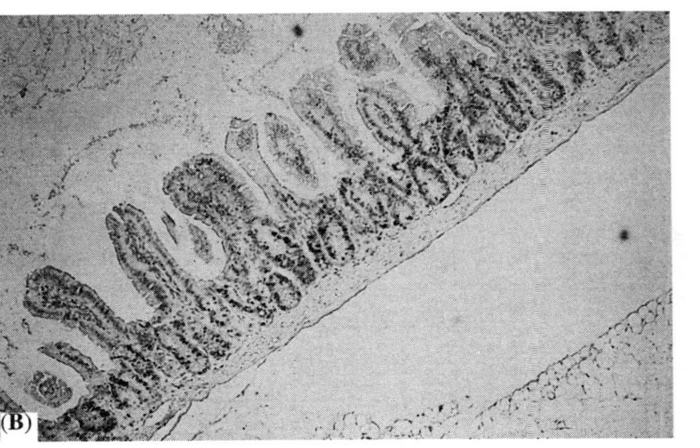

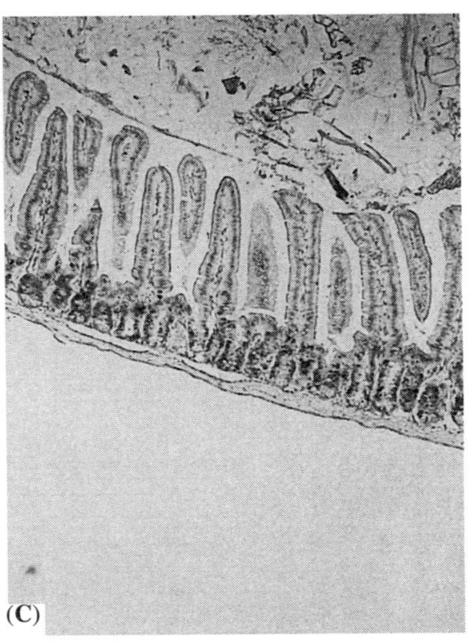

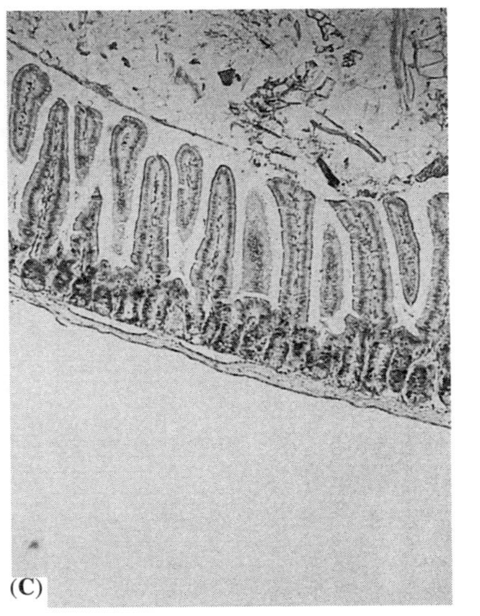

Figure 3 Irradiated B6D2F1 mice either received 80×10^6 B6D2F1 lymphocytes (syngenic control) (**A**) or 80×10^6 C57/BL6 lymphocytes (semi-allogenic) (**B**) without or with 200 μg MR-1 (**C**) each day by i.p. injection. Animals were sacrificed at day 6, 1 h after BrdUr (5 mg/kg bodyweight) was injected, the jejunum was removed and formalin fixed. After paraffin embedding 6–8 μm sections were made and the slides were stained for BrdUr-positive (i.e. proliferating) cells with the BrdUr detection kit (Calbiochem)

important during early activation steps in the pathogenesis of intestinal GvH disease, the OX40–OX40L interaction seems to be crucial for later steps in this pathogenesis. This resembles our own findings concerning B cell differentiation. The *in vivo* application of an anti-OX40 antibody did not prevent antigen-specific (early) IgM response in the course of a T cell-dependent humoral immune response[23]. However, it significantly blocked the secretion of antigen-specific IgG and IgA (later steps of B cell differentiation). In contrast, the application of anti-gp39 during a T cell-dependent humoral immune response totally prevented B cell activation and differentiation[6]. Thus, in conclusion, the OX40–OX40L interaction seems to be important for later steps in the differentiation of B cells and T cells, whereas the CD40–CD40L interaction is crucial for earlier steps.

ACKNOWLEDGEMENT

We acknowledge the superb technical assistance of Maren Dirks. The study was supported by a grant of the Deutsche Forschungsgemeinschaft (STU 157/3–1).

References

1. Guy-Grand D, Vassalli P. Gut injury in mouse graft-versus-host reaction. J Clin Invest. 1986;77:1584–1595.
2. Schwartz RH. A cell culture model for T lymphocyte clonal anergy. Science. 1990;248: 1349–1354.
3. Möller G. Accessory molecules in the immune response. Immunol Rev. 1996;153:1–223.
4. Smith CA, Farrah T, Goodwin RG. The TNF receptor superfamily of cellular and viral proteins: activation, costimulation and death. Cell. 1994;76:959–962.
5. van Kooten C, Banchereau J. Functional role of CD40 and its ligand. Int Arch Allergy Immunol. 1997;113:393–399.
6. Foy TM, Shepherd DM, Durie FH, Aruffo A, Ledbetter JA, Noelle RJ. Prolonged suppression of the humoral immune response by an antibody to the ligand for CD40, gp39. J Exp Med. 1993;178:1567–1575.
7. Noelle RJ. CD40 and its ligand in host defense. Immunity. 1995;4:415–419.
8. Roy M, Aruffo A, Ledbetter J, Lindsley P, Kehry M, Noelle RJ. Studies on the interdependence of gp39 and B7 expression and function during antigen-specific immune responses. Eur J Immunol. 1995;256:596–603.
9. Stüber ER, Strober W, Neurath MF. Blocking the CD40L–CD40 interaction in vivo specifically inhibits the priming of Th1-T cells. J Exp Med. 1996;183:693–698.
10. Cella M, Scheidegger D, Palmer-Lehmann K, Lane P, Lanzavecchia A, Alber G. Ligation of CD40 on dendritic cells triggers production of high levels of IL-12 and enhances T cell stimulatory capacity. J Exp Med. 1996;184:747–752.
11. Noelle RJ, Roy M, Shepherd DM, Stamenkovic I, Ledbetter JA, Aruffo A. A 39-kDa protein on activated helper T cells binds to CD40 and transduces the signal for cognate activation of B cells. Proc Natl Acad Sci USA. 1992;89:6550–6554.
12. Rus V, Svetic A, Nguyen P, Gause WC, Via CS. Kinetics of Th1 and Th2 cytokine production during early course of acute and chronic murine graft-versus-host disease. J Immunol. 1995;155:2396–2406.
13. Stüber E, Neurath M, Calderhead D, Fell HP, Strober W. Crosslinking of OX40-ligand, a member of the NGF/TNF family of cytokines, induces proliferation and differentiation in murine splenic B cells. Immunity. 1995;2:507–521.
14. Cayabyab M, Phillips JH, Lanier L. CD40 preferentially costimulates activation of CD4+ T lymphocytes. J Immunol. 1994;152:1523–1531.
15. Durie FH, Foy TM, Masters SM, Laman JD, Noelle RJ. The role of CD40 in the regulation of humoral and cell mediated immunity. Immunol Today. 1994;15:406–411.

16. Foy TM, Durie FH, Noelle RJ. The expanding role of CD40 and its ligand, gp39, in immunity. Semin Immunol. 1994;6:259–266.
17. Shu U, Kiniwa CY, Wu C et al. Activated CD4 T cells induce interleukin-12 production by monocytes via CD40–CD40L interaction. Eur J Immunol. 1995;25:1125–1128.
18. Kato T, Hakamda R, Yamane N, Nariuchi R. Induction of IL-12 p40 messenger RNA expression and IL-12 production of macrophages via CD40–CD40L interaction. J Immunol. 1996;156:3932–3938.
19. Durie FH, Aruffo A, Ledbetter JA et al. Antibody to the ligand to CD40, gp39, blocks the occurrence of the acute and chronic forms of graft-vs-host disease. J Clin Invest. 1994;94:1333–1338.
20. Williamson E, Garside P, Bradley JA, More IAR, Mowat AM. Neutralizing IL-12 during induction of murine acute graft-versus-host disease polarizes the cytokine profile toward a Th2-type alloimmune response and confers long term protection from disease. J Immunol. 1997;159:1208–1215.
21. Williamson E, Garside P, Bradley JA, Mowat AM. IL-12 is a central mediator of acute graft-versus-host disease in mice. J Immunol. 1996;157:689–699.
22. Stüber E, von Freier A, Marinescu D, Fölsch UR. Involvement of OX40-OX40L interactions in the intestinal manifestations of the murine acute graft-versus-host disease. Gastroenterology. 1998; in press.
23. Stüber E, Strober W. The T cell–B cell interaction via OX40–OX40L is necessary for the T cell dependent humoral immune response. J Exp Med. 1996;183:979–990.

15
Concepts in the treatment of experimental granulomatous colitis with Th1 inhibitory therapeutic modalities

I. J. FUSS, T. MARTH, W. STROBER and M. NEURATH

INTRODUCTION

Inflammatory bowel disease (IBD) encompasses Crohn's disease (CD) and ulcerative colitis, the prototypes of chronic inflammatory diseases of the gastro-intestinal tract in humans[1,2]. Recently, various animal models of chronic intestinal inflammation have been established that will probably provide new insights into the pathogenesis of IBD. These include rats carrying transgenes of HLA-B27 and β_2-microglobulin[3] and mice in which the genes for interleukin IL-2[4], IL-10[5], $G_{i\alpha2}$[6], and the α or β chain of the T-cell receptor[7] have been inactivated by homologous recombination. In addition, a Th1-mediated granulomatous colitis model has been established by the adoptive transfer of normal CD45Rb[hi] T cells from BALB/c to recipient SCID mice[8]. As such, these models provide an excellent opportunity to study the immunopathogenesis and possible treatment of these idiopathic diseases. One additional model is TNBS colitis, a chronic colitis in mice induced by the intra-rectal administration of trinitrobenzene sulphonic acid (TNBS). In this chapter we shall discuss our recent studies of this model and show how these studies have led to new insights into the immunological mechanisms underlying CD.

CHARACTERISTICS OF TNBS COLITIS

TNBS is a classical skin contactant, i.e. a chemical compound that induces delayed hypersensitivity reactions when applied to the skin because it haptenates body proteins with trinitrophenyl (TNP) groups and renders such self-protein immunogenic to the immune system. Thus, as shown in Figure 1, when TNBS is introduced into the colon of susceptible mice via intra-rectal instillation, it induces T cell-mediated immune response in the colonic mucosa, in this case

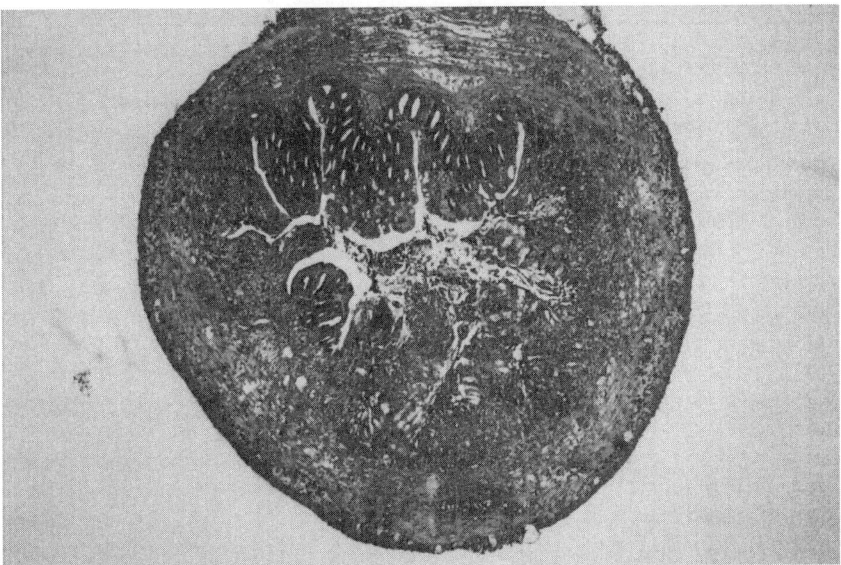

Figure 1 Histological analysis of the colon in mice with TNBS-induced colitis. Photomicrograph of HE-stained cross-section (× 50) of a colon of a SJL/J mouse with TNBS-induced colitis

leading to a massive mucosal inflammation characterized by the dense infiltration of T cells and macrophages throughout the entire wall of the large bowel[9]. Moreover, this histopathological picture is accompanied by the clinical picture of progressive weight loss (wasting), bloody diarrhoea, rectal prolapse and large-bowel wall thickening; in short, a pattern not dissimilar to that seen in human CD.

One important difference between skin contact hypersensitivity and TNBS colitis induced by application of TNBS is that in the skin the reaction is self-limited, whereas in the colon the reaction is persistent. This is probably due to the fact that the immune cells called forth by TNBS cross-react with ubiquitous mucosal antigens, i.e. antigens that exist in the bacterial microflora, and thus continue to be stimulated even after the TNP haptenated proteins have disappeared. Evidence in support of this view is several-fold. First, if lamina propria T cells in a mouse with TNBS colitis are transferred to a naïve mouse they cause mild but definite colitis in the recipients; since antigen is not transferred with such T cells this reaction is probably due to cross-reactivity[10]. Second, as will be evident from the discussion from Dr Strober (Chapter 10), colitis can be induced in IL-2-deficient mice merely by systemic injection of TNP-KLH; suggesting that T cells stimulated by TNP can traffic to the gut where they encounter cross-reactive antigens and induce colitis. Third and finally, it has recently been shown that T cells from mice with TNBS colitis proliferate in response to exposure to their own flora, whereas normal mice do not[11]. This finding implies that, in the normal situation, a mouse is 'tolerant' to its own flora and such tolerance is broken in TNBS colitis.

IMMUNOLOGICAL CHARACTERIZATION OF TNBS COLITIS

In our initial studies of TNBS colitis we sought to characterize the types of T cells that differentiate in the colon in response to TNBS stimulus[9]. We thus extracted purified CD4[+] T cells from the colon and spleen of mice with TNBS colitis and then stimulated the extracted cells with polyclonal stimulants such as anti-CD3/anti-CD28, to determine their capacity to secrete cytokines. In such studies a predominance of interferon gamma (IFN-γ) secretion would be indica-

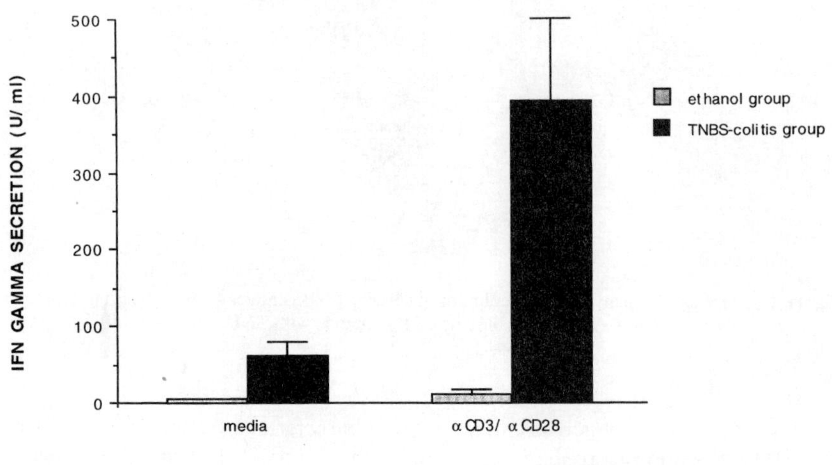

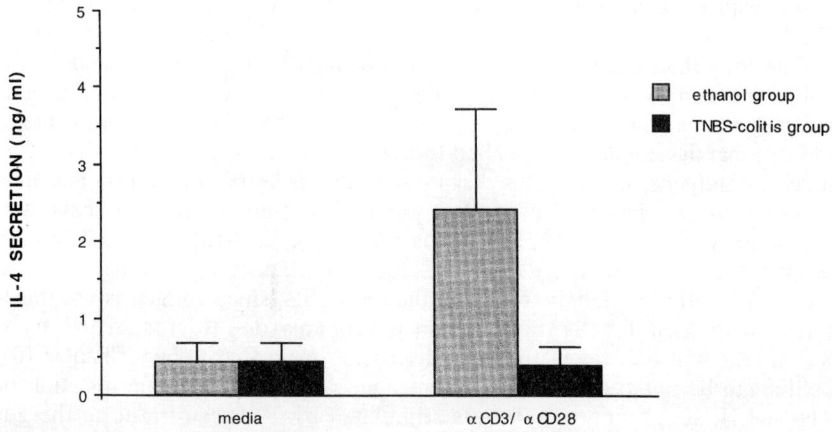

Figure 2 Cytokine production of stimulated and unstimulated LP CD4[+] T cells in TNBS-induced colitis. LP CD4[+] T cells were isolated from TNBS and control ethanol-treated mice on day 7, cultured for 2 days in the absence or presence of anti-CD3 and anti-CD28 and culture supernatants were analysed for concentration of IFN-γ and IL-4. Data represent three independent experiments done in triplicate. Standard errors are indicated

tive of a Th1 T cell response, whereas that of IL-4 secretion would be indicative of a Th2 T cell response. As shown in Figure 2, we found that the T cells in the TNBS colitis lesions produce greatly increased amounts of IFN-γ and decreased amounts of IL-4 following stimulation *in vitro* (as compared to T cells in controls), a clear indication that in TNBS colitis the relevant immune response is in fact a Th1 T cell reaction.

If TNBS colitis is indeed a Th1 T cell-mediated inflammation, as suggested by the findings described above, it should be associated with increased production of the cytokine that plays a central role in Th1 T cell differentiation, IL-12. We therefore performed *in-situ* immunohistological studies in which tissues from mice with and without TNBS colitis were stained with fluorochrome-labelled antibodies specific for IL-12 (as well as control antibodies). With this approach we showed that TNBS colitis is characterized by the presence of vastly increased amounts of tissue-associated IL-12, strongly implying that IL-12 synthesis is increased in the inflamed tissue. These results, plus those obtained from studies recounted below showing that anti-IL-12 abrogates TNBS colitis, provide very solid evidence that TNBS colitis is an IL-12-driven Th1 T cell-mediated inflammation.

On the basis of the above information, TNBS colitis is best explained by the immunological mechanism depicted in Figure 3, which can be described as follows: in the first step of the process the application of TNBS to the rectal mucosa results in the presentation of TNP to TNP-specific (and cross-reactive) T cells, which as a result become activated and express the CD40L, signalling molecule; the latter, via its interaction with the CD40 molecule on the antigen-presenting cells (APC), then allow the T cells to back-stimulate the APC to produce IL-12. In the next step of the process, the IL-12 produced by APC induces T cells in the lamina propria to undergo Th1 T cell differentiation and

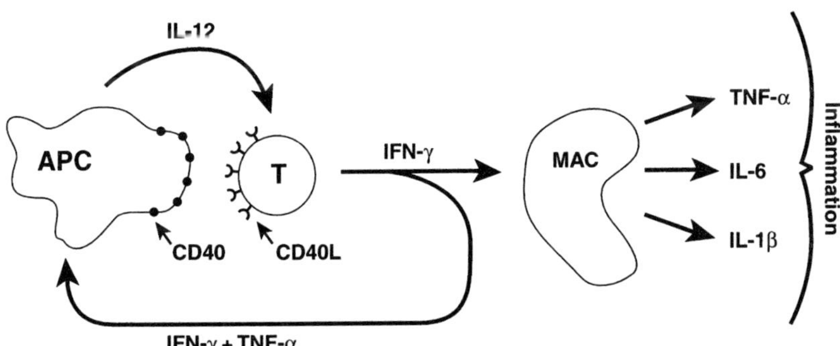

Figure 3 Activated T cells expressing CD40 ligand (CD40L) interact with CD40 on antigen-presenting cells (APC) and thereby induce APC production of the key Th1 inductive cytokine IL-12. IL-12 acts on the interacting T cells to induce IFN-γ which, in turn, induces macrophages to produce TNF-α and other pro-inflammatory cytokines necessary for inflammation. IFN-γ and TNF-α also act together to further stimulate IL-12 production in a positive feedback loop. Anti-TNF-α interrupts this inflammatory cascade by either decreasing the inflammatory potential of the secreted pro-inflammatory cytokines or by interrupting the positive feedback loop. Alternatively, anti-TNF-α has a direct effect on Th1 T cells which express TNF-α on their surface

thus cells which secrete IFN-γ and tumour necrosis factor alpha (TNF-α). The latter, in turn, bring about two effects: on the one hand these cytokines act 'up-stream' on APC to induce increased amounts of IL-12, and thus to magnify the Th1 T cell reaction: on the other hand these cytokines act 'downstream' on macrophages to induce the latter to produce a host of pro-inflammatory cytokines such as IL-1β, IL-6 and TNF-α. Finally, these latter substances cause the influx of cells giving rise to the inflammation of TNBS colitis.

TREATMENT OF TNBS COLITIS

One of the predictions of this proposed sequence of events underlying TNBS colitis is that the latter should be treatable by the systemic administration of antibodies (or other agents) that interfere with the sequence at any one of several stages; in particular it should be treatable by the systemic administration of anti-IL-12. To formally test this possibility we administered anti-IL-12 monoclonal antibody (hybridoma clone C17.8) to mice either at the same time as TNBS was administered per rectum or 3 weeks following such administration. As shown in Figure 4, these treatment regimens were remarkably effective in that they either completely prevented the development of TNBS colitis (when given at the time of induction of the disease) or led to dramatic resolution of the TNBS colitis (when given when the lesion was fully developed). These studies, in showing that a murine model resembling CD is treatable with anti-IL-12, imply that CD,

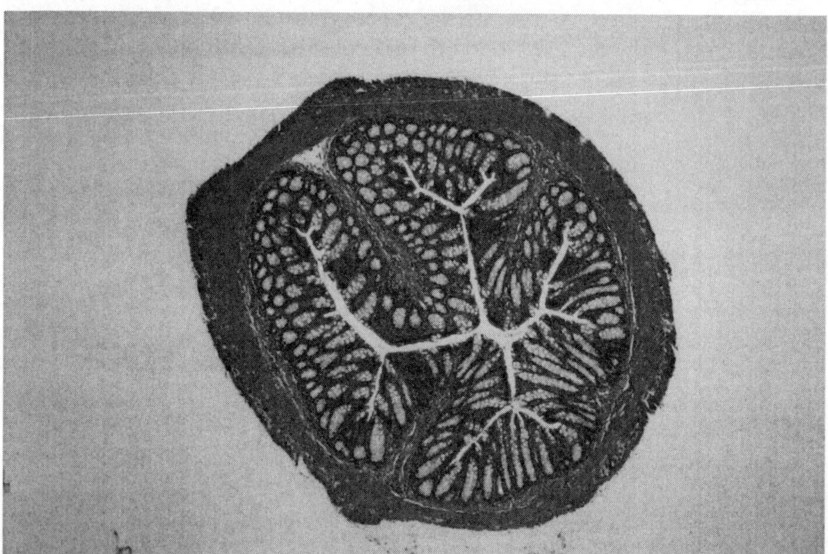

Figure 4 Histological analysis of the colon in mice with TNBS-induced colitis given anti-IL-12. Photomicrograph of HE-stained cross-section ($\times$ 50) of a colon of a SJL/J mouse with TNBS-induced colitis after treatment with anti-IL-12 antibodies. A striking reduction in inflammatory activity is evident

also an apparently Th1-mediated disease process, is also treatable in this fashion (see Chapter 23 by Dr Parronchi).

While the blocking of IL-12 activity with anti-IL-12 may be an efficient way of interrupting the Th1 T cell activation pathway necessary for TNBS colitis, it is certainly not the only way the latter can be accomplished. As indicated above, the critical APC–T cell interactions leading to Th1 T cell differentiation require T cell expression of CD40L on activated T cells and signalling of APC via CD40 for production of IL-12. Thus, it is theoretically possible to interfere with Th1 T cell differentiation by blocking the CD40L–CD40 interaction. To test this possibility we administered anti-CD40L antibody to mice at the time of TNBS colitis induction with intra-rectal TNBS administration[12]. Such treatment did indeed prevent colitis induction as well as the increased IFN-γ production in the lamina propria associated with colitis, and thus a second avenue is available for the prevention of TNBS colitis. Whether anti-CD40L can also be used to treat ongoing TNBS colitis, as can anti-IL-12, awaits further study.

Another way the Th1 pathway can be experimentally thwarted in the context of the TNBS colitis model would be to inhibit more distal inflammatory cytokine effects, either by the administration of anti-IFN-γ or anti-TNF-α[13,14]. In studies relevant to this possibility we found that anti-IFN-γ also inhibited the development of colitis, although such inhibition was not as effective as that achieved with anti-IL-12[14]. Thus, while prevention of TNBS colitis was inhibitable with a single injection of anti-IL-12, prevention of colitis with anti-IFN-γ required multiple injections and was, in general, not as complete. In addition, whereas mice cured by colitis with anti-IL-12 were not subject to re-induction of colitis with sub-colitis-inducing doses of TNBS, mice cured of colitis with anti-IFN-γ were subject to such colitis induction. This suggests that anti-IL-12-treated mice no longer have cells reactive with colitis, whereas anti-IFN-γ-treated mice have such cells. Important confirmation of this possibility has recently come from the observation that mice with TNBS colitis treated with anti-IL-12 display large numbers of apoptotic cells in the inflamed colons, whereas the same mice treated with anti-IFN-γ display only modest numbers of apoptotic cells at this site. Overall, then, these studies strongly suggest that the efficacy of anti-IL-12 in TNBS colitis is due to the fact that the antibody not only neutralizes IL-12 but also rids the body of the disease-causing Th1 T cells.

An additional means of treatment has involved the blockage of the multi-faceted cytokine, TNF-α. TNF-α can mediate its inflammatory effects in many ways. As an early regulator of inflammation it can synergize with IFN-γ to up-regulate the production of IL-12[15]. It can also influence inflammatory responses distally at the mucosal level through activation of intestinal enzymes, i.e. collagenase, and the release of inflammatory mediators which can increase intestinal permeability, i.e. arachidonic acid[16,17]. These inflammatory mediators can in turn lead to tissue injury, disruption of mucosal tissue and further exposure of LP T cells to antigen challenge and immune-mediated responses.

Therefore researchers have selected to target this TNF-α response in many different fashions. Our laboratory has shown that established murine TNBS colitis can be effectively treated by the intraperitoneal administration of mono-clonal antibody to TNF-α[13]. In these studies, treatment of TNBS colitis induced mice with murine antibodies to TNF-α led to both an improvement in wasting disease and resolution of macroscopic signs of colitis. This improvement correlated with the decreased production of TNF-α at the mRNA level as well as the decreased synthesis *in vitro* of pro-inflammatory cytokines such as IL-1β and IL-6. In related studies we have also demonstrated that the intra-rectal administration of an anti-sense oligonucleotide molecule can effectively down-regulate TNBS-induced colitis. This specific therapy functions to block the local synthesis of the p65 subunit of nuclear factor-$\kappa\beta$ (NF-$\kappa\beta$) a key regulatory transcription factor necessary for TNF-α transcription[18]. In these studies, local enema treatment with an anti-sense oligonucleotide molecule directed against the p65 NF-$\kappa\beta$ subunit led to both the clinical and histological improvement in established TNBS colitis. The down-regulation of p65 protein expression also correlated with the decreased *in-vitro* production of pro-inflammatory cytokines such as IL-1β, IL-6 and TNF-α. Taken together, these studies indicate the important role of TNF-α in the pathogeneisis of chronic intestinal inflammation, and suggest the potential value of therapies directed at this arm of the inflammatory process.

CONCLUDING REMARKS

In recent human treatment trials directed at TNF-α, the systemic administration of a chimaeric monoclonal antibody to TNF-α to CD patients has led to marked improvement in the majority of treated patients[19,20]. This finding, and the studies in mice, are promising, but whether this form of therapy will ultimately prove useful in the long term still remains uncertain. It may be that, in time, Crohn's inflammatory process will become independent of TNF-α, as has been the experience in the treatment of some rheumatoid arthritis patients with anti-TNF-α[21].

The previous observation of an increased IL-12 response leading to a dysregulated Th1 T cell response[9–12,14], makes this treatment a more desirable modality. As mentioned, IL-12 plays a major role in the generation of the Th1 T cell response; therefore anti-IL-12 can counteract this dysregulated response[22]. As mentioned above, reports from our laboratory have demonstrated that administration of antibodies to IL-12 not only abrogates the development of a Th1-mediated inflammatory response but can lead to apoptosis of the activated Th1 T cell within the lesional tissue[9,14]. These findings indicate that IL-12 is necessary not only for the development of the Th1 T cell, but also for its continued viability. These factors therefore suggest that neutralization of IL-12 effects in the inflammatory process may be one of the important means of dealing with the Th1 response found in CD patients. On this basis, treatment trials of CD patients with a humanized anti-IL-12 antibody are currently being developed at the National Institutes of Health.

As a final note, the better understanding of these immunological mechanisms that control intestinal inflammation allows us a more advantageous position with regard to the ultimate treatment of such disease states as Crohn's disease.

References

1. Podolsky D. Inflammatory bowel disease. N Engl J Med. 1995;325:928–36.
2. Strober W, Neurath M. Immunological diseases of the gastrointestinal tract. In: Rich RR, editor, Clinical Immunology. St Louis: Mosby; 1995;1401–1428.
3. Hammer R, Maika S, Richardson J, Tang Y, Taurog J. Spontaneous inflammatory disease in transgenic rats expressing HLA-B27 and human β2m: an animal model of HLAB-27-associated human disorders. Cell. 1990;63:1099–1109.
4. Sadlack B, Merz H, Schorle H, Schimpl A, Feller C, Horvak I. Ulcerative colitis-like disease in mice with a disrupted interleukin-2 gene. Cell. 1993;75:253–62.
5. Kühn R, Löhler D, Rennick D, Rajewsky K, Müller W. Interleukin-10-deficient mice develop chronic enterocolitis. Cell. 1993;75:263–77.
6. Rudolf U, Finegold M, Rich S et al. Ulcerative colitis and adenocarcinoma of the colon in Gα12-deficient mice. Nature Gen. 1995;10:143–9.
7. Mombaerts P, Mizoguchi E, Grusby M, Glimcher L, Bahn A, Tonegawa S. Spontaneous development of inflammatory bowel disease in T cell receptor mutant mice. Cell. 1993;75: 275–88.
8. Powrie F, Leach M, Mauze S, Menon S, Caddle L, Coffman R. Inhibition of Th1 responses prevents inflammatory bowel disease in SCID mice reconstituted with CD45Rb^{hi}CD4$^+$ T cells. Immunity. 1994;1:553–65.
9. Neurath M, Fuss I, Kelsall B, Stüber E, Strober W. Antibodies to IL-12 abrogate established experimental colitis in mice. J Exp Med. 1995;182:1281–90.
10. Neurath M, Fuss I, Kelsall B, Presky D, Waegall W, Strober W. Experimental granulomatous colitis in mice is abrogated by induction of TGF-β-mediated oral tolerance. J Exp Med. 1996;183:2605–16.
11. Duchmann R, Schmitt E, Knolle P, Meyer zum Buschenfelde KH, Neurath M. Tolerance toward resident intestinal flora in mice is abrogated in experimental colitis and restored by treatment with interleukin-10 or antibodies to interleukin-12. Eur J Immunol. 1996;26:934–8.
12. Stuber E, Strober W, Neurath M. Blocking the CD40L–CD40 interaction *in vivo* specifically prevents the priming of T helper 1 cells through the inhibition of interleukin 12 secretion. J Exp Med. 1996;183:693–8.
13. Neurath M, Fuss I, Pasparakis M et al. Predominant pathogenic role of tumor necrosis factorα in experimental colitis in mice. Eur J Immunol. 1997;27:1743–50.
14. Fuss IJ, Marth T, Pearlstein G, Neurath MF, Strober W. Anti-interleukin-12 regulates apoptosis of activated Th1 T cells in murine experimental granulomatous (TNBS) colitis. Gastroenterology. 1997;112:A978.
15. Veta C, Kawajumi H, Fujiwara H, Miyagawa T, Kida H, Ohmoto Y. Interleukin-12 activates human gamma delta T cells: synergistic effect of tumor necrosis factor-alpha. Eur J Immunol. 1996;26:3066–73.
16. Brynskov J, Nielson OH, Ahnfelt-Ronne I, Bendtzen K. Cytokines and their natural regulation in inflammatory bowel disease: a review. Dig Dis. 1994;12:290.
17. Dayer JM, Beutler B, Cerami A. Cachectin/tumor necrosis factor stimulates collagenase and prostaglandin E$_2$ production by human synovial cells and dermal fibroblasts. J Exp Med. 1985;162:2163–8.
18. Neurath MF, Pettersson S, Meyer zum Buschenfelde KH, Strober W. Local administration of antisense phosphorothioate oligonucleotides to the p65 subunit of NF-$\kappa\beta$ abrogates established experimental colitis in mice. Nature Med. 1996;2:998–1004.
19. van Dullemen HM, van Deventer SJ, Hommes DW et al. Treatment of Crohn's disease with anti-tumor necrosis factor chimeric monoclonal antibody (cA2). Gastroenterology. 1995;109: 129–34.
20. Targan S, Hanauer SB, van Deventer SJ et al. A short-term study of chimeric monoclonal antibody cA2 to tumor necrosis factor α for Crohn's disease. N Engl J Med. 1997;337:1029–35.
21. Firestein GS, Zvaifler NJ. Anticytokine therapy in rheumatoid arthritis. N Engl J Med. 1997;337:195–7.
22. Trinchieri G. Interleukin-12: a cytokine produced by antigen-presenting cells with immunoregulatory function in the generation of T-helper cells type 1 and cytotoxic lymphocytes. Blood. 1994;4:4008–14.

16
TNF-induced matrix metalloproteinase production in gut inflammation

S. L. F. PENDER and T. T. MACDONALD

INTRODUCTION

There is increasing evidence that pro-inflammatory cytokines such as interleukin (IL)-1β, IL-6 and tumour necrosis factor-α (TNF-α) play a crucial role in inflammatory bowel disease (IBD)[1-3]. TNF-α, which is mainly produced by monocytes, macrophages and T cells, also plays a key role in tissue injury in other inflammatory and autoimmune diseases, such as septic shock and rheumatoid arthritis when produced in excess[4-6]. In Crohn's disease (CD), serum TNF-α concentrations are moderately increased[7]. TNF-α-positive cells can be detected by immunohistochemistry throughout the mucosa, and elevated numbers of TNF-α-secreting cells are present in single cell suspensions of mucosal biopsies[1,2]. TNF-α-immunoreactive cells are also elevated in the gut in ulcerative colitis, but in this case the increase is restricted to the lamina propria[2]. High concentrations of TNF-α can be detected in stools of children with active inflammatory bowel disease[8], and isolated mononuclear cells from patients with IBD secrete more TNF-α than cells from control patients[3]. Therefore anti-TNF-α could be a possible treatment for IBD.

ANTI-TNF-α TREATMENT IN CROHN'S DISEASE

Several studies have addressed the potential efficacy of anti-TNF-α treatment in CD (reviewed in Ref. 9). Treatment of patients with severe steroid refractory CD with a TNF-α antibody (cA2) resulted in a rapid decrease in the CD activity index, remarkable healing of mucosal ulcers, complete clinical remission and few side effects[10]. Recently, a single infusion of cA2 antibody therapy has been shown to be efficacious in inducing remission in CD in a placebo controlled, double blind, multicentre trial[11].

The mechanism by which anti-TNF-α therapy inhibits inflammation in CD is unknown. The antibodies may be neutralizing soluble TNF-α in the interstitial fluids. Alternatively, the antibody most widely used, cA2, is of the IgG1 isotype and may bind membrane bound TNF-α and fix complement. Thus there is a possibility that the therapeutic effect is not due to TNF-α neutralization but is brought about by the cytotoxic killing of membrane TNF-positive T cells and macrophages, thereby lowering the concentrations of all tissue cytokines. In this regard another TNF-α antibody of the IgG4 isotype, which is unlikely to fix complement, appears to be less effective in CD than the cA2 antibody[12]. Underlying all of this is the lack of knowledge of the mechanisms by which increased concentrations of TNF-α cause tissue injury in the gut.

ANTI-TNF TREATMENT IN THE HUMAN FETAL SMALL INTESTINE MODEL OF ENTEROPATHY

We have used human fetal tissue to study cytokine mediated gut inflammation (Figure 1). In this *ex vivo* system, lamina propria T cells in explant cultures of human fetal small intestine are activated directly with mitogens or super-antigens[13–15]. Pokeweed mitogen (PWM) activates virtually all mucosal T cells whereas *Staphylococcus aureus* enterotoxin B (SEB) activates mucosal Vβ3$^+$ T cells. PWM-activated lamina propria T cells in the explants secrete IL-2 and IFN-γ, and adjacent macrophages become class II$^+$, CD25$^+$ and secrete TNF-α[13,14,16]. T cell activation by SEB requires its presentation by class II MHC molecules[17,18] which are abundant on accessory cells in the fetal lamina propria[19]. The consequence of T cell activation is predictable and results in tissue injury. The mucosal destruction induced by PWM and the less severe villous atrophy and crypt hyperplasia caused as a result of SEB activation of T cells are both associated with degradation of lamina propria extracellular matrix (ECM) and the production of matrix metalloproteinases (MMP)[20–22].

The fetal gut system differs from clinical intestinal inflammation in many ways. The human fetal gut model obviously lacks the complexity seen *in vivo* since it lacks blood-borne inflammatory cells. Although T cell-mediated[13–15] it is a relatively speedy response compared with the chronic immune activation seen in CD. Tissue injury can manifest as villous atrophy and crypt cell hyperplasia or as severe injury with complete mucosal destruction similar to that seen in severe graft-versus-host disease and late stage intestinal allograft rejection[13,14]. PWM-induced tissue injury is almost completely inhibited by cyclosporin A and FK506[14], indicating that injury is T cell-mediated and not due to the non-specific toxic effects of the lectin. Nevertheless, in both CD and in the fetal gut system, the role of T$_H$1 cells appears to be of major importance as high concentrations of both interferon-γ (IFN-γ) protein and mRNA expression are seen in PWM-stimulated explant cultures. IL-4 concentrations are almost unchanged (Table 1)[2,23,24]. Therefore we believe that the fetal gut model gives important insights into the pathways by which activated T cells, macrophages and stromal cells interact during mucosal cell-mediated immune responses. The final mediators of tissue injury in the fetal gut explant model appear to be MMP, especially stromelysin-1.

MMP are a group of Ca^{2+}-activated, Zn^{2+}-containing neutral endopeptidases which are secreted and activated extracellularly and can degrade all class of

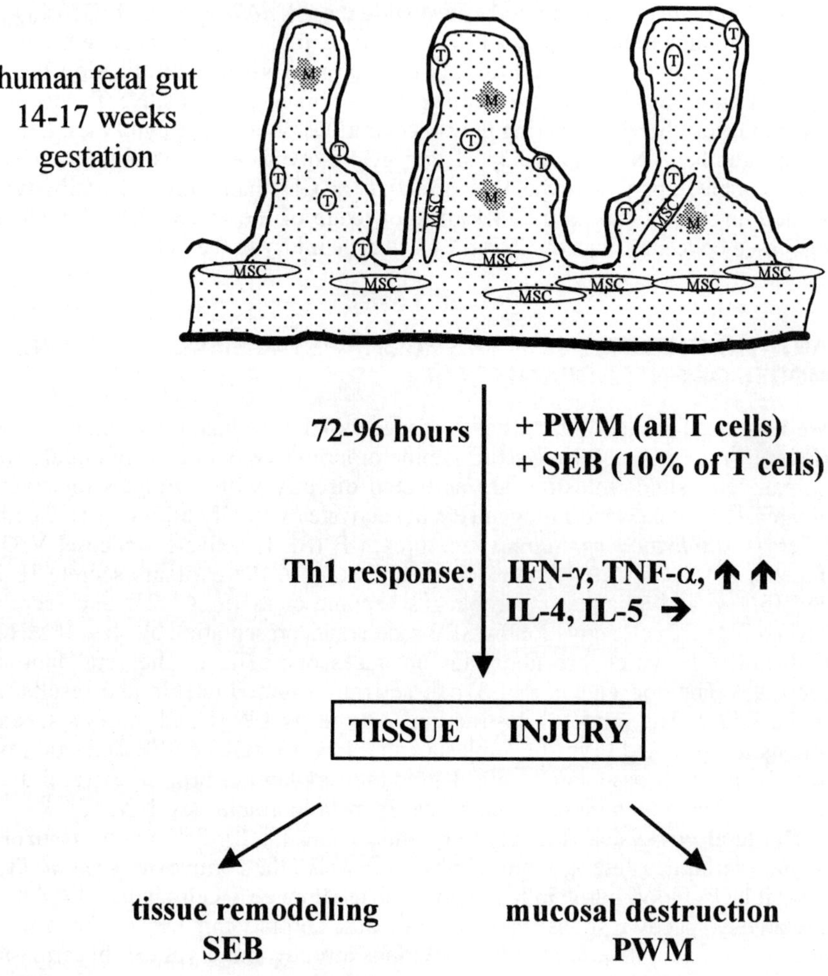

Figure 1   Schematic diagram of human fetal gut model

Table 1   Concentration of TNF-α, IFN-γ and IL-4 in day 3 fetal gut explant culture supernatants.

	TNF-α	*IFN-γ (pg/ml)*	*IL-4*
Control	3.63 ± 1.90	401.61 ± 125.79	5.65 ± 3.60
PWM	42.73 ± 6.92	5846.05 ± 856.40	12.32 ± 0.43
Fold increase	12×	13×	2×

ECM. The extracellular activity of MMP is regulated by tissue inhibitors of metalloproteinases (TIMP), secreted by the same cell types that produce MMP[25–27]. When stromal cells from fetal intestine are stimulated *in vitro* with IL-1β or TNF-α they produce extremely large amounts of MMP[21]. Therefore a possible therapeutic effect of anti-TNF-α therapy is to interrupt this pathway of tissue injury and prevent mucosal matrix degradation.

Recently, we used a soluble TNF-α receptor (TNFR)–human IgG fusion protein to attempt to inhibit injury and MMP production in the fetal gut model. This TNFR–IgG fusion protein consists of the extracellular portion of human p55 TNFR linked to the hinge, CH2 and CH3 domains of human IgG1 heavy chain[28]. The TNF-α binding affinity of TNFR–IgG is 75–100 pM[28,29]. This TNFR–IgG is more potent than anti-TNF-α mAb in protecting against rat endotoxic shock *in vivo*[28,30] and its ability to neutralize the activity of endogenous TNF-α in murine listeriosis is 10-fold that of anti-TNF-α mAb TN3-19.12[31].

Production of TNF-α protein and mRNA in PWM-stimulated human intestinal explants

Following activation of lamina propria T cells with PWM, there was a 10-fold increase in TNF-α protein in day 3 PWM-stimulated explant culture supernatants compared with unstimulated controls (Table 1). Competitive quantitative PCR showed that T cell activation induced a significant increase in TNF-α transcripts in the fetal gut explants as well as a large increase in IFN-γ transcripts (Table 2).

Effects of TNFR–IgG fusion protein in human fetal gut explant culture

In two separate experiments, PWM (10 μg/ml) produced severe tissue injury with complete mucosal destruction in 100% of the explants. If TNFR–IgG was added at the onset of the cultures along with the PWM, about 93% of the explants were morphologically normal. The addition of TNFR–IgG at 10 μg/ml dramatically inhibited tissue injury, and villus morphology was retained even though there was some crypt hypertrophy. Control normal human IgG had no effect on tissue injury.

TNFR–IgG fusion protein inhibits the production MMP

Activation of lamina propria T cells results in increased concentrations of MMP in the organ culture supernatants and inhibition of their enzymatic activity ameliorates injury[21]. In control supernatants, collagenase, stromelysin-1 and

Table 2 Number of TNF-α and IFN-γ transcripts (per μg total RNA) measured by quantitative competitive reverse transcriptase–PCR in day 1 human fetal gut explants. (ND = not detectable)

	TNF-α	IFN-γ
Control	ND	ND
PWM	14 048	27 200 000

TIMP-1 were detectable at low levels by western blotting. T cell activation with PWM resulted in increased amounts of both the inactive and active forms of collagenase and stromelysin-1, and increased amounts of the inactive forms of gelatinase B and increased TIMP-1. Normal human IgG had no inhibitory effect on PWM-induced MMP production. However TNFR–IgG produced a slight decrease in collagenase, gelatinase B and TIMP-1 immunoreactivity, but markedly reduced stromelysin-1 (Figure 2).

TNF-α (1 ng/ml) causes an increase in interstitial collagenase, stromelysin-1 and TIMP-1 production by mucosal mesenchymal cells (MSC). When graded doses of TNFR–IgG were added along with the TNF-α, significant inhibition of collagenase, stromelysin-1, gelatinase B and TIMP-1 was seen, even at 10 ng/ml. Gelatinase A was unaffected[32]. As a specificity control, IL-1β was

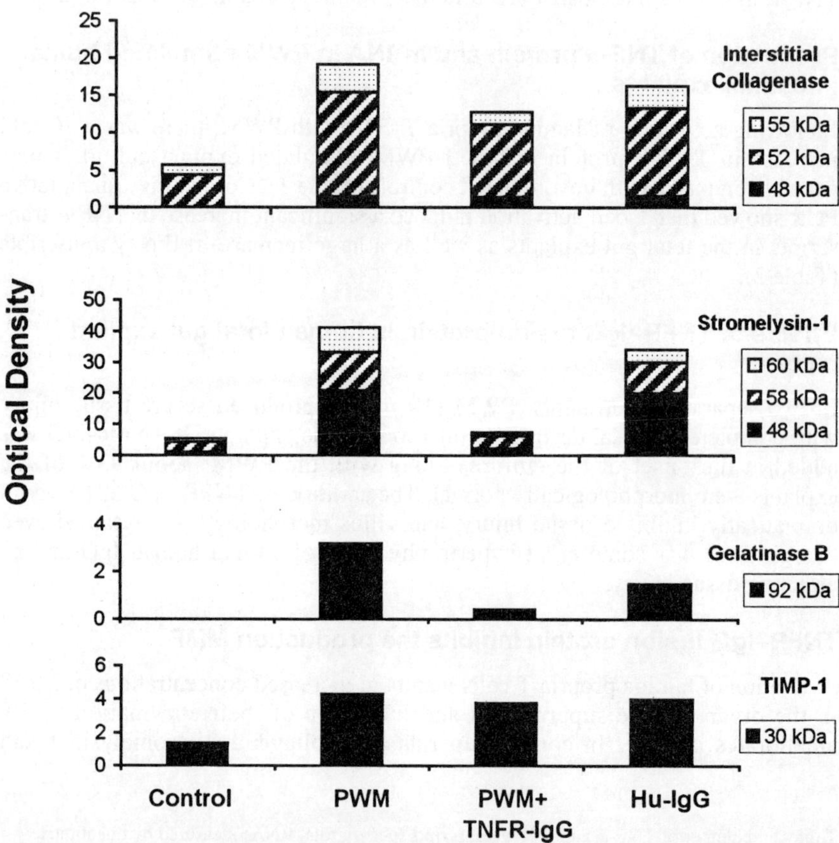

Figure 2 Effect of TNFR–IgG fusion protein on MMP and TIMP-1 production in PWM-stimulated human fetal small intestine explants. TNFR–IgG fusion protein and normal human IgG (10 μg/ml) were added at the onset of culture. Supernatants were collected after 3 days of culture, concentrated 6- to 7-fold, and analysed by western blotting. The bands of latent forms and active forms of MMP were scanned and plotted. The example shown is representative of four separate experiments

also investigated. It also produced an increase in MMP, but had less effect on TIMP-1. However in the presence of graded doses of TNFR–IgG, IL-1β-induced MMP production was unaltered.

POSSIBLE MECHANISM

TNFR–IgG can prevent the severe tissue injury which occurs following lamina propria T cell activation with PWM in explant cultures of human fetal small intestine. There is no evidence that the TNFR–IgG had any unexpected immuno-suppressive effects since neither TNF-α nor IFN-γ transcripts was reduced (data not shown), and therefore we can attribute its effects to neutralization of the TNF-α within the tissue. Whether this occurs by binding soluble TNF-α trimers or membrane-bound molecules is unknown. However we can probably exclude complement-mediated destruction of TNF-α secreting cells since the explants were cultured in serum-free medium.

Elevated concentrations of TNF-α were present in organ culture supernatants following activation of lamina propria T cells with PWM. This TNF-α probably originates from lamina propria T cells[33] or tissue macrophages activated by T cell products. In patients with IBD the majority of the TNF-α-secreting cells are monocytes recently extravasated from the blood[34], and there is no *a priori* reason why resident macrophages should not make TNF-α, especially in the fetus where there are marked differences between the Class II$^+$ MHC cells compared with postnatal intestine[19]. In any case, the cellular source of the TNF-α is probably less important than its functional consequences since in IBD, TNF-α has been detected in epithelial cells, fibroblasts, neutrophils, mast cells, eosinophils, Paneth cells and macrophages[35]. How many of these cell types produce meaningful amounts is unknown.

TNF-α markedly up-regulates interstitial collagenase and stromelysin-1 production by mucosal MSC[21], as it does with MSC from other tissues[36–40]. *In vitro* experiments using MSC lines isolated from human fetal gut showed that the addition of very low doses of TNFR–IgG (10 ng/ml) were effective at inhibiting TNF-α-induced interstitial collagenase and stromelysin-1 production. The increase in MMP was also seen in the culture supernatants of explants treated with PWM, in which there was extensive mucosal injury, confirming previous studies[21]. When the TNFR–IgG was added there was a marked reduction in stromelysin-1 and gelatinase B, but a much smaller reduction in collagenase and gelatinase A. We consider it highly probable that the reduction in stromelysin-1 is the reason for the maintenance of structural integrity in the PWM-stimulated explants co-cultured with TNFR–IgG. In previous studies we have added recombinant gelatinase A and B, stromelysin-1 and interstitial collagenase to explants and only stromelysin is able to cause tissue injury at low concentrations. In addition, a stromelysin/gelatinase inhibitor is much more effective than a collagenase inhibitor in preventing injury[21]. We therefore suggest that a major role for TNF-α in gut injury is the reduction of stromelysin-1 production by stromal cells. It is also worthy of comment that although interstitial collagenase was markedly increased in PWM-stimulated explants, it was only minimally decreased when TNFR–IgG was added. This suggests that stromelysin-1 is more important than interstitial collagenase in this model and also that it is not TNF-α causing the elevated collagenase but another factor, such as IL-1β.

One of the puzzles in interpreting the therapeutic effects of anti-TNF-α therapy in CD as a specific inhibitor of TNF-α is that the treatment should have no effect on other pro-inflammatory cytokines such as IL-1β, unless one evokes a complex feedback loop whereby TNF-α promotes the production of other cytokines. IL-1β concentrations are markedly elevated in IBD[41], and in rabbit colitis IL-1 receptor antagonist (IL-1RA) is highly effective at preventing gut injury[42]. Studies in man have revealed an imbalance of IL-1β/IL-1RA ratios[43,44] in the gut in IBD as well as elevated concentrations of PAF, IL-6, IL-8, IL-15, etc[45]. There have, however, been no reported clinical studies on the use of IL-1RA in IBD. Even if one neutralizes TNF-α one would expect that local IL-1β would also act on mucosal MSC to increase stromelysin-1 production and maintain tissue injury. However this does not appear to be the case, either in fetal gut explants or in patients, so perhaps in the tissue microenvironment there is sufficient IL-1RA to inhibit IL-1β, despite the altered ratios.

ACKNOWLEDGEMENTS

This work was supported by the Wellcome Trust, Special Trustees of the St. Bartholomew's Hospital (London, UK) and the Crohn's in Childhood Research Association. This study received ethical approval from the Hackney and District Health Authority, London.

References

1. Murch SH, Braegger CP, Walker-Smith JA, MacDonald TT. Location of tumour necrosis factor alpha by immunohistochemistry in chronic inflammatory bowel disease. Gut. 1994;34:1705–1709.
2. Breese EJ, Michie CA, Nicholls SW et al. Tumor necrosis factor alpha-producing cells in the intestinal mucosa of children with inflammatory bowel disease. Gastroenterology. 1994;106:1455–1466.
3. Reinecker HC, Steffen M, Witthoeft T et al. Enhanced secretion of tumour necrosis factor-alpha, IL-6, and IL-1-beta by isolated lamina propria mononuclear cells from patients with ulcerative colitis and Crohn's disease. Clin Exp Immunol. 1993;94:174–181.
4. Beutler B, Cerami A. The biology of cachectin/TNF-a primary mediator of the host response. Annu Rev Immunol. 1989;7:625–655.
5. Beutler B, Grau GE. Tumor necrosis factor in the pathogenesis of infectious diseases. Crit Care Med. 1993;21:S423.
6. Weil D. What's new about tumor necrosis factors? Eur Cytokine Netw. 1992;3:347–351.
7. Murch SH, Lamkin VA, Savage MO, Walker-Smith JA, MacDonald TT. Serum concentrations of tumour necrosis factor alpha in childhood chronic inflammatory bowel disease. Gut. 1991;32:913–917.
8. Braegger CP, Nicholls S, Murch SH, Stephens S, MacDonald TT. Tumour necrosis factor alpha in stool as a marker of intestinal inflammation. Lancet. 1992;339:89–91.
9. van Deventer SJH. Tumour necrosis factor and Crohn's disease. Gut. 1997;40:443–448.
10. van Dullemen HM, van Deventer SJ, Hommes DW et al. Treatment of Crohn's disease with anti-tumor necrosis factor chimeric monochlonal antibody (cA2). Gastroenterology. 1995;109:129–135.
11. Targan SR, Hanauer SB, van Deventer SJH et al. A short-term study of chimeric monoclonal antibody cA2 to tumor necrosis factor α for Crohn's disease. N Engl J Med. 1997;337:1029–1035.
12. Stack WA, Mann SD, Roy AJ et al. Randomised control trial of CDP571 antibody to tumor necrosis factor-α in Crohn's disease. Lancet. 1997;349:521–524.

13. MacDonald TT, Spencer J. Evidence that activated mucosal T cells play a role in the pathogenesis of enteropathy in human small intestine. J Exp Med. 1988;167:1341–1349.

14. Lionetti P, Breese E, Braegger CP, Murch SH, Taylor J, MacDonald TT. T cell activation can induce either mucosal destruction or adaptation in cultured human fetal small intestine. Gastroenterology. 1993;105:373–381.

15. Lionetti P, Spencer J, Breese EJ, Murch SH, Taylor J, MacDonald TT. Activation of mucosal Vβ3+ T cells and tissue damage in human small intestine by the bacterial superantigen, *Staphylococcus aureus* enterotoxin B. Eur J Immunol. 1993;23:664–668.

16. Monk T, Spencer J, Cerf-Bensussan N, MacDonald TT. Stimulation of mucosal T cells in situ with anti-CD3 antibody: location of the activated T cells and their distribution within the mucosal micro-environment. Clin Exp Immunol. 1988;74:216–222.

17. Fraser JD. High-affinity binding of staphylococcal enterotoxin A and B to HLADR. Nature. 1989;339:221–223.

18. Komisar JL, Small-Harris S, Tseng J. Localization of binding sites of Staphylococcal enterotoxin B (SEB), a superantigen for HLA-DR by inhibition with sythetic peptides of SEB. Infect Immun. 1994;62:4775–4780.

19. Spencer J, MacDonald TT, Isaacson PG. Heterogeneity of non-lymphoid cells expressing HLA-D region antigens in human fetal gut. Clin Exp Immunol. 1987;67:415–424.

20. Pender SLF, Lionetti P, Murch SH, Wathen N, MacDonald TT. Proteolytic degradation of intestinal mucosal extracellular matrix following lamina propria T cell activation. Gut. 1996;39:284–290.

21. Pender SLF, Tickle SP, Docherty AJP, Howie D, Wathen NC, MacDonald TT. A major role of matrix metalloproteinases in T cell injury in the gut. J Immunol. 1997;158:1582–1590.

22. Pender SLF, Breese EJ, Günther U et al. Suppression of T cell mediated injury in human gut by interleukin-10: role of matrix metalloproteinases. Gastroenterology. 1998;155:573–583.

23. Fuss IJ, Neurath M, Boirivant M et al. Disparate CD4+ lamina propria (LP) lymphokine secretion profiles in inflammatory bowel disease. Crohn's disease LP cells manifest increased secretion of IFN-gamma, whereas ulcerative colitis LP cells manifest increased secretion of IL-5. J Immunol. 1996;157:1261–1270.

24. Parronchi, P, Romagnani P, Annunziato F et al. Type 1 T-helper cell predominance and interleukin-12 expression in the gut of patients with Crohn's disease. Am J Pathol. 1997;150:823–832.

25. Woessner JF, Jr. Matrix metalloproteinases and their inhibitors in connective tissue remodelling. FASEB J. 1991;5:2145–2154.

26. Matrisian LM. The matrix-degrading metalloproteinases. Bioessays. 1992;14:455–463.

27. Birkedal-Hansen H, Moore WGI, Bodden MK et al. Matrix-metalloproteinases: a review. Crit Rev Oral Biol Med. 1993;4:197–250.

28. Ashkenazi A, Marsters SA, Capon DJ et al. Protection against endotoxic shock by a tumor necrosis factor receptor immunoadhesin. Proc Natl Acad Sci USA. 1991;88:10535–10539.

29. Loetscher H, Gentz R, Zulauf M et al. Recombinant 55-kDa tumor necrosis factor (TNF) receptor. Stoichiometry of binding to TNF alpha and TNF beta and inhibition of TNF activity. J Biol Chem. 1991;266:18324–18329.

30. Jin H, Yang R, Marsters SA et al. Protection against rat endotoxic shock by p55 tumor necrosis factor (TNF) receptor immunoadhesin: comparison with anti-TNF monoclonal antibody. J Infect Dis. 194;170:1323–1326.

31. Haak-Frendscho M, Marsters SA, Mordenti J et al. Inhibition of TNF by a TNF receptor immunoadhesin. Comparison to an anti-TNF monoclonal antibody. J Immunol. 1994;152:1347–1353.

32. Pender SLF, Fell JMC, Chamow SM, Ashkenazi A, MacDonald TT. A p55 tumor necrosis factor (TNF) receptor immunoadhesin prevents T cell-mediated intestinal injury by inhibiting matrix metalloproteinase production. J Immunol. 1998;160:4098–4103.

33. Targan SR, Deem RL, Liu M, Wang S, Nel A. Definition of a lamina propria T cell responsive state. Enhanced cytokine responsiveness of T cells stimulated through the CD2 pathway. J Immunol. 1995;154:664–675.

34. Rugtveit J, Nilsen EM, Bakka A, Carlsen H, Brandtzaeg P, Scott H. Cytokine profiles differ in newly recruited and resident subsets of mucosal macrophages from inflammatory bowel disease. Gastroenterology. 1997;112:1493–1505.

35. Beil WJ, Weller PF, Peppercorn MA, Galli SJ, Dvorak AM. Ultrastructural immunogold localization of subcellular sites of TNF-alpha in colonic Crohn's disease. J Leukocyte Biol. 1995;58:284–298.

36. Dayer JM, Beutler B, Cerami A. Cachetic/tumor necrosis factor stimulates collagenase and prostaglandin E2 production by human synovial cells and dermal fibroblasts. J Exp Med. 1985;162:2163–2168.
37. Meikle MC, Atkinson SJ, Ward RV, Murphy G, Reynolds JJ. Gingival fibroblasts degrade type l collagen films when stimulated with tumor necrosis factor and interleukin 1: evidence that breakdown is mediated by metalloproteinases. J Periodontal Res. 1989;24:207–214.
38. Ito A, Sato T, Iga T, Mori Y. Tumor necrosis factor bifunctionally regulates matrix metallo-proteinase and tissue inhibitor of metalloproteinase (TIMP) production by human fibroblasts. FEBS Lett. 1990;269:93–95.
39. Jasser MZ, Mitchell PG, Cheung HS. Induction of stromelysin-1 and collagenase synthesis in fibrochondrocytes by tumor necrosis factor-alpha. Matrix Biol.1994;14:241–249.
40. Galis ZS, Muszynski M, Sukhova GK, Simon-Morrissey E, Libby P. Enhanced expression of vascular matrix metalloproteinases induced in vitro by cytokines and in regions of human atherosclerotic lesions. Ann NY Acad Sci. 1995;748:501–507.
41. Mahida YR, Wu K, Jewell DP. Enhanced production of interleukin-1β by mononuclear cells isolated from mucosa with active ulcerative colitis or Crohn's disease. Gut. 1989;30:835–838.
42. Cominelli F, Nast CC, Duchini A, Lee M. Recombinant interleukin-1 receptor antagonist blocks the proinflammatory activity of endogenous interleukin-1 in rabbit immune colitis. Gastro-enterology. 1992;103:65–71.
43. Casini-Raggi V, Kam L, Chong YJ, Fiocchi C, Pizarro TT, Cominelli F. Mucosal imbalance of IL-1 and IL-1 receptor antagonist in inflammatory bowel disease. A novel mechanism of chronic intestinal inflammation. J Immunol. 1995;154:2434–2440.
44. Hyams JS, Fitzgerald JE, Wyzga N et al. Relationship of interleukin-1 receptor antagonist to mucosal inflammation in inflammatory bowel disease. J Pediatr Gastroenterol Nutr. 1995;21:419–425.
45. Sartor RB. Current concepts of the etiology and pathogenesis of colitis and Crohn's disease. Gastroenterol Clin North Am. 1995;24:475–507.

Section IV
Mechanisms of inflammatory disease 2: Role of luminal constituents, bacterial flora, and specific agents in inflammation

17
The role of bacterial flora in experimental models of intestinal inflammation

C. VELTKAMP and R. B. SARTOR

INTRODUCTION

Crohn's disease (CD) and ulcerative colitis (UC), collectively referred to as inflammatory bowel disease (IBD), result from a loss of immunoregulation probably caused by genetic and environmental factors[1]. Recently developed rodent models of intestinal inflammation allow the characterization of the influence of genetic alterations as well as exogenous factors in the development of chronic intestinal inflammation.

Observations in rodent models of inducible and spontaneously developing colitis provide strong evidence that resident enteric bacteria can induce and perpetuate chronic intestinal inflammation[2] (Table 1). Evidence supporting stimulation of inflammation by normal bacteria comes from observations that chronic inflammation in animal models preferentially occurs in the distal ileum and colon, which contain the highest load of predominantly anaerobic bacteria (10^{8-9} and 10^{10-12} colonies/g, respectively)[3]. The consistent and selective occurrence of colitis, without inflammation in most other organs where bacterial colonization is minimal, is the best evidence that colonic luminal bacteria provide the persistent stimulus to drive chronic inflammation[4].

Table 1 Experimental evidence implicating resident enteric bacteria in the pathogenesis of intestinal inflammation in rodent models

1. Inflammation occurs in areas of highest luminal bacterial concentrations.
2. Induction and perpetuation of inflammation by purified bacterial products (PG–PS, LPS).
3. Small bowel bacterial overgrowth induces and reactivates extraintestinal inflammation.
4. Attenuation of colitis and gastritis by caecal excision or bypass.
5. Prevention and treatment of intestinal and systemic inflammation by antibiotics.
6. Germ-free (sterile) environment attenuates acute injury and prevents chronic inflammation.
7. Increased cellular and humoral immune responses to endogenous enteric bacteria.

PG-PS, peptidoglycan-polysaccharide polymers; LPS, lipopolysaccharide

Table 2 The influence of the normal luminal bacterial environment on inflammation in animal models

Model	Species	SPF	Germ-free	Antibiotics
Indomethacin	Rat	Acute SB, colonic and gastric ulcers, chronic SB ulcers	Attenuated acute, absent chronic	⇓ by metronidazole, tetracycline
Carrageenan	Guinea pig	Caecal inflammation	No colitis	⇓ by metronidazole, clindamycin
HLA-B$_{27}$ transgenic	Rat	Gastritis, colitis, arthritis	No GI or joint inflammation	⇓ by metronidazole, vancomycin/ imipenem
CD45RB^{hi} → SCID	Mouse	Colitis	No colitis	⇓ by streptomycin and bacitracin
IL-2$^{-/-}$	Mouse	Colitis, gastritis, hepatitis	Absent-attenuated inflammation	ND
IL-10$^{-/-}$	Mouse	Colitis, gastritis	No inflammation	⇓ by metronidazole, cipro, vancomycin/ imipenem
TCR$\alpha^{-/-}$	Mouse	Colitis	No inflammation	ND

SB, small bowel; GI, gastrointestinal; ND, not done; ⇓, attenuation of disease.

The absence or attenuation of disease in animals raised in germ-free facilities or treated with antibiotics (Table 2) provides direct evidence that bacteria play an important role in intestinal inflammation[4,5]. Interestingly, not all bacteria have the same potential to induce and perpetuate inflammation[6]. In some rodent models certain bacterial strains have a preferential ability to induce chronic inflammation[7,8]. Other bacteria may be neutral or even able to diminish the inflammation[9,10].

The present review summarizes evidence that enteric pathogens or bacterial flora have an aetiological or contributory role in experimental animal models of chronic intestinal inflammation.

CHEMICALLY INDUCED COLITIS

Continuous administration of 5% acid-degraded *carrageenan* in the drinking water leads to ulceration of the large intestine and the colon in guinea pigs[11]. The inducing agent used in this model is a sulphated polysaccharide, often used as a thickening agent in food products. Bacteria are important for the development of disease since germ-free guinea pigs treated in an identical manner do not develop colitis[8]. Treatment with metronidazole prevents ulcerations[12], suggesting a role for anaerobes in this model. Selective bacterial colonization studies indicate that *Bacteroides vulgatus* preferentially induces colitis in this model[8,13]. Monoassociation of germ-free guinea pigs with *B. vulgatus* along with carrageenan feeding produces ulceration, but, in absence of the chemical agent, the organism does not cause any lesions[14]. Interestingly, the immunization of guinea pigs with outer membrane from *B. vulgatus* further enhances colonic inflammation in this model[15].

Subcutanous administration of the NSAID *indomethacin* produces inflammation of the distal jejunum, proximal ileum and colon in a dose-dependent fashion in rats. Initial epithelial damage[16] and genetically determined host susceptibility of different rat strains[17] are pathogenetic factors in this model. Ubiquitous luminal bacteria and bacterial products play an important role in the pathogenesis of the disease. Germ-free littermates develop only attenuated acute inflammation and lack chronic enteritis and periportal hepatic inflammation[18]. Feeding of bacterial polymers worsens intestinal ulcers[19]. In contrast, treatment with metronidazole and tetracycline attenuates the inflammation in this model[20].

Another chemical that induces acute and chronic colitis in mice, rats and hamsters[21,22] is *dextran sulphate sodium* (DSS). Mice treated orally with DSS develop a mild to moderate left-sided colitis characterized by focal areas of inflammation and crypt abscesses. Dieleman *et al.*[23] showed that the acute phase of DSS-induced colitis is not dependent on T or B lymphocytes since it is also inducible in SCID mice, which lack these cells. The earliest change seen after DSS treatment is a loss of crypts[22]. The role of luminal bacteria in this model is controversial: metronidazole and ciprofloxacin prevent inflammation, whereas imipenem and vancomycin can treat established colitis[24]. However, Bylund-Fellenius *et al.*[25] showed that DSS-induced colitis is more severe in germ-free mice than in mice with a normal microbial environment.

PG–PS ENTEROCOLITIS

Bacterial cell wall polymers such as lipopolysaccharide (LPS, endotoxin) and peptidoglycan-polysaccharide polymers (PG–PS) can cause colitis in susceptible hosts[26,27]. PG–PS is the primary structural component of cell walls of nearly all bacteria. Enterocolitis, associated in the chronic phase with fibrosis, arthritis, hepatic granulomas and anaemia, results when PG–PS derived from group A streptococci (PG-APS) is injected into the intestine of rats[28,29]. Acute intestinal inflammation develops at the site of subserosal injection in Lewis, Sprague-Dawley, Buffalo and Fischer rats. In contrast chronic granulomatous, fibrotic enterocolitis spontaneously reactivates only in Lewis rats and to a lesser extent in Sprague-Dawley rats[30]. Non-MHC genes must be responsible for this different susceptibility because Lewis and Fischer rats are MHC identical. Lewis rats differ from Fischer rats in that the immune responsiveness is overly aggressive in Lewis rats. They have a defective hypothalamic-pituitary-adrenal axis response to cytokines and bacterial products[31], resulting in an inadequate peripheral corticosteroid response. It has also been shown that the plasma kallikrein-kinin pathway is activated in Lewis rats after intestinal PG-APS injections whereas no activation was detected in the low-responding Buffalo rats[29]. As in all other animal models, the chronic phase of the inflammation is T cell dependent because it does not occur in T-lymphocyte-deficient rats and is prevented by cyclosporin-A[32].

Sterile luminal PG–PS polymers also potentiate colitis induced by *acetic acid* and enteritis caused by *indomethacin*[19,33], indicating that nonviable bacterial products in the lumen can perpetuate intestinal inflammation. Conversely, Lewis rats raised in a sterile environment do not develop chronic intestinal inflammation after subcutaneous indomethacin injection[18].

ANIMAL MODELS WITH SPONTANEOUSLY DEVELOPING COLITIS

Bacteria are likely to play a role in the colitis which develops spontaneously around the third to fourth week of life in *C3H/HeJ* Bir mice: this is the time when bacterial colonization of the gut occurs. The caecum and right colon develop a mild inflammation which resolves by 10–12 weeks of age[34]. Perianal ulcerations also occur in these mice, accompanied by increased levels of interleukin-4 (IL-4), IgG1, IgE and also IgG2a[35]. C3H/HeJ Bir mice have a high frequency of serum antibodies to antigens of the normal enteric bacterial flora[36]. Recently, it has been shown that CD4+ T cells from mice with colitis respond *in vitro* to enteric bacteria but not to food or epithelial antigens and they have a T_H1 profile of lymphokines[37]. Bacteria-responsive CD4+ T cells transfer colitis to SCID mice, which is a direct demonstration of their involvement in the pathogenesis of intestinal inflammation in this animal model.

Rats with an *overexpression of the human HLA-class I molecule HLA-B27 together with β_2 microglobulin* present a well studied animal model of intestinal inflammation. Transgenic rats, especially females, spontaneously develop gastroduodenitis, colitis, arthritis and spondylitis[38]. Diarrhoea develops between 5 and 20 weeks of age and is the earliest clinical manifestation. Arthritis usually follows the onset of colitis by several weeks[38,39]. In contrast to conventionally raised rats, germ-free rats develop neither intestinal inflammation nor arthritis[7,40]. These results emphasize the pathogenic role of bacteria in this animal model. Rath *et al.*[7] showed that B27 transgenic rats develop active colitis and gastritis within 1 month of exposure to specific pathogen-free bacteria and implicated resident anaerobic flora by demonstrating a protective effect of metronidazole on colitis and gastritis[41]. Reconstitution studies show that *B. vulgatus* is uniquely capable of inducing colitis in HLA-B27 transgenic rats[7]. Several other bacteria, including *E. coli*, *Peptostreptococcus*, *Eubacteria* and *Group D streptococci* did not influence inflammation in this model. Importantly, these studies indicate that not all bacteria have the same capacity to induce colitis.

Selective *gene targeting that deletes IL-10* in mice leads to a chronic intestinal inflammation with the duodenum, proximal jejunum and proximal colon being most severely affected[42]. Inflammation probably occurs due to the missing regulatory function of IL-10 as a potent inhibitor of macrophages and T_H1 lymphocytes. The important role of the intestinal bacterial flora as a modulator of the immune response is shown by the fact that IL-10-deficient mice raised under SPF conditions develop inflammation limited to the colon and germ-free mice have no evidence of colitis and immune system activation[43]. Adult germ-free mice develop caecal inflammation as early as 1 week after colonization with specific pathogen free bacteria. Administration of broad-spectrum antibiotics to IL-10 knockout mice has a beneficial effect both on the onset and the progression of the intestinal inflammation[44]. Total caecal bacterial concentrations were 1–2 logs fewer in vancomycin/imipenem-treated animals than in untreated animals, which points to the total luminal bacterial load as an important factor for initiation and perpetuation of colonic inflammation in this model.

Recent studies have shown that colonization of IL-10 deficient mice with *Lactobacillus plantarum* attenuates established colitis[9]. These results are in agreement with Madsen *et al.*[10], who showed that native *Lactobacillus* sp. prevents colitis in this model and suggest a potential role for probiotic therapy in human IBD.

Sadlack *et al.*[45] showed similar responses to resident enteric bacteria in *IL-2 knockout mice*. Animals kept in a conventional environment developed normally during the first 3–4 weeks of age, but then soon showed severe autoimmune anaemia with a mortality rate of 50% in the first 9 weeks. Surviving animals developed chronic aggressive colonic and hepatobiliary inflammation beginning between 6 and 15 weeks of age. The disease was progressive, leading to death within 10–25 weeks. Even this severe disease was completely absent in IL-2-deficient mice raised in a germ-free facility[45]. Contractor *et al.*[46] showed that although their germ-free IL-2 knockout animals were colitis free, lymphoid hyperplasia, autoimmunity and compromised intestinal intraepithelial lymphocyte development still occurred. Consequently these data demonstrate that colitis in SPF mice depends upon the presence of intestinal bacterial flora. However, bacterial and dietary antigens present in dead bacteria in the autoclaved rodent food seem to be sufficient to cause inflammation, since germ-free IL-2 knockout animals in our own gnotobiotic facility showed mild focal intestinal inflammation[47].

Mice deficient in either α or β chain of the T cell receptor (TCR) spontaneously develop colitis and a progressive wasting syndrome by 3–4 months of age, which results in death by 6–9 months of age[48]. Small bowel and other organs are not involved in the disease. The histological features together with the selective involvement of the large intestine are reminiscent of human UC. The exact pathological mechanism in this experimental model is not known, but this model has a unique activation of T_H2 lymphocytes[49]. Bacteria play an important role in this model since mice fail to develop colitis in the absence of a microbial environment[50]. It is of special interest that although SPF animals develop colitis with a high level of penetrance, colonization of germ-free mice with a limited bacterial spectrum consisting of *Lactobacillus plantarum, Streptococcus faecalis, S. faecium*, and/or *E. coli* does not cause intestinal inflammation[50]. These observations underline the hypothesis that not all bacteria are important in chronic intestinal inflammation but that a specific organism or group of organisms normally presented in the gut is responsible for the induction of colitis in susceptible hosts.

Severe combined immune deficiency (SCID) mice have a spontaneous genetic mutation in receptor recombination (T cell receptor, immunoglobulin genes) that results in a T and B cell defect with a deficiency of both cell lines. These mice have an innate immune system, however, and remain healthy if kept in SPF facilities. The SCID mouse is ideal to study the function of subsets of immune cells by adoptive cell transfer into these mice. Transfer of CD4+ T cells expressing high levels of CD4+, CD45RB[hi] subsets results in a disease manifested by chronic intestinal inflammation, involving mainly the colon, and a wasting syndrome[51,52]. Interestingly, transfer of the entire unfractionated CD4[+] population does not result in disease, nor does transfer of the reciprocal subset expressing low levels of the CD45RB molecule (CD4[+], CD45RB[lo])[51–54]. The function of CD4[+], CD45RB[lo] was further clarified by experiments showing that cotransfer of the CD4[+], CD45RB[lo] or of the whole CD4 T cells along with the disease inducing CD4[+], CD45RB[li] T cell subsets prevent disease. Antibiotic treatment with bacitracin and streptomycin ameliorated the wasting syndrome[54], suggesting a role of the gut bacterial flora in the development of disease. In SCID mice that have significantly reduced numbers of enteric bacteria wasting and colitis are significantly attenuated[55]. It has been shown recently that optimal engraftment of intestinal T cells required bacterial flora, as the number of mucosal lymphocytes was greatly reduced in SCID recipients with reduced flora[56].

Terhorst and colleagues have demonstrated that *over-expression of the CD3ε chain* in mice results in a block of prothymocyte development resulting in a complete T cell depletion and lack of thymus development[57]. When these Tgε26 mice are transplanted with bone marrow from normal donor animals they develop a wasting syndrome and colitis 4–8 weeks after transplantation[58]. Activated T cells are found in the large intestine of sick animals and transfer of mesenteric lymph node cells from sick animals into unreconstituted Tε26 mice leads to similar inflammation. CD4 T cells from sick Tgε26 mice can also transfer disease to Rag-2[−/−] mice. On the other hand, bone marrow from Rag 2[−/−] or TCR[−/−] mice fails to induce colitis in Tgε 26 mice. From these experiments it can be concluded that T cells mediate the disease in this experimental model. Transplant of a neonatal thymus prior to bone marrow transfer prevents disease, suggesting that colitis is the result of the lack of negative thymic selection of aggressive CD4[+] T lymphocytes. Our preliminary unpublished data suggest that the intestinal bacteria present the antigenetic stimulus that activates the abnormal T cell population, because germ-free animals seem to be disease free.

SUMMARY

There is a wide range of susceptibility factors in different rodent models of intestinal inflammation which might in part resemble the aetiological heterogeneity in human IBD. Nevertheless, an overwhelming body of experimental evidence indicates that the normal resident intestinal bacterial flora provides the antigenic stimulus that leads to colitis in susceptible hosts.

Absence of colitis in germ-free animals argues against the possibility of an autoimmune aetiology suggested in some models and shows that bacteria are either the necessary antigenic stimulus or provide adjuvant-like stimulation of the immune response. Monoassociation and exposure of germ-free animals to various 'cocktails' of bacteria provides the possibility to find out which dominant bacterial stimuli provide the antigenic drive for inflammation. Existing data suggest that these stimuli might be different in separate animal models and might therefore be different in genetic subsets of patients. Future studies will be required to identify potential mechanisms by which luminal bacteria and bacterial constituents initiate and sustain chronic, immune-mediated intestinal inflammation in genetically susceptible hosts (Table 3).

Table 3   Potential mechanisms of mucosal immune activation

1. Activation of resident macrophages and dendritic cells (cytokine secretion, APC activity)
2. Antigen-specific stimulation of T lymphocytes
3. Antigen-specific humoral immune responses
4. Induction of autoimmune responses (molecular mimicry, adjuvant effects)
5. Disruption of the mucosal barrier (cytolytic or mucolytic enzymes, metabolic toxins)
6. Modulation of immunoregulatory cell function

References

1. Sartor RB, Pathogenesis and immune mechanisms of chronic inflammatory bowel diseases. Am J Gastroenterol. 1997;92:5S.
2. Sartor RB. Microbial factors in the pathogenesis of Crohn's disease, ulcerative colitis and experimental intestinal inflammation. In: Kirsner JB, Shorter RG (eds). Inflammatory Bowel Disease, 4th edn. Baltimore: Williams & Wilkins, 1995:96–124.
3. Simon GL, Gorbach S. Normal alimentary tract microflora. In: Blaser MJ, Smith PD, Ravdin JL, Greenberg HB, Guerrant RL (eds). Infections of the GI tract. New York: Raven Press, 1995:53–69.
4. Sartor RB. Insights into the pathogenesis of inflammatory bowel disease provided by new rodent models of spontaneous colitis. Inflam Bowel Dis. 1995;1:64–75.
5. Schultz M, Sartor RB. Aberrant host responses to luminal bacteria in the pathogenesis of chronic intestinal inflammation. In: Ernst PB, Michetti P, Smith PD (eds). The Immunobiology of *H. pylori*: From Pathogenesis to Prevention. Philadelphia: Lippincott-Raven, 1997:167–182.
6. Sartor RB. Enteric microflora in IBD: pathogens or commensals? Inflamm Bowel Dis. 1997;3:230–235.
7. Rath HC, Herfarth HH, Ikeda JS et al. Normal luminal bacteria, especially *Bacteroides* species, mediate chronic colitis, gastritis, and arthritis in HLA-B27/humanβ_2 microglobulin transgenic rats. J Clin Invest. 1996;4:945–953.
8. Onderdonk AB, Franklin ML, Cisneros RL. Production of experimental ulcrative colitis in gnotobiotic guinea pigs with simplified microflora. Infect Immun. 1981;4:225–231.
9. Schultz M, Veltkamp C, Dieleman LA, Wyrick PB, Tonkonogy SL, Sartor RB. Continuous feeding of *Lactobacillus plantarum* attenuates established colitis in interleukin-10 deficient mice. Gastroenterology. 1998;114:A1081.
10. Madsen KL, Taverni MM, Doyle JSG, Fedorak RN. *Lactobacillus* sp prevents development of enterocolitis in interleukin-10 gene deficient mice. Gastroenterology. 1997;112:A1030.
11. Watt J, Marcus R. Carrageenan induced ulceration of the large intestine in the guinea pig. Gut. 1991;12:164–171.
12. Onderdonk AB, Hermos JA, Drink JI, Battlett JG. Protective effect of metronidazole in experimental ulcerative colitis. Gastroenterology. 1978;74:521–526.
13. Oestreicher P, Nielsen ST, Rainsford KD. Inflammatory bowel disease induced by combined bacterial immunization and oral carrageenan in guinea pigs. Model development, histopathology, and effects of sulfasalazine. Dig Dis Sci. 1991;36:461–470.
14. Onderdonk AB, Bronson R, Cisneros RL. Comparison of *Bacteroides vulgatus* strains in the enhancement of experimental ulcerative colitis. Infect Immun. 1987;55:835–836.
15. Breeling JL, Onderdonk AB, Cisneros RL, Kasper DL. *Bacteroides vulgatus* outer membrane antigens associated with carrageenan-induced colitis in guinea pigs. Infect Immun. 1988;56:1754–1759.
16. Elson CO, Sartor RB, Tennyson GS, Riddell RH. Experimental models of inflammatory bowel disease. Gastroenterology. 1995;109:1344–1367.
17. Sartor RB. Susceptibility of inbred rat strains to intestinal inflammation induced by indomethacin. Gastroenterology. 1992;102:A690.
18. Sartor RB. Absolute requirement for ubiquitous luminal bacteria in the pathogenesis of chronic intestinal inflammation. Gastroenterology. 1994;106:A767.
19. Davis SW, Holt LC, Sartor RB. Luminal bacteria and bacterial polymers potentiate indomethacin-induced intestinal injury in the rat. Gastroenterology. 1990;98:A444.
20. Yamada T, Deitch E, Specian RD, Perry MA, Sartor RB, Grisham MB. Mechanisms of acute and chronic intestinal inflammation induced by indomethacin. Inflammation. 1993;17:641–662.

21. Okayasu I, Hatakeyama S, Yamada M, Ohkusa T, Inagaki Y, Nakaya R. A novel method in the induction of reliable experimental acute and chronic ulcerative colitis in mice. Gastroenterology. 1990;98:694–702.

22. Cooper HS, Murthy SNS Shah RS, Sedergran DJ. Clinicopathologic study of dextran sulfate sodium experimental murine colitis. Lab Invest. 1993;69:238–249.

23. Dieleman LA, Ridwan BU, Tennyson GS, Beagley DW, Bucy RP, Elson CO. Dextran sulfate sodium-induced colitis occurs in severe combined immunodeficient mice. Gastroenterology. 1994;107:1643–1652.

24. Rath HC, Schultz M, Dieleman LA et al. Selective vs broad spectrum antibiotics in the prevention and treatment of experimental colitis in two rodent models. Gastroenterology. 1998;114:A1067.

25. Bylund-Fellenius A-C, Landstroem E, Acelsson L-G, Midtvedt T. Experimental colitis induced by dextran sulphate in normal and germfree mice. Microb Ecol Health Dis. 1994;7:207–215.

26. Chadwick VS, Anderson RP. Microorganisms and their products in inflammatory bowel disease. In: MacDermott RP (ed): Inflammatory Bowel Disease. Elsevier: New York, 1992:241–258.

27. Schwab JH. Phlogistic properties of peptidoglycan-polysaccharide polymers from cell walls of pathogenic and normal-flora bacteria which colonize humans. Infect Immun. 1993;61: 4535–4539.

28. Sartor RB Cromartie WJ, Powell DW, Schwab JH. Granulomatous enterocolitis in rats by purified bacterial cell wall fragments. Gastroenterology. 1985;89:587–595.

29. Sartor RB, De La Cadena RA, Green KD et al. Selective kallikrein-kinin system activation in inbred rats differentially susceptible to granulomatous enterocolitis. Gastroenterology. 1996;110: 1467–1481.

30. McCall RD, Haskill S, Zimmerman EM et al. Tissue interleukin-1 and interleukin-1 receptor antagonist expression in enterocolitis in resistant and susceptible rats. Gastroenterology. 1994;106:960–972.

31. Sternberg EM, Hill JM, Chrousos GP et al. Inflammatory mediator-induced hypothalamic-pituitary-adrenal activation is defective in streptococcal cell wall arthritis-susceptible Lewis rats. Proc Natl Acad Sci USA. 1989;86:2374–2378.

32. Sartor RB, Bender DE, Allen JB et al. Chronic experimental enterocolitis and extraintestinal inflammation are T lymphocyte dependent. Gastroenterology. 1993;104:A775.

33. Sartor RB, Bond TM, Schwab JH. Systemic uptake and intestinal inflammatory effects of luminal bacterial cell wall polymers in rats with acute colonic injury. Infect Immun. 1988;56: 2101–2108.

34. Sundberg JP, Elson CO, Bedigian HL, Birkenmeier EH. Spontaneous, heritable colitis in a new substrain of C3H/HeJ mice. Gastroenterology. 1994;107:1726–1735.

35. Tonkonogy SL, Sartor RB. Immune system activation in C3H/HeJBir mice exhibiting spontaneous perianal ulceration. Inflamm Bowel Dis. 1997;3:10–19.

36. Brandwein SL, McCabe RP, Cong Y et al. Spontaneously colitic C3H/HeJBir mice demonstrate selective antibody reactivity to antigens of the enteric bacterial flora. J Immunol. 1997;159: 44–52.

37. Cong BY, Brandwein SL, McCabe RP et al. CD4$^+$ T cells reactive to enteric bacterial antigens in spontaneously colitic C3H/JeJBir mice: increased T helper cell type 1 response and ability to transfer disease. J Exp Med. 1998;187:855–864.

38. Hammer RE, Maika SD, Richardson JA, Tang JP, Taurog JD. Spontaneous inflammatory disease in transgenic rats expressing HLA-B27 and human beta 2m: an animal model of HLA-B27-associated human disorders. Cell. 1990;63:1099–1112.

39. Taurog JD, Maika SD, Simmons WA, Braban M, Hammer RE. Susceptibility to inflammatory disease in HLA-B27 transgenic rat lines correlates with the level of B27 expression. J Immunol. 1993;150:4168–4178.

40. Taurog JD, Richardson JA, Croft JT et al. The germfree state prevents development of gut and joint inflammatory disease in HLA-B27 transgenic rats. J Exp Med. 1994;180:2359–2364.

41. Rath HC, Bender DE, Holt LC et al. Metronidazole attenuates colitis in HLA-B27/β2-m trangenic (TG) rats: a pathogenic role for anaerobic bacteria. Clin Immunol Immunopathol. 1995;76 (suppl):S45.

42. Kuehn R, Loehler J, Rennick D, Rejewski K, Mueller W. Interleukin-10-deficient mice develop chronic enterocolitis. Cell. 1993;75:263–274.

43. Sellon R, Tonkonogy SL, Schultz M, Sartor RB. Absence of gastritis and colitis in germ free IL-10 knockout mice. Gastroenterology. 1997;112:A1088.

44. Braat H, Kieleman LA, Sellon RK, Schultz M, Sartor RB. Effects of antibiotics on the initiation and perpetuation of colitis in the IL-10 ko mice. Gastroenterology. 1998;114:A1081.
45. Sadlack B, Merz H, Schorle H, Schimpl A, Feller AC, Horak K. Ulcerative colitis-like disease in mice with a disrupted interleukin-2 gene. Cell. 1993;75:253–261.
46. Contractor NV, Bassiri H, Reya T et al. Lymphoid hyperplasia, autoimmunity, and compromised intraepithelial lymphocyte development in colitis-free gnotobiotic IL-2-deficient mice. J Immunol. 1998;160:385–394.
47. Schultz M, Sellon RK, Tonkonogy SL, Balish E, Sartor RB. IL-2 deficient mice raised under germfree conditions develop delayed mild focal intestinal inflammation and progressive loss of B cells. Gastroenterology. 1997;112:A1086.
48. Mombaerts P, Mizoguchi E, Grusby MJ, Glimcher LH, Bhan AK, Tonegawa S. Spontaneous development of inflammatory bowel disease in T cell receptor mutant mice. Cell. 1993;75: 275–282.
49. Mizoguchi E, Mizoguchi A, Bhan AK. Role of cytokines in the early stages of chronic colitis in TCR alpha-mutant mice. Lab Invest. 1997;76:385–397.
50. Dianda L, Hanby AM, Wright NA, Sebesteny A, Hayday AC, Owen MJ. T cell receptor-$\alpha\beta$-deficient mice fail to develop colitis in the absence of a microbial environment. Am J Pathol. 1997;150:91–97.
51. Powrie F, Leach MW, Mauze S, Caddle LB, Coffman RL. Phenotypically distinct subsets of CD4[+] T cells induce or protect from chronic intestinal inflammation in C.B-17 scid mice. Int Immunol. 1993;5:1461–1471.
52. Morrissey PJ, Charrier K, Braddy S, Liggitt D, Watston JD. CD4 T cells that express high levels of CD45RB induce wasting disease when transferred into congenic severe combined immuno-deficient mice. Disease development is prevented by cotransfer of purified CD4[+] T cells. J Exp Med. 1993;178:273–4.
53. Powrie F, Correa-Oliveira R, Mauze S, Coffman RL. Regulatory interactions between CD45RB[high] and CD45RB[low] CD4[+] T cells are important for the balance between protective and pathogenic cell-mediated immunity. J Exp Med. 1994;179:589–600.
54. Morrissey PJ, Charrier K. Induction of wasting disease in SCID mice by the transfer of normal CD4[+]/CD45RB[hi] T cells and the regulation of this autoreactivity by CD4[+]/CD45RB[lo] T cells. Res Immunol. 1994;145:357–362.
55. Aranda R, Sydora BC, McAllister PL et al. Analysis of intestinal lymphocytes in mouse colitis mediated by transfer of CD4[+], CD45RB[high] T cells to SCID recipients. J Immunol. 1997;158: 3464–3473.
56. Camerini V, Sydora BC, Aranda R et al. Generation of intestinal mucosal lymphocytes in SCID mice reconstituted with mature, thymus-derived T cells. J Immunol. 1998;160:2608–2618.
57. Hollander GA, Wang B, Nichogiannopoulou A et al. Developmental control point in induction of thymic cortex regulated by a subpopulation of prothymocytes. Nature. 1995;373:350–353.
58. Hollander GA, Simpson SJ, Mizoguchi E et al. Severe colitis in mice with aberrant thymic selection. Immunity. 1995;3:27–38.

18
Role of normal intestinal flora

R. DUCHMANN

INTRODUCTION

The normal gastrointestinal (GI) microflora represents a complex ecosystem and comprises 10 times more bacteria than the body contains cells. In the adult individual, the vertical and horizontal composition of the microflora along the intestinal canal is remarkably organized and the result of an orderly and successive colonization process. The mechanisms of colonization are very complex and therefore difficult to sort out, but there is reason to believe that in addition to purely microbiological influences, the immune system and the genetics of an individual are important contributing factors. In the healthy individual, bacteria from the GI microflora sustain normal functions of the host, protect it against colonization by pathogenic bacteria and are important for the normal development of the host immune system and GI morphology. Thus, the intestinal flora normally exerts a variety of beneficial effects and offers effective protection against the development of inflammatory diseases. However, under conditions when either the normal flora or the host is disturbed, inflammatory diseases may ensue. Abnormal metabolic, microbiological and immunological interactions between the normal GI flora and the host can all contribute to mechanisms of inflammatory disease.

THE FLORA WITHIN THE HUMAN GI TRACT

Definition of gastrointestinal flora

Today, the cosmos of microorganisms that normally inhabit the GI tract is generally referred to as the indigenous flora or normal flora. Definitions of the gastrointestinal flora generally appreciate the fact that the gastrointestinal flora is not a random assortment of bacteria, but results from a co-evolutionary process which involves both microbial and host factors. As recently reviewed by Berg[1], the indigenous flora was described by Dubos *et al.*[2] in 1965 as comprising three types of microorganisms: first, ubiquitous microorganisms that were present during the evolution of an animal and therefore colonize the GI tract of all members of a particular animal species (autochthonous flora); second, microorganisms that are so ubiquitous in a local environment that they colonize the GI tract of all members of a particular community, but which are not necessarily present in all communities of a given animal species (normal flora), and lastly, microorganisms that are acquired accidentally and are able to persist in tissues of at least some members of a community (true pathogens). Twelve years later, Savage redefined the gastrointestinal flora by distinguishing microorganisms present in all normal adults of an animal species (autochthonous flora) from those which only transiently colonize an intestinal habitat and need not be present in a larger number of members of that species (allochthonous or transient flora).

Organization of normal intestinal microflora in the human GI tract

The normal intestinal microflora shows a striking level of vertical and horizontal organization. Thus, in human adult individuals, characteristic population levels are maintained in defined regions along the alimentary canal. In the oral cavity about 200 different bacterial species are present. Some of these bacteria are involved in the pathogenesis of dental plaque[3], an important medical problem and a major source of morbidity and health care expenses[4]. The oesophagus is usually devoid of bacteria and the stomach, duodenum and jejunum generally contain only relatively small numbers of mostly acid tolerant bacteria. These bacteria are thought to represent a transient flora made up by bacteria which were taken up orally and survived the acid milieu in the stomach. Among the bacteria found in the upper GI tract, *H. pylori* may form a notable exception. Clearly pathogenic in some individuals, *H. pylori* colonizes the stomach of more than half the adult population in the world and also seems to exert effects that are beneficial for the host[5]. Whether *H. pylori* should therefore be regarded a member of the normal flora is currently under discussion.

In the ileum, which represents a transition zone to the colon, the number of bacteria and bacterial species rises sharply, reaching its maximal complexity of 10^{10}–10^{11} bacteria/g and > 400 species in the colon. The terminal ileum and colon are affected most often in inflammatory bowel disease (IBD), suggesting that components of the normal flora may be important in IBD pathogenesis[6].

Most of our current knowledge on the composition of the normal intestinal flora within the alimentary canal has been generated from studies of faecal or luminal flora. Luminal flora, however, resides in but one of several horizontally oriented habitats (Figure 1), which may differ considerably from each other[7,8]. Colonization of habitats closer to the bowel wall is likely to be influenced by characteristics of the specific mucus which overlies the intestinal epithelium or the deeper layers within the intestinal crypts of Lieberkühn[1]. Here cryptdins, a fascinating group of recently described peptides with potent antimicrobial activity produced by Paneth cells, may further shape the bacterial colonization process[9]. In addition, special bacterial characteristics may be required to allow direct bacterial adherence to the epithelial cell or even invasion of the bowel wall. New techniques for the definition of intramural bacteria, which may be especially important for the induction of mucosal immune responses, are now available. Since the intestinal flora is thus diversified, investigations into abnormalities involved in the pathogenesis of a disease will only be meaningful if the relevant habitat is selected for study.

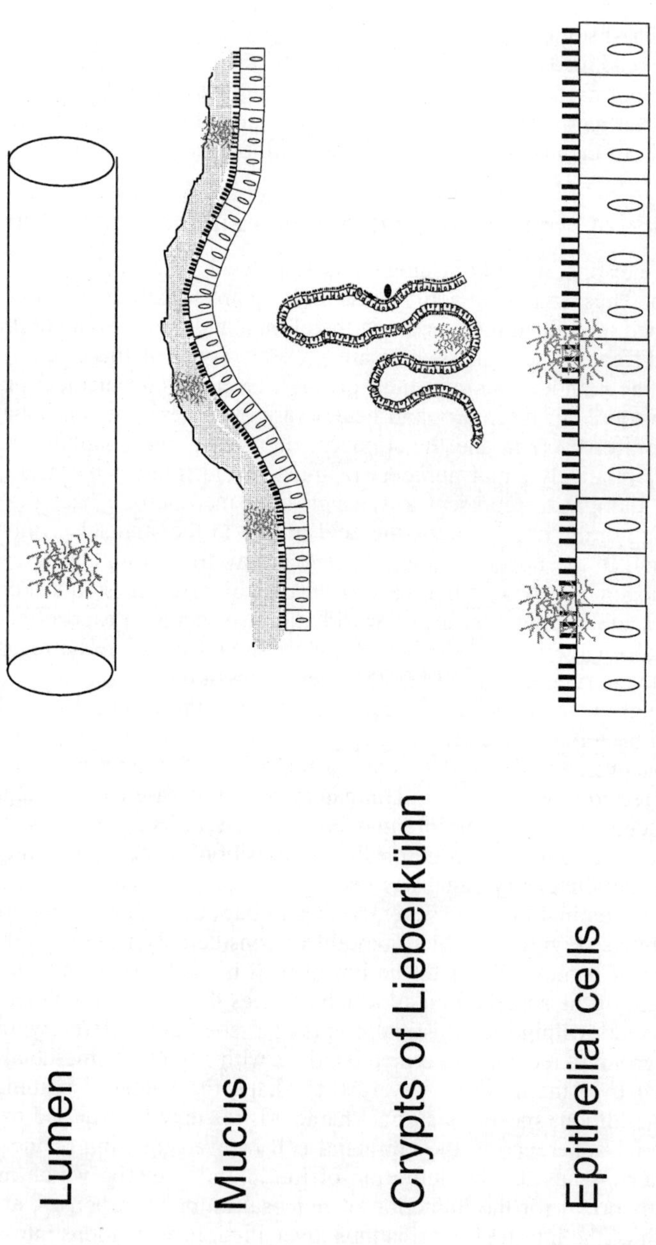

Figure 1 **Major horizontal bacterial habitats.** The normal intestinal microflora shows a striking level of vertical and horizontal organization. Individual habitats may have specific functions for intestinal physiology and disease pathogenesis.

INTESTINAL FLORA IN HEALTH AND DISEASE

Protective influences of the normal flora

One group of protective influences of the normal intestinal flora is related to its metabolic activity, which has been estimated to be potentially equal to that of the human liver[1]. Metabolic activities include the synthesis of vitamins (K and B complex), the metabolism of bile acid and the anaerobic microbial fermentation of polysaccharides which results in the production of significant amounts of short-chain fatty acids (SCFA). SCFA, and especially *n*-butyrate, represent a major fuel among the substrates available to the human colonic mucosa[10] and may, therefore, have positive effects on intestinal barrier function. Consistent with this putative beneficial role, irrigation with SCFA or butyrate alone has been shown to improve inflammation in diversion colitis or distal ulcerative colitis[11,12].

In addition to its metabolic effects, the normal flora has the ability to prevent pathogenic bacteria from colonizing the alimentary canal and causing disease. Competition for epithelial adhesion receptors, competition for carbon and energy sources or the production of antimicrobial substances are important factors mediating this colonization resistance (Figure 2). For example, *bifido-bacteria* inhibit the association of enterotoxigenic, enteropathogenic, diffusely adhering *Escherichia coli* and *Salmonella typhimurium* strains with enterocytes and inhibit epithelial invasion by enteropathogenic *E. coli, Yersinia pseudo-tuberculosis,* and *S. typhimurium* strains[13]. Bifidobacteria also excrete anti-microbial substances[14] and reduce the incidence of acute diarrhoea and rotavirus

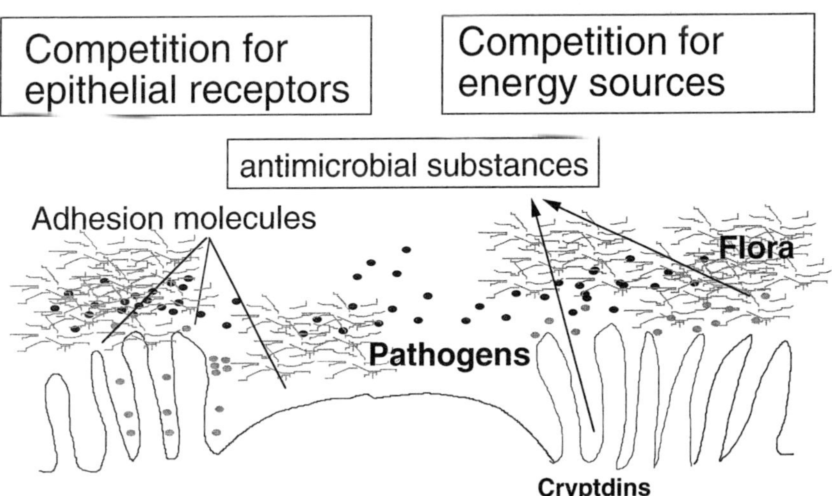

Figure 2 Colonization resistance. Competition between normal flora and pathogenic bacteria for epithelial adhesion receptors, carbon and energy sources and the production of cryptdins or other antimicrobial substances can prevent pathogenic bacteria from stably colonizing the intestinal tract. Enhancing the concentration of protective bacteria within the intestinal flora may thus be useful for prevention or treatment of inflammatory intestinal disorders.

shedding in infants[15,16]. Clearly, diminished concentrations of protective bacteria may facilitate disease induction by pathogenic bacteria[17]. Enhancing the concentrations of protective bacteria within the intestinal flora may be of therapeutic benefit in the prevention or treatment of inflammatory intestinal disorders[18–21].

Inflammatory influences of the normal flora

Passage of viable bacteria from the GI tract to the mesenteric lymph nodes and to other organs is defined as bacterial translocation (Figure 3). Whereas a low level of translocation can be seen in healthy individuals, increased bacterial translocation with systemic spread seems to play a central role in the pathogenesis of the systemic inflammatory response syndrome (SIRS), which may progress to multi-organ failure and death[22]. Increased bacterial translocation may occur in immunocompromised individuals (immunosuppressive treatment, cancer, AIDS, etc), patients with physical damage to their intestinal barrier (ischaemia/reperfusion injury, endotoxin or haemorrhagic shock) or patients who develop intestinal overgrowth following disruption of their GI ecology (oral antibiotics, protein malnutrition, shock)[1].

Bacteria from the normal intestinal flora are also implicated in the pathogenesis of intestinal inflammation and arthritis[23]. *Bacteroides vulgatus* has recently been identified as a critical bacterium mediating chronic colitis, gastritis, and arthritis in HLA-B27/human β_2-microglobulin transgenic rats[24]. The same bacterium was shown to play an essential role in the pathogenesis of carrageenan-induced colitis in guinea pigs[25,26]. The reason for the increased capacity of *B. vulgatus* to induce intestinal inflammation in these animal models is unknown and may include immunological and non-immunological causes. *Bacteroides* spp. and Enterobacteriaceae are known to cause synergistic infec-

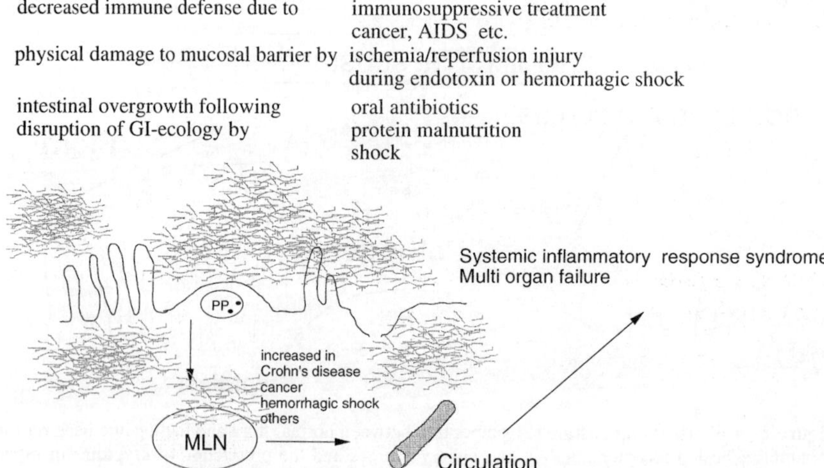

Figure 3 Bacterial translocation. In certain clinical situations, passage of viable bacteria from the GI tract may be pathologically increased, contributing to substantial morbidity and mortality.

tions, possibly due to the capacity of *Bacteroides* spp. to inhibit phagocytosis of Enterobacteriaceae and to suppress specific immune functions[27]. In addition, *Bacteroides fragilis* enterotoxin may cause augmented internalization of selected strains of enteric bacteria that preferentially adhere to exposed enterocyte lateral surface[28].

INTESTINAL FLORA AND THE IMMUNE SYSTEM

The intestinal flora, an important endogenous immune modifier

Studies in germ-free animals and subsequent reconstitution experiments (Figure 4) clearly demonstrate the importance of the intestinal flora for the development of a normal intestinal immune morphology and function[29–33]. Interestingly, in these studies the intestinal flora was required for the full development of both immunizing[30] and tolerizing[31–33] intestinal immune functions. While the mechanisms by which the intestinal flora interacts with the intestinal immune system are still incompletely understood, there is now ample evidence from clinical investigations and a variety of animal models of IBD which all indicate that the intestinal flora represents a crucial endogenous stimulus to induce and maintain chronic intestinal inflammation in the susceptible host[21,34].

Selecting the intestinal microflora and the immune response to it

As mentioned above, the microflora shows a remarkable vertical and horizontal organization. In addition, its composition is not transient, but follows an orderly and successive colonization process which usually begins during birth, and reaches a stable expression shortly thereafter. The factors which influence the selection and relative stability of the intestinal flora within a given individual are not well understood. However, several studies suggest that, in addition to microbiological influences, the immune system and the genetics of an individual are important contributing factors.

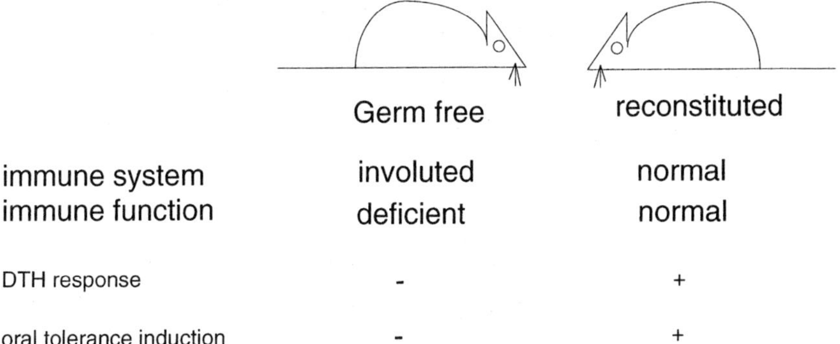

Figure 4 The normal intestinal flora is an important immune modifier. Studies in germ free animals and subsequent reconstitution experiments demonstrate that the intestinal flora is important for the development of a normal intestinal immune morphology and function.

Indicating that selection of the resident faecal flora is under genetic control, Van de Merwe *et al.* found that faecal floras of monozygotic twin siblings were much more alike than those of dizygotic twin siblings[35]. Another study performed by a Russian group and determining the variability of the qualitative and quantitative characteristics on the levels of both genera and individual microbial species in healthy members of 10 complete families (altogether 50 persons) confirmed a strong genetic determination[36]. Extending the prior observations that the intestinal flora contains bacteria that are found in all members of an animal species, which led to the definition of an autochthonous flora, these data indicate a further diversification and specification of the intestinal flora on the individual level.

Joining genes and the immune system in the selection process, Foo *et al.* not only found that there is a selective unresponsiveness to autochthonous *Bacteroides* spp. in adult mice but also demonstrated cross-reaction between autochthonous *Bacteroides* spp. and intestinal tissue of neonatal mice (i.e., self-antigen)[37,38]. This cross-tolerization between self-antigens and antigens from normal intestinal flora indicates that tolerance of an individual to his own intestinal flora may share aspects of self-tolerance. Supporting the idea that immune tolerance or unresponsiveness may provide an advantage for bacteria to stay, specific humoral immunological unresponsiveness to autochthonous flora in mice was also reported by Berg *et al.*[39] In addition, data from Van der Waaij

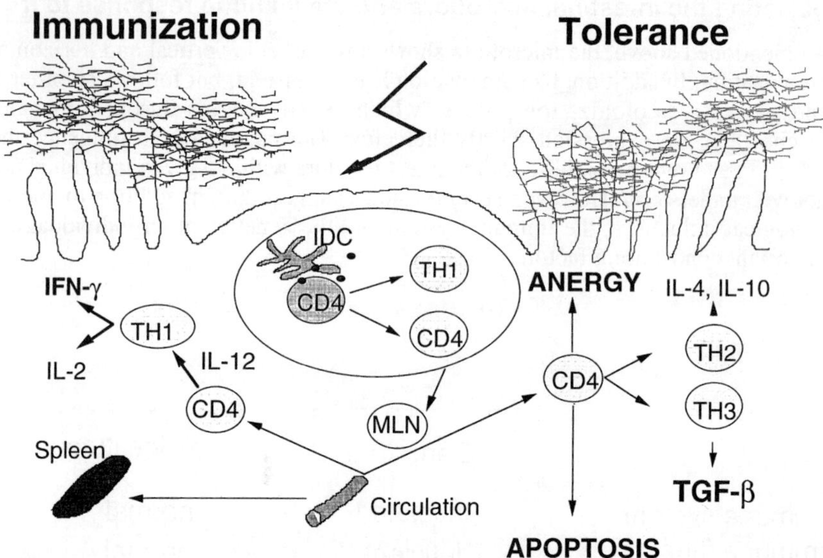

Figure 5   Loss of tolerance to normal intestinal flora. Under normal circumstances, CD4+ T cell responses to discrete bacterial antigens seem to result in some form of immune tolerance. This immune tolerance may be mediated by T cell anergy, apoptosis or the induction of T cells producing regulatory cytokines like IL-4, IL-10 and TGF-β. In chronic intestinal inflammation, however, CD4+ T cells seem to be dysregulated. Among many different possible causes for such an immune dysregulation, IL-12-mediated induction of high IFN-γ producing CD4+ T cells may be a common pathway, leading to immunization to normal intestinal flora and ultimately chronic intestinal inflammation.

determining the level of Ig coating of anaerobic bacteria in human faeces[40] as well as studies by our own group[41] indicate that humoral and cellular immune non-responsiveness to 'self-intestinal flora' also occurs in humans.

Loss of tolerance to antigens from the normal intestinal flora (Figure 5), indicated by increased humoral[42–44] and cellular[41–45] immune responses to intestinal flora in IBD patients, has been implicated as a mechanism of IBD pathogenesis[46]. Although the mechanisms of tolerance induction to antigens from the normal intestinal flora are not well understood, they may at least in part be similar to the tolerance elicited by luminal antigens from ingested dietary products or other sources[47,48]. Restoration of tolerance to self-intestinal flora by antibodies to interleukin-12 (IL-12) in a mouse model of IBD[49] suggests that IL-12 is not only an important counter-regulator of transforming growth factor-β (TGF-β) mediated oral tolerance[50,51] but also counter-regulates tolerance to normal intestinal flora.

CONCLUSION

A highly delicate and complex system of checks and balances is required to ensure that the potent metabolic, microbiological and immunological effects of the normal intestinal flora are used in a way that is beneficial to the host. Current data would suggest that host genes and the host immune system influence selection of bacteria for the intestinal flora so that it is not only tailored to the animal species but also to the individual host. Abnormal immune responses to normal flora in the genetically susceptible host have been shown to provide the major inflammatory stimulus in IBD. A better understanding of the rules that govern the interactions between the host and the intestinal flora will offer new insights into the mechanism of intestinal inflammatory diseases and may provide the basis for new treatment strategies.

References

1. Berg RD. The indigenous gastrointestinal microflora. Trends Microbiol. 1996;4:430–435.
2. Dubos R, Schaedler RW, Costello R, Hoet P. Indigenous, normal, and autochthonous flora of the gastrointestinal tract. J Exp Med. 1965;122:67–76.
3. Bowden GH. Does assessment of microbial composition of plaque/saliva allow for diagnosis of disease activity of individuals? Community Dent Oral Epidemiol. 1997;25:76–81.
4. Bowen WH. Defense mechanisms in the mouth and their possible role in the prevention of dental caries: a review. J Oral Pathol. 1974;3:266–278.
5. Blaser MJ. *Helicobacter pylori*: costs of commensalism. Gut. 1997;41(Suppl 3), A:01.03.
6. Sartor RB. Role of the intestinal microflora in pathogenesis and complications. In: Schölmerich J, Kruis W, Goebell H, Hohenberger W, Gross V (eds). Inflammatory Bowel Diseases: Pathophysiology as Basis of Treatment. Lancaster: Kluwer Academic, 1992:175–187.
7. Nelson D, Mata L. Bacterial flora associated with the human gastrointestinal mucosa. Gastroenterology. 1970;58:56–61.
8. Peach S, Drasar B, Hawley P, Hill M, Marks C. Mucosal flora of the human colon. Gut. 1975;16:824.
9. Boman HG. Peptide antibiotics and their role in innate immunity. Annu Rev Immunol. 1995;13:61–92.
10. Roediger W. Role of anaerobic bacteria in the metabolic welfare of the colonic mucosa in man. Gut. 1980;21:793–798.
11. Harig JM, Soergel KH, Komorowski RA, Wood CM. Treatment of diversion colitis with short chain fatty acid irrigation. N Engl J Med 1989;320:23–28.

12. Scheppach W, Sommer H, Kirchner T et al. Effect of butyrate enemas on the colonic mucosa in distal ulcerative colitis. Gastroenterology. 1992;103:51–56.
13. Bernet MF, Brassart D, Neeser JR, Servin AL. Adhesion of human bifidobacterial strains to cultured human intestinal epithelial cells and inhibition of enteropathogen-cell interactions. Appl Environ Microbiol. 1993;59:4121–4128.
14. Gibson GR, Wang X. Regulatory effects of bifidobacteria on the growth of other colonic bacteria. J. Appl Bacteriol. 1994;77:412–420.
15. Biavati B, Castagnoli P, Crociani F, Trovatelli LD. Species of the *Bifidobacterium* in the feces of infants. Microbiologica. 1984;7:341–345
16. Saavedra JM, Bauman NA, Oung I, Perman JA, Yolken RH. Feeding of *Bifidobacterium bifidum* and *Streptococcus thermophilus* to infants in hospital for prevention of diarrhoea and shedding of rotavirus. Lancet. 1994;344:1046–1049.
17. Tvede M, Rask-Madsen J. Bacteriotherapy for chronic relapsing *Clostridium difficile* diarrhoea in six patients. Lancet. 1989;5:1156–1160.
18. Mao Y, Nobaek S, Kasravi B et al. The effects of *Lactobacillus* strains and oat fiber on methotrexate induced enterocolitis in rats. Gastroenterology. 1996;111:334–344.
19. Bernet MF, Brassart D, Neeser JR, Servin AL. *Lactobacillus acidophilus* LA1 binds to cultured human intestinal cell lines and inhibits cell attachment and cell invasion by enterovirulent bacteria. Gut. 1994;35:483–489.
20. Sartor RB. Treating IBD by altering luminal contents: rationale and response. In: Rachmilewitz D (ed). Inflammatory Bowel Diseases. Lancaster: Kluwer Academic, 1994:177–191.
21. Duchmann R, Neurath M, Märker-Hermann E, Meyer zum Büschenfelde K-H. Immune responses towards intestinal bacteria–current concepts and future perspectives. Zeits Gastroenterol. 1997;35:285–294.
22. American College of Chest Physicians/Society of critical care medicine consensus conference. Definitions for sepsis and organ failure and guidelines for the use of innovative therapies in sepsis. Crit Care Med. 1992;20:864.
23. Gaston JSH. Pathogenic role of gut inflammation in the spondylarthropathies. Curr Opin Rheumatol. 1997;9:302–307.
24. Rath HC, Herfarth HH, Ikeda JS et al. Normal luminal bacteria, especially bacteroides species, mediate chronic colitis, gastritis, and arthritis in HLA-B27/human β2 microglobulin transgenic rats. J Clin Invest. 1996;98:945–953.
25. Onderdonk AB, Franklin ML, Cisneros RL. Production of experimental ulcerative colitis in gnotobiotic guinea pigs with simplified microflora. Infect Immun. 1981;32:225–231.
26. Onderdonk AB, Cisneros RL, Bronson RT. Enhancement of experimental ulcerative colitis by immunization with *Bacteroides vulgatus*. Infect Immun. 1983;42:783–788.
27. Rodloff AC, Widera P, Ehlers S et al. Suppression of blastogenic transformation of lymphocytes by *Bacteroides fragilis* in vitro and in vivo. Int J Med Microbiol. 1990;274:406–416.
28. Wells CL, van de Westerlo E, Jechorek RP, Feltis BA, Wilkins TD, Erlandsen SL. *Bacteroides fragilis* enterotoxin modulates epithelial permeability and bacterial internalization by HT. 29 enterocytes. Gastroenterology. 1996;110:1429–1437.
29. Simon GL, Gorbach SL. Intestinal flora in health and disease. Gastroenterology. 1984;86:174–193.
30. MacDonald TT, Carter PB. Requirement for a bacterial flora before mice generate cells capable of mediating the delayed hypersensitivity reaction to sheep red blood cells. J Immunol. 1979;122:2624–2629.
31. Wannemuehler MJ, Kiyono H, Babb JL, Michalek SM, McGhee JR. Lipopolysaccharide (LPS) regulation of the immune response: LPS converts germfree mice to sensitivity to oral tolerance induction. J Immunol. 1982;129:959–965.
32. McGhee JR, Kiyono H, Michalek SM, Babb JL, Rosenstreich DL, Mergenhagen SE. Lipopolysaccharide (LPS) regulation of the immune response: T lymphocytes from normal mice suppress mitogenic and immunogenic responses to LPS. J Immunol. 1980;124:1603–1611.
33. Sudo N, Sawamura S, Tanaka K, Aiba Y, Kubo C, Koga Y. The requirement of intestinal bacterial flora for the development of an IgE production system fully susceptible to oral tolerance induction. J Immunol. 1997;159:1739–1745.
34. Sartor RB. Microbial agents in the pathogenesis, differential diagnosis and complications of inflammatory bowel diseases. In: Blaser MJ, Smith PD, Ravdin JI, Greenberg HB, Guerrant RL (eds). Infections of the Gastrointestinal Tract. New York: Raven Press, 1995:435–458.

35. Van de Merwe JP, Stegeman JH, Hazenberg MP. The resident fecal flora is determined by genetic characteristics of the host. Implications for Crohn's disease? Antonie van Leeuwenhook. 1983;49:119–124.

36. Vorob'ev AA, Nesvizhskii-Iu V, Budanova EV, Inozemtseva-LO. The population genetic aspect of the intestinal microbiological phenotype in healthy humans. Zh Mikrobiol Epidemiol Immunobiol. 1995;4:30–35.

37. Foo MC, Lee A. Immunological response of mice to members of the autochthonous intestinal microflora. Infect Immun. 1972;6:525–532.

38. Foo MC, Lee A. Antigenic cross-reaction between mouse intestine and a member of the autochthonous microflora. Infect Immun. 1974;9:1066–1069.

39. Berg R, Savage D. Immune response of specific pathogen-free and gnotobiotic mice to antigens of indigenous and non-indigenous microorganisms. Infect Immun. 1975;11:320–329.

40. Van der Waaij LA, Limburg PC, Mesander G, Van der Waaij D. In vivo IgA coating of anaerobic bacteria in human faeces. Gut. 1996;38:348–354.

41. Duchmann R, Kaiser I, Hermann E, Mayet W, Ewe K, Meyer zum Büschenfelde KH. Tolerance exists towards resident intestinal flora but is broken in active inflammatory bowel disease. Clin Exp Immunol. 1995;102:448.

42. Chao LP, Steele J, Rodrigues C et al. Specificity of antibodies secreted by hybridomas generated from activated B cells in the mesenteric lymph nodes of patients with inflammatory bowel disease. Gut. 1988;29:35–40.

43. Macpherson A, Khoo UY, Forgacs I, Philpott-Howard J, Bjarnason J. Mucosal antibodies in inflammatory bowel disease are directed against intestinal bacteria. Gut. 1996;38:365–375.

44. van der Waaij LA, Kroese FGM, Jansen PLM, Visser A, Hunter JO. Anaerobic bacteria in feces of patients with IBD are coated with immunoglobulins: Loss of immunological tolerance? Gut. 1997;41A:P161A.

45. Duchmann R, Märker-Hermann E, Meyer zum Büschenfelde KH. Bacteria-specific T-cell clones are selective in their reactivity towards different enterobacteria or *H. pylori* and increased in inflammatory bowel disease. Scand J Immmunol. 1996;44:71–79.

46. Duchmann R, Neurath MF, Meyer zum Büschenfelde KH. Responses to self and non-self intestinal microflora in health and inflammatory bowel disease. Res Immunol. 1997;148:589–594.

47. Mowat AM. The regulation of immune responses to dietary protein antigens. Immunol Today. 1987;8:93–98.

48. Weiner HL. Oral tolerance: immune mechanisms and treatment of autoimmune diseases. Immunol Today. 1997;18:335–343.

49. Duchmann R, Schmitt E, Knolle P, Meyer zum Büschenfelde KH, Neurath M. Tolerance towards resident intestinal flora in mice is abrogated in experimental colitis and restored by treatment with interleukin-1 antibodies to interleukin-12. Eur J Immunol. 1996,26:934 938.

50. Neurath MF, Fuss I, Kelsall B, Pretsky DH, Waegell W, Strober W. Experimental granulomatous colitis in mice is abrogated by induction of TGF-β-mediated oral tolerance. J Exp Med. 1996;183:2605–2616.

51. Marth T, Stober W, Kelsall BL. High dose oral tolerance in ovalbumin TCR-transgenic mice: systemic neutralization of IL-12 augments TGF-beta secretion and T cell apoptosis. J Immunol. 1996;157:2348–2357.

19
Local regulatory mechanisms in *Helicobacter pylori* infection

P. B. ERNST

INTRODUCTION

The specific causes of inflammatory bowel disease (IBD) have remained elusive. Thus, one is obliged to use surrogate models in an attempt to identify mechanisms that may have general relevance. Infection with *H. pylori* provides an ideal opportunity to study the role of the host response in gastrointestinal disease. It is a lifelong infection that gives rise to a chronic inflammation in all infected individuals. The more severe sequelae of infection, such as peptic ulcer and gastric cancer, only arise in a minority of patients. This allows one to study events in the host response and environment that may modulate outcome of infection, two important variables that affect the development of other gastrointestinal diseases. The fact that more than 50% of the world population is infected with *H. pylori* for life provides ample opportunity to study the pathogenesis of this infection in humans. More importantly for immunologists, this disease provides a rare opportunity to study antigen-specific responses in the digestive tract.

Although *H. pylori* is virtually the only species of bacteria that resides in the stomach, it took until 1984 for its significance to modern medicine to begin to be appreciated[1]. As there are more than 400 species of bacteria in the colon, only about 10–15% of which have ever been grown, any specific microbial aetiology for inflammatory bowel disease may not be identified for some time. This leaves *H. pylori* as one of the few models with which to study the interaction between gastrointestinal immune responses and microbial flora in the pathogenesis of chronic inflammation.

INDUCTION OF IMMUNE AND INFLAMMATORY RESPONSES IN THE GASTROINTESTINAL TRACT

The induction of immune responses in the intestinal tract has been extensively reviewed elsewhere[2–4]. Briefly, lymphoid aggregates in the Peyer's patches are believed to be the primary inductive site for T and B cell responses in the intestine. Various cytokines have been shown to direct the differentiation of B cells into IgA-producing cells while others expand the number of IgA-producing cells and IgA secretion. These cytokines include transforming growth factor-β (TGF-β), interleukin (IL)-4, IL-5, IL-6 and IL-10. This panel of cytokines is produced by T cells associated with the T_H2 subset of helper T cells. Stimulated T and B lymphoblasts are believed to exit the Peyer's patches and seed other areas of the intestine as well as more remote mucosal tissues, including the salivary glands and the respiratory and urogenital tracts. This model implies that lymphocytes from Peyer's patches would also seed the stomach; however, there is no direct evidence that this occurs. In fact, in the absence of gastric inflammation, very few T and B cells are found in the gastric mucosa.

T_H2 cells satisfy the criterion of selecting for protective mucosal IgA responses while inhibiting cell-mediated immunity. The mucosal inflammation in association with a persistent exposure to antigen intimates that T_H1 cells predominate in the inflamed stomach and subvert the strategy of developing protection without inflammation.

REGULATION OF T_H CELL DIFFERENTIATION

Following exposure to infection, the host produces an acute inflammatory response that contributes to the recruitment and activation of cells that can present antigen to T cells. These antigen-presenting cells, in turn, stimulate adjacent T cells. *H. pylori* has been shown to be a modest T cell mitogen *in vitro* and in fact, it may even inhibit some T cell responses[5]. It is possible that one of several molecules expressed by *H. pylori*, including proteases, interfere with antigen presentation and T cell activation. However, the striking accumulation of T cells in the gastric mucosa during infection with *H. pylori* speaks to the fact that T cells are recruited and activated *in vivo*. MHC-restricted, *H. pylori*-specific T cell clones have been derived from both the peripheral blood and gastric mucosa of infected individuals[6]. Furthermore, *H. pylori* induces interferon-γ (IFN-γ) production from peripheral blood leukocytes[7] as well as those isolated from the gut[5]. In addition, IFN-γ-producing cells are increased in the gastric mucosa during infection[8-10]. Importantly, these studies also suggest that very few IL-4 producing T_H2 cells are found in the gastric mucosa before or after the induction of inflammation. It should be noted that the IFN-γ-producing cells predominate in the absence of infection as well as in response to gastritis due to aetiologies other than *H. pylori*[8,10]. Therefore, this response may reflect the influence of the gastric microenvironment on helper T cell selection.

The selection of T_H1 and T_H2 cells is largely controlled by their interaction with antigen-presenting cells. The production of IL-10, IL-12 and IL-18 can select for T_H2 (IL-10) and T_H1 cells (IL-12 and IL-18). We have shown that live *H. pylori* preferentially induces IL-12 and that IL-12 predominates over IL-10 in gastric biopsies[9]. This would be consistent with the increase in IFN-γ that was reported previously. Interactions between antigen-presenting cells and T cells mediated via adhesion molecules can also control T_H cell differentiation. These interactions are now being defined in the stomach and appear to be increased in response to infection.

It is not clear whether T_H1 responses, which select for cell-mediated immunity, are in the best interest of the host in its attempt to clear an extracellular infection. T_H2 responses have been directly implicated in mucosal protection as well as split tolerance – that is, enhanced IgA responses in association with suppressed cell-mediated immunity. T_H1 cells and the associated cell-mediated immunity may be tolerable but an overwhelming T_H1 response, in combination with host genetics, specific strains of bacteria as well as other environmental factors, could combine to contribute to ulcerogenesis.

CONTRIBUTION OF T_H1 CELLS TO AUTOIMMUNITY IN THE STOMACH

The immune response has evolved to protect the host from infection. In the case of the mucosal tissues, the host further discriminates between pathogens and commensal flora. This is achieved by an apparent inhibition of immune responses to enteric commensal organisms. However, an inappropriate response in certain individuals to commensal flora may occur. Thus, a failure in immune regulation such that the host mounts an excessive immune response to flora that persist in the lumen, such as *H. pylori*, may lead to tissue damage on a scale equivalent to classical autoimmune diseases. This notion is supported by a report describing the development of colitis in mice following the ablation of the gene coding for IL-10, a cytokine which selects for T_H2 responses[11]. This disease appears to be driven by luminal bacteria as animals maintained in an environment free of commensal flora do not develop colitis. The evidence that T_H1 cells may be increased relative to T_H2 cells during *H. pylori* infection suggests that a marked skewing in this response may lead to disease as implicated in the pathogenesis of more classical autoimmune diseases[12]. These observations suggest that the difference in gastric disease associated with *H. pylori* infection may be partially attributed to the magnitude of the host response.

The first suggestion that *H. pylori* may cause a bona fide autoimmune response was based on evidence that monoclonal antibodies directed against *H. pylori* could recognize an epitope on the gastric epithelium of mice and humans. Administration of these antibodies to mice resulted in gastritis and caused mild erosions[13]. More recently, it has been shown that antibodies to *H. pylori* lipopolysaccharide cross-react with antigens on epithelial cells[14]. IgM antibodies produced from immortalized B cells obtained from the gastric mucosa have also been shown to recognize the gastric epithelium[15]. Other evidence suggests that B cells within a maltoma express a repertoire that recognizes a determinant shared by both IgA and IgM[16]. Thus, antibodies within the gastric mucosa may recognize epithelial cells or act as rheumatoid factors. This may lead to immune complex-mediated disease that could directly damage the epithelium. If this hypothesis is correct, then future studies may show activated complement adjacent to damaged epithelium.

The presence of T_H1 cells and IFN-γ production are likely to lead to immuno-physiological interactions that directly promote tissue damage. For example, IFN-γ alters epithelial barrier function in intestinal cell lines[17]. Other cytokines, including TNF-α, can collaborate with IFN-γ to alter epithelial cell IL-8 gene expression[18].

INDUCTION OF APOPTOSIS IN GASTRIC EPITHELIAL CELLS

It has been well established that the epithelium of the digestive tract turns over every 4–6 days. Previously, it was believed that the proliferative zone provided cells for this renewal and, in turn, these progenitors differentiate and migrated up towards the villous or gastric gland before being extruded into the lumen. With the development of an assay to measure DNA damage by histochemical techniques, investigators have shown that apoptosis occurs in the epithelium of the healthy digestive tract[19,20]. This suggests that the process of cell loss is regulated, and disruption in either the proliferation or removal of epithelial cells could lead to aberrations in epithelial cell function.

Moss and colleagues[21] were the first to report that apoptosis in gastric epithelial cells *in situ* was increased during infection with *H. pylori*. This observation was followed by other reports describing the increase in apoptosis[22,23]. Another study by Jones *et al.* has confirmed increased epithelial apoptosis in gastric biopsies from *H. pylori* infected patients that also decreased after successful eradication therapy[23]. The frequency of epithelial apoptosis was significantly lower in other forms of gastritis or non-inflamed mucosa in this study. More recently, one study suggested that apoptosis in gastric epithelium was affected by the strain of *H. pylori*. More specifically, individuals infected with cagA-expressing strains reportedly had normal levels of apoptosis while those infected with strains lacking cagA had increased levels of apoptosis[24]. At first glance, these observations appear somewhat incongruous since most individuals are infected with strains expressing cagA and thus, the reports documenting an increase in apoptosis probably included subjects infected with cagA-positive strains. Moreover, another report has suggested that apoptosis is increased in the gastric epithelium during all forms of gastritis tested, including gastritis due to NSAID usage and graft-versus-host disease[23]. Germane to this discussion, strains expressing cagA are associated with increased cytokine responses which themselves can promote apoptosis[25,26]. Therefore, in order to address this apparent paradox one should consider the nature of the inflammatory response in the gastric mucosa during infection.

MECHANISMS BY WHICH CYTOKINES ENHANCE *H. PYLORI*-MEDIATED APOPTOSIS

Direct effects

The study of apoptosis has exploded in the context of the immunopathogenesis of several diseases, and one can simply scan the literature to make several predictions on what may transpire in the gastric mucosa. As suggested above, one of the cytokines induced during infection with *H. pylori*, TNF-α[27], has been widely studied as a potent stimulus of apoptosis. TNF-α can bind to either of two TNF receptors, one of which often directly signals the induction of apoptosis in the cell bearing the TNF receptor. Studies by Behar[28] as well as Wagner[29,30], have shown that TNF-α alone can induce apoptosis in a variety of gastric epithelial cell lines. The mechanistic basis for this response has yet to be dissected as the TNF receptor and signalling mechanisms associated with gastric epithelial cells remain to be described.

IFN-γ is a cytokine produced by T_H1 cells in healthy or inflamed gastric mucosa[8,10]. However, during infection with *H. pylori*, these IFN-γ-producing T cells are increased in number and are highly activated. Thus, the local concentration of this cytokine is increased. Again Behar and Wagner have independently shown that INF-γ has the ability to induce apoptosis in gastric epithelial cells[28,30], albeit at lower levels than TNF-α.

Additional intercellular interactions between epithelial cells and T cells mediated by Fas–Fas ligand interactions may also contribute to apoptosis of epithelial cells. This process may be important in regulating cell death and preventing cancer but it could also induce breaks in the epithelial barrier that induce erosions that may lead to ulcers.

Enhancement of *H. pylori*-mediated apoptosis

In addition to the induction of apoptosis by inflammatory mediator, *H. pylori* itself also induces this response. While *H. pylori*, TNF-α and IFN-γ can stimulate apoptosis alone, gastric epithelial cells are exquisitely sensitive to combinations of these cytokines and *H. pylori*. Over a 48 h period, both cell recovery and viability of gastric epithelial cells plummet after being exposed to *H. pylori* and IFN-γ, *H. pylori* and TNF-α or a combination of *H. pylori*, IFN-γ and TNF-α[28,30]. Since all of these factors are present during infection with *H. pylori*, then it seems most likely that the opportunity exists for these interactions to occur *in vivo*. This is supported by recent evidence showing that both TNF and IFN-γ-producing cells can be detected immunohistochemically next to gastric epithelial cells (C. Lindholm, personal communication).

Effects of cytokines on *H. pylori* binding

Although these observations suggest an important role for cytokines in regulating apoptosis in gastric epithelial cells, some definition of a mechanism would help in relating *in vitro* observations to events *in vivo*. In a recent set of experiments, the binding of *H. pylori* was enhanced after treatment of gastric epithelial cells with IFN-γ[31]. Although this does not prove how cytokines increase *H. pylori*-induced apoptosis, this approach has provided an important tool to understand the molecular basis for this response.

In order to evaluate whether an increase in binding of the bacteria was indeed responsible for the increase in apoptosis, we attempted to identify a host cell receptor for *H. pylori* and then to determine whether this receptor could signal the induction of apoptosis in the gastric epithelial cells[31]. *H. pylori* was incubated with solubilized membrane proteins from radiolabelled gastric epithelial cells. Subsequently, the adherent material was eluted and separated by electrophoresis. Using this approach, class II MHC molecules were identified as potential receptors for *H. pylori*. To confirm this, cells with and without class II

MHC molecules were tested for their ability to bind *H. pylori*: the majority of the binding was shown to be associated with the presence of class II MHC.

To investigate whether class II MHC might induce apoptosis after binding *H. pylori*, gastric epithelial cells were exposed to antibodies to class II MHC and examined for apoptosis. The results showed that apoptosis was induced. Moreover, *H. pylori* was only able to induce apoptosis in cells bearing the class II MHC molecules and both *H. pylori* binding and the induction of apoptosis could be blocked with specific antibodies to class II MHC. Thus, class II MHC can serve as a receptor for *H. pylori* and signal the induction of apoptosis.

Since IFN-γ, and other cytokines including IL-1 and TNF-α, can increase the expression of class II MHC on gastric epithelial cells, it is possible to put all of the observations together into a unifying hypothesis. Cytokines induced during infection, such as IFN-γ, can increase the expression of class II MHC which in turn, bind *H. pylori* and signal the induction of apoptosis. If this model is correct, then it should be supported by observation *in vivo*. Evidence in support of this model includes the increase in IFN-γ-producing cells in juxtaposition with infected epithelial cells *in situ*; the presence of class II MHC molecules on the apical surface of gastric epithelial cells, and reports that class II MHC haplotype may affect rates of infection and the manifestation of gastric disease associated with *H. pylori* infection.

Another interesting aspect of the induction of apoptosis in gastric epithelial cells is that it is relatively slow. In some experimental systems, other cells, such as T cells, can undergo apoptosis within 12–18 h of stimulation. However, evidence to date suggests that this process takes approximately 48 h in gastric epithelial cells. Since the apoptotic gastric epithelial cells are generally detected within the superficial epithelium *in situ*, these observations suggest that the process may be initiated during the time gastric epithelial cells migrate towards the lumen from the proliferative zone. The neck of the gastric gland is highly enriched for immune and inflammatory cells as well as the expression of class II MHC[32,33]. These observations imply that class II MHC is up-regulated by these inflammatory cells in the neck and through the binding of *H. pylori* to class II as well as the effects of cytokines and other mediators on the gastric epithelium, apoptosis is triggered in the neck. Subsequently, the process will develop and be detectable as the cells approach the superficial epithelium.

THE PREVENTION OF APOPTOSIS BY CYTOKINES

The preceding discussion suggests that cytokines may promote apoptosis; however, in the regulation of this response, both an increase or decrease are possible. It is well established that several molecules, including bcl-2 and bcl-x, can protect a cell from the induction of apoptosis. The expression of bcl-2 has been associated with the differential susceptiblity of enterocytes to apoptosis[34]. Moreover, it is entirely possible that cytokines, perhaps anti-inflammatory cytokines such as IL-4 and IL-10, increase the expression of these molecules and further regulate apoptosis.

In addition to any direct effect on apoptosis, IL-4 and IL-10 may also antagonize the effects of TNF-α and IFN-γ. Preliminary studies from our laboratory suggest that the IFN-γ-stimulated increase in the expression of class II MHC molecules may be inhibited and, in so doing, cytokine-enhanced, *H. pylori*-induced apoptosis may be impaired. These interactions remain to be confirmed. It is important to note that levels of IL-10 and IL-4 are low in the gastric tissue during infection. However, these anti-inflammatory cytokines may be induced with immunization and provide a mechanism to decrease gastric inflammation, bacterial colonization and epithelial cell apoptosis.

SIGNIFICANCE OF INCREASED APOPTOSIS IN THE GASTROINTESTINAL EPITHELIUM

Based on the model described above, apoptosis in gastric epithelial cells is very dependent on the immune/inflammatory response associated with *H. pylori* infection. If apoptosis can contribute to a compromise in the epithelial barrier that facilitates the development of peptic ulceration, then one would predict that strains that are associated with the most inflammation would be associated with peptic ulcer. In fact, strains of *H. pylori* expressing cagA have been associated with greater cytokine and inflammatory cell responses and peptic ulcer. Moreover, these strains are also associated with higher bacterial loads supporting the notion that the inflammatory response increases colonization, perhaps by increasing the expression of receptors for the bacteria. It is also possible that the epithelial damage induced during this infection overwhelms the capacity of the tissue to heal. Thus, replacement of epithelial cells with metaplastic cells may favour malignant transformation – an outcome that is shared with subjects with ulcerative colitis.

STRATEGIES IN IMMUNOTHERAPY

Current evidence suggests that an excessive T_H1 response driven by *H. pylori* would favour IFN-γ production, the development of cell mediated immunity and a set of conditions that contribute to the onset of epithelial damage. This damage may be direct, through the recognition of immunogenic peptides presented by the epithelial cells, or by the transient or permanent expression of epitopes that are recognized by antibodies produced during infection. If this model is correct, then immunological intervention that shifts the T cell response from T_H1 to T_H2 may favour the development of IgA responses and protective immunity in asso-ciation with a decrease in tissue damage. This notion is supported since IgA antibodies recognizing urease are sufficient to provide protection in an animal model[35]. In addition, protective immunity can be achieved since immunization of mice with *H. pylori* antigens, in combination with cholera toxin as an adjuvant, provides protection against a challenge with *H. felis* or *H. pylori*[36–38] (reviewed in Ref. 39). These data further support our hypothesis since cholera toxin boosts the T_H2 cell response and IgA responses[40]. Thus, qualitatively changing the response through oral immunization provides a tremendous opportunity for prevention as well as a complement to therapy. Future experiments will have to determine the relative strength of the T_H1 and T_H2 cell responses in different stages of gastric disease versus the response induced by the numerous candidate oral vaccines that are being developed.

RELEVANCE TO OTHER FORMS OF CHRONIC INFLAMMATION IN THE DIGESTIVE TRACT

Gastric diseases associated with *H. pylori* infection have many differences from other forms of chronic inflammation. While many manifestations of gastro-intestinal disease reflect the local environment, i.e. the impact of acid and pepsin on a damaged mucosa or the effect of the massive luminal antigenic load in the colon on inflammation, some of the underlying mechanisms may be similar. The role of the host response in regulating the important epithelial barrier may well have more in common in the stomach and colon than there are differences. Similarly, interactions between the host response and flora that further exacerbate epithelial function in the colon may be extremely important in the pathogenesis of inflammatory bowel disease.

SUMMARY

Our understanding of the control of helper T cell differentiation is in its infancy but the general principles that are emerging appear to predict T_H cell differentiation in response to *H. pylori* infection. *H. pylori* induces IL-12 leading to the production of IFN-γ-producing T cells resembling T_H1 cells. The role of IL-18 has yet to be determined. Work in progress is confirming the presence of these cells in the gastric mucosa. Since the infection is not invasive, cell-mediated responses selected by T_H1 cells are ineffective at clearing the infection. Moreover, they can contribute to inflammation and epithelial damage. The increased turnover of epithelial cells may exceed cytoprotective mechanisms and the restorative powers of restitution. This could lead to ulceration as luminal acid and pepsin gain access to the underlying tissue. Since the T cell response is so homogeneously biased towards T_H1 cells, the successful induction of T_H2 cell in the gastric mucosa through vaccination provides a logical and probably highly successful approach to increase host immunity to *H. pylori*.

As a model of other chronic inflammatory diseases of the digestive tract, *H. pylori* offers some interesting insights. With this pathogen, a specific immune response can be measured and its impact on cell biology and the pathogenesis of disease can be evaluated. To date, it has identified novel mechanisms in regulating cytokine responses and the interaction of these on epithelial cell apoptosis. Moreover, the counterbalancing effect between pro-inflammatory and anti-inflammatory cytokines documents the potential detriments and benefits of these host responses. While the biology of the gastric niche differs substantially from elsewhere in the digestive tract, *H. pylori* can still provide a means with which scientists can better understand the pathogenesis of chronic inflammation in the gut.

References

1. Marshall BJ, Warren JR. Unidentified curved bacilli in the stomach of patients with gastritis and peptic ulceration. Lancet. 1984;8390:1311–1315.
2. McGhee JR, Mestecky J, Dertzbaugh MT, Eldridge JH, Hirasawa M, Kiyono H. The mucosal immune system: From fundamental concepts to vaccine development. Vaccine. 1992;10:75–88.
3. Manganaro M, Ogra PL, Ernst PB. Oral immunization: turning fantasy into reality. Int Arch Allergy Appl Immunol. 1994;103:223–233.
4. Ernst PB, Crowe SE, Reyes VE. The immunopathogenesis of gastroduodenal disease associated with *Helicobacter pylori* infection. Curr Opin Gastroenterol. 1995;11:512–518.
5. Fan XJ, Chua A, Shahi CN, McDevitt J, Keeling PWN, Kelleher D. Gastric T lymphocyte response to *Helicobacter pylori* in patients with *H. pylori* colonisation. Gut. 1994;35:1379–1384.
6. Di Tommaso A, Xiang Z, Bugnoli M et al. *Helicobacter pylori*-specific CD4+ T-cell clones from peripheral blood and gastric biopsies. Infect Immun. 1995;63:1102–1106.
7. Tarkkanen J, Kosunen TU, Saksela E. Contact of lymphocytes with *Helicobacter pylori* augments natural killer cell activity and induces production of gamma interferon. Infect Immun. 1993;61:3012–3016.
8. Karttunen R, Karttunen T, Ekre H-PT, MacDonald TT. Interferon gamma and interleukin 4 secreting cells in the gastric antrum in *Helicobacter pylori* positive and negative gastritis. Gut. 1995;36:341–345.
9. Haeberle H, Kubin M, Bamford KB et al. Induction of IL-12 and selection of Th1 cells in the gastric mucosa in response to *H. pylori*. Infect Immun. 1997;65:4229–4235.
10. Bamford KB, Fan XJ, Crowe SE et al. Lymphocytes during infection with *Helicobacter pylori* have a helper 1 (Th1) phenotype. Gastroenterology. 1998;114:482–492
11. Kuhn R, Lohler J, Rennick D, Rajewsky K, Muller W. Interleukin-10-deficient mice develop chronic enterolcolitis. Cell. 1993;75:263–274.
12. Liblau RS, Singer SM, McDevitt HO. Th1 and Th2 CD4+ T cells in the pathogenesis of organ-specific autoimmune diseases. Immunol Today. 1995;16:34–38.
13. Negrini R, Lisato L, Zanella I et al. *Helicobacter pylori* infection induces antibodies cross-reacting with human gastric mucosa. Gastroenterology. 1991;101:437–445.
14. Appelmelk BJ, Simoons-Smit I, Negrini R. Potential role of molecular mimicry between *Helicobacter pylori* lipopolysaccharide and host Lewis blood group antigens in autoimmunity. Infect Immun. 1996;64:2031–2040.
15. Vollmers HP, Dammrich J, Ribbert H et al. Human monoclonal antibodies from stomach carcinoma patients react with *Helicobacter pylori* and stimulate stomach cancer cells in vitro. Cancer. 1994;74:1525–1532.
16. Greiner A, Marx A, Heesemann J, Leebmann J, Schmausser B, Muller-Hermelink HK. Idiotype identity in a MALT-type lymphoma and B cells in *Helicobacter pylori* associated chronic gastritis. Lab Invest. 1994;70:572–578.
17. Madara JL, Stafford J. Interferon-γ directly affects barrier function of cultured intestinal epithelial monolayers. J Clin Invest. 1989;83:724–727.
18. Yasumoto K, Okamoto S, Mukaida N, Murakami S, Mai M, Matsushima K. Tumor necrosis factor α and interferon γ synergistically induce interleukin 8 production in a human gastric cancer cell line through acting concurrently on AP-1 and NF-kappaB-like binding sites of the interleukin 8 gene. J Biol Chem. 1992;267:22506–22511.
19. Hall PA, Coates PJ, Ansari B, Hopwood D. Regulation of cell number in the mammalian gastrointestinal tract: The importance of apoptosis. J Cell Sci. 1994;107:3569–3577.
20. Watson AJM. Necrosis and apoptosis in the gastrointestinal tract. Gut. 1995;37:165–167.
21. Moss SF, Calam J, Agarwal B, Wang S, Holt PG. Induction of gastric epithelial apoptosis by *Helicobacter pylori*. Gut. 1996;38:498–501.
22. Mannick EE, Bravo LE, Zarama G et al. Inducible nitric oxide synthase, nitrotyrosine and apoptosis in *Helicobacter pylori* gastritis: Effect of antibiotics and antioxidants. Cancer Res. 1996;56:3238–3243.
23. Jones NL, Yeger H, Cutz E, Sherman PM. *Helicobacter pylori* induces apoptosis of gastric antral epithelial cells *in vivo*. Gastroenterology. 1996;110:A933.
24. Peek RM, Jr, Moss SF, Tham KT et al. *Helicobacter pylori* cagA+ strains and dissociation of gastrointestinal epithelial cell proliferation from apoptosis. J Natl Cancer Inst. 1997;89:863–868.
25. Peek RM, Jr, Miller GG, Tham KT et al. Heightened inflammatory response and cytokine expression in vivo to cagA+ *Helicobacter pylori* strains. Lab Invest. 1995;73:760–770.

26. Yamaoka Y, Kita M, Sawai N, Imanishi J. *Helicobacter pylori cagA* gene and expression of cytokine messenger RNA in gastric mucosa. Gastroenterology. 1996;110:1744–1752.
27. Crabtree JE, Shallcross TM, Heatley RV, Wyatt JI. Mucosal tumour necrosis factor α and interleukin-6 in patients with *Helicobacter pylori* associated gastritis. Gut. 1991;32:1473–1477.
28. Behar S, Van Houten N, Bamford KB, Reyes VE, Crowe SE, Ernst PB. *H. pylori* induces apoptosis in gastric epithelial cells which is enhanced by cytokines derived from Th1 cells. Gastroenterology. 1996;110:A853.
29. Wagner S, Beil W, Obst B et al. *H. pylori* induces apoptosis in gastric epithelial cells: potentiation by TNF-α and CD95 ligand. Gastroenterolgy. 1997;112:A324.
30. Wagner S, Beil W, Westermann J et al. Regulation of epithelial cell growth by *Helicobacter pylori*: Evidence for a major role of apoptosis. Gastroenterology. 1997;113:1836–1847.
31. Fan XJ, Crowe SE, Behar S et al. The effect of class II MHC expression on adherence of *Helicobacteri pylori* and induction of apopotosis in gastric epithelial cells: a mechanism for Th1 cell-mediated damage. J Exp Med. 1998;187:1659–1669.
32. Valnes K, Huitfeldt HS, Brandtzaeg P. Relation between T cell number and epithelial HLA class II expression quantified by image analysis in normal and inflamed human gastric mucosa. Gut. 1990;31:647–652.
33. Brandtzaeg P, Valnes K, Scott H, Rognum TO, Bjerke K, Baklien K. The human gastrointestinal secretory immune system in health and disease. In: Polak JM, Bloom SR, Wright NA, Butler AG, eds. Basic Science in Gastroenterology: Diseases of the gut. Norwich: Page Bros, 1986:179–200.
34. Merritt AJ, Potten CS, Watson AJM et al. Differential expression of bcl-2 in intestinal epithelia. Correlation with attenuation of apoptosis in colonic crypts and incidence of colonic neoplasia. J Cell Sci. 1995;108:261–271.
35. Blanchard TG, Czinn SJ, Maurer R, Thomas WD, Soman G, Nedrud JG. Urease-specific monoclonal antibodies prevent *Helicobacter felis* infection in mice. Infect Immun. 1995;63:1394–1399.
36. Chen M, Lee A, Hazell S. Immunisation against gastric *Helicobacter* infection in a mouse/*Helicobacter felis* model. Lancet. 1992;339:1120–1121.
37. Michetti P, Corthesy-Theulaz I, Davin C et al. Immunization of BALB/c mice against *Helicobacter felis* infection with *Helicobacter pylori* urease. Gastroenterology. 1994;107:1002–1011.
38. Pappo J, Thomas WD, Kabok Z, Taylor NS, Murphy JC, Fox JG. Effect of oral immunization with recombinant urease on murine *Helicobacter felis* gastritis. Infect Immun. 1995;63:1246–1252.
39. Ghiara P, Michetti P. Development of a vaccine. Curr Opin Gastroenterol. 1995;11:52–56.
40. Xu-Amano DJ, Kiyono H, Jackson RJ et al. Helper T cell subsets for immunoglobulin A responses: Oral immunization with tetanus toxoid and cholera toxin as adjuvant selectively induces Th2 cells in mucosa associated tissues. J Exp Med. 1993;178:1309–1320.

20
Immunodeficiency in Whipple's disease

T. SCHNEIDER, T. MARTH and M. ZEITZ

INTRODUCTION

Whipple's disease, first described by George Whipple[1], is a rare, systemic illness. The bacterial nature of the disease was recognized more than 30 years ago[2,3]. The causative bacterium, recently classified phylogenetically as an actinomycete by polymerase chain reaction (PCR) analysis of bacterial DNA encoding 16S rRNA[4,5] is now called *Tropheryma whippelii*[5]. Only recently Shoedon and co-workers succeeded in isolating and propagating the agent *in vitro*[6]. The disease is usually characterized by arthralgia, diarrhoea and malabsorption/ weight loss. However, it is a systemic illness that can give rise to symptoms relating to nearly every organ system including, in later stages, symptoms related to the central nervous system (CNS)[7]. Prior to the use of antibiotics Whipple's disease was uniformly fatal[8], but most patients are now successfully treated with various antibiotic regimens. Nevertheless, there still exist occasional patients, particularly those with CNS involvement, who have a downhill course in spite of antibiotic therapy[9–11].

The pathogenesis of infection with *T. whippelii* is poorly understood, but host factors, especially immune defects involving T cells and/or macrophages, are suspected of playing a role[12–16]. Recent advances in clinical immunology have demonstrated the importance of interferon-γ (IFN-γ) in the defence against intracellular bacteria and parasites. Several studies *in vitro* and *in vivo* suggest that cytokine signals to monocytes or macrophages by IFN-γ are crucial in the containment and clearance of intracellular bacteria[17,18]. One example of this kind is the discovery that chronic intracellular infection with atypical mycobacteria is associated in certain patients with defects in monocyte production of interleukin (IL)-12 and this, in turn, leads to reduced production of IFN-γ[19]. Indeed, in a recent study Marth and co-workers showed that patients with Whipple's disease also manifest a defect in macrophage production of IL-12 which is similar but not identical to that found in patients with atypical mycobacterial infection[20]. These observations may offer new therapeutic options in treating patients with Whipple's disease.

FINDINGS INDICATING AN IMMUNODEFICIENCY IN PATIENTS WITH WHIPPLE'S DISEASE

Whipple's disease is characterized by periodic acid Schiff (PAS)-positive lamina propria macrophages in the small intestine. This staining corresponds to bacteria[3]. The inability of patients with Whipple's disease to rid themselves of these intracellular bacteria without antibiotic treatment is unexplained, and for more than 30 years investigators have looked for immunological defects in these patients. Peripheral lymphocytopenia is common and reduced proliferation of lymphocytes derived from these patients to mitogenic stimuli such as phytohaemagglutinin (PHA) or concanavalin A (ConA) has been reported[13,21–24]. Furthermore, responses to intracutaneous testing with recall antigens are clearly reduced in these patients[13,22,23]. Impaired bacterial phagocytosis and bacterial degradation by macrophages from patients with Whipple's disease have also been described[14,25]. Some of these disturbances improve in patients after successful treatment.

A more recent study demonstrated a reduced number of cells expressing the complement receptor 3 α-chain (CD11b) in patients with active disease and in patients after successful treatment[16]. Decreased CD4/CD8 ratios were also found in the peripheral blood of patients with active Whipple's disease[16].

As in the case of other intracellular pathogens, the T_H1-driven immune response seems to play a key role in elimination of *T. whippelii*. Theoretically different disturbances in this pathway may be involved. One possibility is a primary macrophage/monocyte defect with disturbed IL-12 production leading

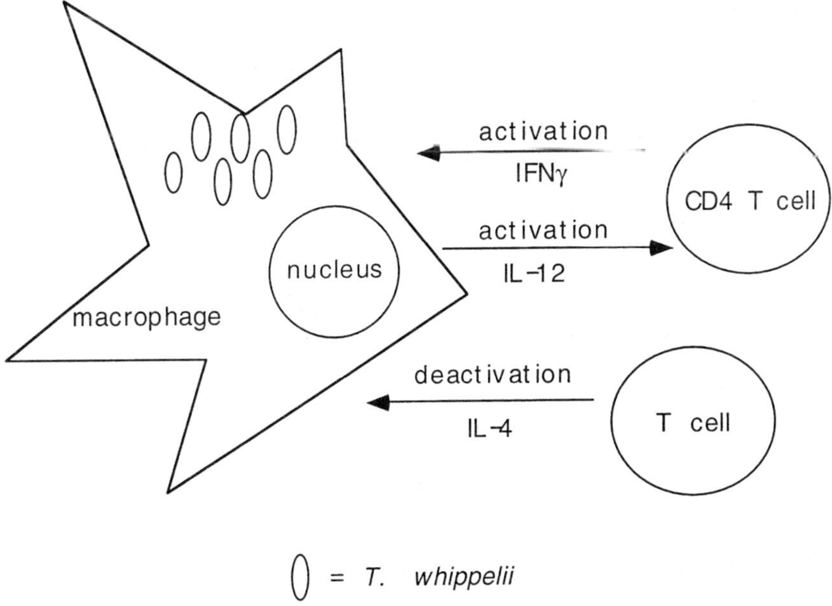

Figure 1 Interaction of macrophages and T cells, which may influence the degradation of *T. whippelii*.

to an impaired T_H1 activation and reduced IFN-γ production, which normally activates macrophages to destroy bacteria or other pathogens in their phagolysosomes by nitric oxide and superoxide production (Figure 1). A second possibility is a primary T-cell defect with reduced and inefficient production of IFN-γ or a dominating T_H2 response with cytokines such as IL-4 and IL-10, which block macrophage activation (Figure 1). A third possibility is the absence or defect of IFN-γ receptor on macrophages/monocytes, as has been described in some families with fatal infections by *Mycobacterium avium* complex, which is closely related to *T. whippelii*.

Indeed some of these defects have been recently described in patients with Whipple's disease.

FINDINGS SUPPORTING A PRIMARY MONOCYTE/MACROPHAGE DEFECT

In favour of the first possibility of a primary macrophage/monocyte defect is a study by Thomas Marth and co-workers who compared IL-12 production of peripheral monocytes isolated by counter flow centrifugation from controls and two patients with Whipple's disease. These cells were then stimulated either with *Staphylococcus aureus* + IFN-γ or with lipopolysaccharides + IFN-γ. In both cases clearly reduced IL-12 production by monocytes isolated from the patients with Whipple's disease was observed[20].

FINDINGS SUPPORTING A PRIMARY T CELL DEFECT

In favour of the second possibility is the recent successful attempt to isolate and propagate *T. whippelii* using IL-4, a T_H2 cytokine, to deactivate macrophages[6], indicating that a shift from a T_H1 to a T_H2 immune response may facilitate the replication of *T. whippelii*. We observed a reduction of IFN-γ production by mononuclear cells isolated from a patient with Whipple's disease compared to controls[26]. Interestingly this phenomenon improved after successful elimination of *T. whippelii*, indicating that bacterial factors probably contribute to the observed immunodeficiency in patients with Whipple's disease.

PRACTICAL CONSEQUENCES

If activation of macrophages is crucial to the elimination of *T. whippelii*, why not include IFN-γ in the treatment of refractory Whipple's disease? A patient with a more than 10-year history of antibiotic-refractory Whipple's disease, who was finally successfully treated with IFN-γ, is described. This patient was continuously treated with antibiotics in an attempt to eradicate the bacterium. Despite this therapy he had many relapses. In 1995, involvement of central nervous system was documented by the presence *T. whippelii*-specific DNA and PAS-positive cells in the cerebrospinal fluid. At this time point the decision was made to start combined therapy consisting of trimethoprim-sulphamethoxazole supplemented with recombinant human IFN-γ. Three weeks after initiation of

IFN-γ administration the patient recovered from clinical symptoms. Six months later *T. whippelii*-specific DNA and PAS-positive cells were no longer found in the cerebrospinal fluid. However, duodenal biopsy continued to reveal PAS-positive cells and *T. whippelii*-specific DNA. The dose of IFN-γ was increased and 4 months later the PCR analysis of duodenal biopsy for detection of *T. whippelii*-specific DNA was negative. Combined therapy was discontinued after 16 months, and the patient remains without symptoms[26].

CONCLUSIONS

Whipple's disease is a rare chronic illness due to infection with a bacterium which is able to replicate within macrophages. Despite successful antibiotic treatment in most of the patients, some, particularly those with central nervous system (CNS) involvement, have a downhill course suggesting an immunological defect. Investigations over the last 30 years have indicated an impaired cell mediated immune response by demonstrating a reduction of lymphocyte proliferation after stimulation with mitogens such as PHA and ConA, a reduced reactivity to intracutaneous testing with recall antigens, and reduced phagocytosis and degradation of bacteria in macrophages. As in the case of other intracellular pathogens the T_H1 driven immune response seems to play a key role in elimination of *T. whippelii*. Theoretically, different disturbances in this pathway may be involved in Whipple's disease: recently some defects in this pathway have been described which may have an influence on the treatment of the Whipple's disease, particularly in those with antibiotic-resistant disease. There may be a pre-existing immunodeficiency with an imbalance in the T_H1/T_H2 activities or a primary macrophage/monocyte defect in patients with Whipple's disease. On the other hand, factors produced by *T. whippelii* may block one or more steps in macrophage stimulation and activation. Whatever the mechanism, immunomodulatory therapy with IFN-γ, especially in antibiotic-refractory cases of Whipple's disease, seems to contribute to elimination of the agent.

References

1. Whipple GH. A hitherto undescribed disease characterized by deposits of fat and fatty acids in the intestinal and mesenteric lymphatic tissues. Bull Johns Hopkins Hosp. 1907;18:382–391.
2. Cohen AS, Holt PR, Isselbacher KJ. Ultrastructural abnormalities in Whipple's disease. Proc Soc Exp Biol Med. 1960;105:411–414.
3. Yardley JH, Hendrix TR. Combined electron and light microscopy in Whipple's disease: demonstration of 'bacillary bodies' in the intestine. Bull Johns Hopkins Hosp. 1961;109:80–98.
4. Wilson KH, Blitchington R, Frothingham R, Wilson JA, Phylogeny of the Whipple's-disease-associated bacterium. Lancet. 1991;338:474–475.
5. Relman DA, Schmidt TM, MacDermott RP, Falkow S. Identification of the uncultured bacillus of Whipple's disease. N Engl J Med. 1992;327:293–301.
6. Schoedon G, Goldenberger D, Forrer R et al. Deactivation of macrophages with interleukin-4 is the key to the isolation of *Tropheryma whippelii*. J Infect Dis. 1997;176:672–677.
7. Fleming JL, Wiesner RH, Shorter RG. Whipple's disease: clinical, biochemical, and histopathologic features and assessment of treatment in 29 patients. Mayo Clin Proc. 1988;63:539–551.
8. Paulley JW. A case of Whipple's disease (intestinal lipodystrophy). Gastroenterology. 1952;22:128–133.

9. Feurle GE, Volk B, Waldherr R. Cerebral Whipple's disease with negative jejunal histology. N Engl J Med. 1979;300:907–908.
10. Feldman M, Hendler RS, Morrison EB. Acute meningoencephalitis after withdrawal of antibiotics in Whipple's disease. Ann Intern Med. 1980;93:709–711.
11. Keinath RD, Merrell DE, Vliestra R, Dobbins WOI. Antibiotic treatment and relapse in Whipple's disease. Long-term follow-up of 88 patients. Gastroenterology. 1985;88:1867–1873.
12. Maizel H, Ruffin JM, Dobbins WO. Whipple's disease: a review of 19 patients from one hospital and a review of the literature since 1950. Medicine. 1970;49:175–205.
13. Martin FF, Vilseck J, Dobbins WOI, Buckley CEI, Tyor MP. Immunological alterations in patients with treated Whipple's disease. Gastroenterology. 1972;63:6–18.
14. Bjerkness R, Odegaard S, Bjerkvig R, Borkje B, Laerum OD. Whipple's disease: demonstration of a persisting monocyte and macrophage dysfunction. Scand J Gastroenterol. 1988;23:611–619.
15. Ectoers N, Geboes K, Rutgeerts P, Delabie J, Desmet V, Janssens J. RFD7-RFD9 coexpression by macrophages points to T cell macrophage interaction deficiency in Whipple's disease. Gastroenterology. 1992;106:A676.
16. Marth T, Roux M, von Herbay A, Meuer SC, Feurle GE. Persistent reduction of complement receptor 3 α-chain expressing mononuclear blood cells and transient inhibitory serum factors in Whipple's disease. Clin Immunol Immunopathol. 1994;72:217–226.
17. Holland SM, Eisenstein EM, Kuhns DB et al. Treatment of refractory disseminated non-tuberculous mycobacterial infection with interferon gamma. N Engl J Med. 1994;330:1348–1355.
18. Gallin JI, Farber JM, Holland SM, Nutman TB. Interferon-γ in the management of infectious disease. Ann Intern Med. 1995;123:216–224.
19. Frucht DM, Holland SM. Defective monocyte costimulation for INF-γ production in familial disseminated Mycobacterium avium complex infection: abnormal IL-12 regulation. J Immunol. 1996;157:411–416.
20. Marth T, Neurath M, Cuccherini BA, Strober W. Defects of monocyte interleukin 12 production and humoral immunity in Whipple's disease. Gastroenterology. 1997;113:442–448.
21. Maxwell JD, Ferguson A, McCay AM, Imrie RC, Watson WC. Lymphocytes in Whipple's disease. Lancet. 1968;1;887–889.
22. Groll A, Valberg LS, Simon JB, Eidinger D, Wison D, Forsdyke DR. Imunological defect in Whipple's disease. Gastroenterology. 1972;63:943–950.
23. Feurle GE, Dörken B, Schöpf E, Lenhard V. HLA-B27 and defects in the T-cell system in Whipple's disease. Eur J Clin Invest. 1979;9:385–389.
24. Kirkpatrick PM, Kent SP, Mikas A, Pritchett P. Whipple's disease: A case report with immunological studies. Gastroenterology. 1978;75:297–301.
25. Gupta S, Pinching AJ, Onwubalili J, Vince A, Evans DJ, Hodgson HJF. Whipple's disease with unusual clinical, bacteriologic, and immunologic findings. Gastroenterology. 1986;90:1286–1289.
26. Schneider T, Stallmach A, von Herbay A, Marth T, Strober W, Zeitz M. Treatment of refractory Whipple's disease with interferon gamma. Ann Intern Med. 1998; in press.

21
Interferon-γ induces necrosis in the small intestines of mice following peroral infection with *Toxoplasma gondii*

O. LIESENFELD, J. KOSEK, J. S. REMINGTON and Y. SUZUKI

INTRODUCTION

Remarkable differences in mortality following acute infection with the obligate intracellular protozoan parasite, *Toxoplasma gondii*, have been observed among inbred strains of mice[1-3]. Whereas multiple genes, including those linked to the H-2 complex, were found to be involved in regulation of resistance against death following infection, the mechanism(s) which underlies the differences in mortality among inbred strains of mice following the infection is unknown. We therefore analysed the mechanism(s) that underlies the remarkable difference in susceptibility to peroral infection with *T. gondii* in genetically resistant and susceptible strains of mice.

EXPERIMENTAL RESULTS

C57BL/6 mice all died 7–13 days following peroral infection with 100 cysts of the low-virulent ME49 *T. gondii* strain, whereas all BALB/c mice survived ($p < 0.001$; Fig. 1)[4]. Of interest is that C57BL/6 mice appeared healthy until 5 days after infection. Thereafter, they quickly developed piloerection, became huddled, and lost mobility. Histological examination of brains, hearts, lungs, spleens and large intestines 7 days after infection revealed no inflammatory changes in either strain of mouse (there were higher numbers of inflammatory foci in livers of C57BL/6 compared to BALB/c mice) but severe necrosis of the villi and mucosal cells was observed in ilea of susceptible C57BL/6 and not in resistant BALB/c mice (Table 1)[4]. Numbers of tachyzoites were significantly higher in the ilea of C57BL/6 mice than in BALB/c mice at the same time (Table 1)[4]. Since there were areas of necrosis without tachyzoites, suggesting that tachyzoites are not involved in development of necrosis, and since we

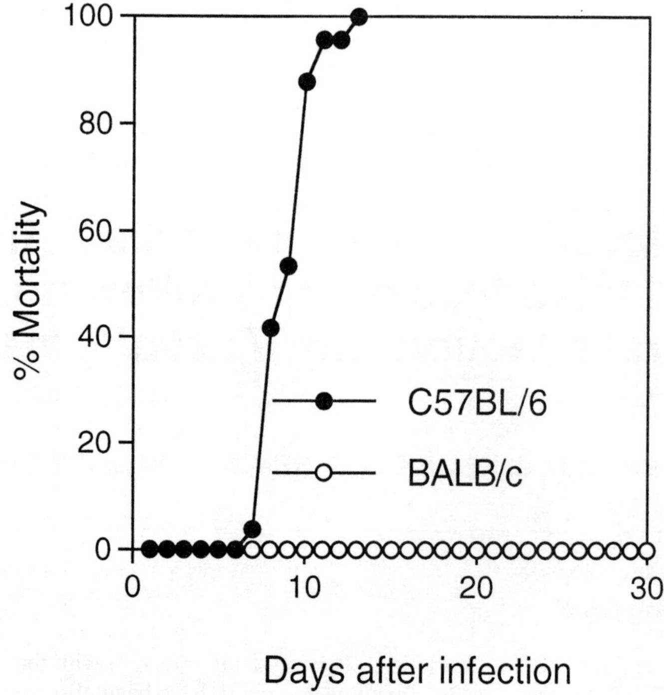

Figure 1   Mortality in C57BL/6 and BALB/c mice following peroral infection with 100 cysts of the ME49 *T. gondii* strain (adapted from reference 4, with permission)

Table 1   Necrosis and numbers of parasitophorous vacuoles containing tachyzoites in the ilea of C57BL/6 and BALB/c mice following peroral infection with *T. gondii*[a]

Days after infection	Strain of mouse	Length of ileum with necrosis (cm) (H&E stain)	Number of parasitophorous vacuoles/cm of ileum (immunoperoxidase stain)
3	BALB/c	0	0
	C57BL/6	0	0
5	BALB/c	0	0
	C57BL/6	0	12.1 ± 18.9
7	BALB/c	0	14.9 ± 22.5
	C57BL/6	10.5 ± 0.5[b]	265 ± 16.1[c]

[a] Table adapted from reference 4, with permission.
[b] $p < 0.004$ versus BALB/c mice at the same time point.
[c] $p < 0.0001$ versus BALB/c mice at the same time point.

observed a significant decrease in CD4[+] T cells in Peyer's patches only in infected C57BL/6 mice (data not shown), we examined the role of T cells in resistance against death due to infection in both strains of mice using athymic nude mice. BALB/c-background athymic nude mice all died whereas euthymic control BALB/c mice all survived ($p < 0.0001$)[4]. C57BL/6-background athymic nude mice survived significantly longer than euthymic control C57BL/6 mice ($p = 0.0007$), although both strains died of acute infection, indicating that the presence of T cells predisposes to early death in genetically susceptible C57BL/6 mice following infection whereas these cells confer protection against death in resistant BALB/c mice. Seven days after infection, necrosis in the ilea was observed in the control but not the athymic C57BL/6 mice. However, fewer tachyzoites were observed in the ilea of the former than the latter mice[4]. These results indicate that necrosis in the ilea of C57BL/6 mice was not due to destruction of tissue by tachyzoites but rather was mediated by T cells. Neither control nor athymic BALB/c mice developed necrosis of the ilea. To determine whether α/β or γ/δ T cells are critical for development of necrosis, α/β T cell-deficient, γ/δ T cell-deficient and control mice, which have the H-2[b] haplotype as do C57BL/6 mice, were perorally infected with the ME49 strain and their intestines examined histologically 7 days later. Necrosis of the villi and mucosal cells was observed in the ilea of the γ/δ T cell-deficient and control mice but not in the α/β T cell-deficient mice (Fig. 2), indicating that α/β but not γ/δ T cells are required for development of necrosis in the ilea following infection[4]. Furthermore, severe necrosis was observed in wide areas of the ilea of β2-microglobulin-deficient mice, which lack CD8[+] T cells (Fig. 2) and control mice (Fig. 2)[4]. In contrast, necrosis was not observed in the small intestines of MHC class II-deficient mice, which lack CD4[+] T cells (Fig. 2). Thus, CD4[+] T cells induce necrosis of the ilea in genetically susceptible mice following infection.

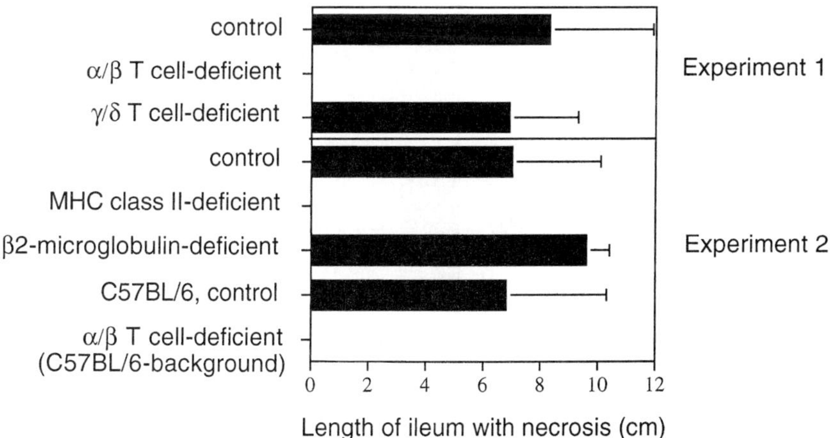

Figure 2 Length of the ileum with necrosis in mutant mice deficient in different T cell subsets following peroral infection with *T. gondii* (adapted from reference 4, with permission)

IFN-γ is known to be critical for resistance against death of BALB/c mice following peroral infection with *T. gondii*[5,6]. Therefore, we examined the effect of anti-IFN-γ mAb on mortality and time to death in C57BL/6 mice by treatment of mice with 2 mg anti-IFN-γ mAb every 5 days beginning 1 day before infection. BALB/c mice treated with anti-IFN-γ mAb all died by day 12 whereas 91% of control treated BALB/c mice survived ($p = 0.0014$)[4]. C57BL/6 mice treated with anti-IFN-γ mAb all died significantly earlier than control treated mice which all died by day 15 ($p = 0.0023$)[4]. These results indicate that IFN-γ plays a protective role in resistance against death in C57BL/6 mice, although the protective effect was partial and all mice died by day 15 of infection. Because C57BL/6 mice developed signs of illness between 5 and 6 days after infection, we performed a separate experiment to examine the role of IFN-γ in resistance against death of these mice during this stage of their infection using treatment of C57BL/6 mice with anti-IFN-γ mAb at 5, 7 and 9 days after infection. In contrast to the results obtained when treatment with anti-IFN-γ mAb was begun 1 day before infection, mice treated with anti-IFN-γ mAb 5, 7, and 9 days following infection survived significantly longer than control mice ($p = 0.0012$)[4]. These results indicate that IFN-γ predisposed to death in C57BL/6 mice through its action during the time when the mice developed clinical signs of the infection. Histological studies revealed that whereas mice treated with control IgG had severe necrosis of the villi in most parts of the ilea (Fig. 3), those treated with anti-IFN-γ mAb did not have such areas of necrosis (Fig. 3)[4]. The numbers of parasitophorous vacuoles containing tachyzoites in the ilea did not differ between mice treated with control

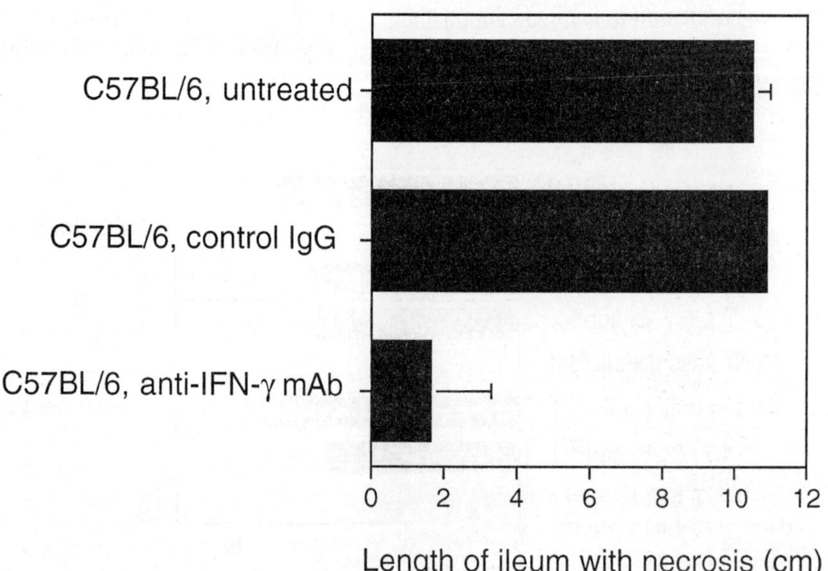

Figure 3 Effect of treatment with anti-IFN-γ mAb on development of necrosis in the ilea of C57BL/6 mice following peroral infection with *T. gondii* (adapted from reference 4, with permission)

IgG and those treated with anti-IFN-γ mAb[4]. These results demonstrate that development of necrosis in the ilea was mediated by IFN-γ.

Our studies reveal a requirement for CD4[+] T cells and IFN-γ for development of necrosis in the ilea of C57BL/6 mice which die following peroral infection with *T. gondii*. Along with the protective role for T cells and IFN-γ in resistant BALB/c mice these results indicate that a single cytokine, IFN-γ, plays a critical role in the mechanisms that determine early death or survival of inbred strains of mice after peroral infection with *T. gondii*. Further analysis of the mechanism(s) of development of necrosis in the small intestine in genetically susceptible C57BL/6 mice will provide important information for better understanding of the genetic susceptibility to infection with *T. gondii*. Since CD4[+] T cells and IFN-γ have been reported to be involved in development of intestinal pathology in the colon in different murine models of inflammatory bowel disease[7–9], information generated from *T. gondii*-infected mice may also be valuable for understanding of the immunopathogenesis of inflammatory diseases in the intestine in general.

ACKNOWLEDGEMENTS

We thank Nhung Nguyen for her excellent technical assistance. This work was supported by a grant from Japan Immunoresearch Laboratories Co. Ltd., and in part by U. S. Public Health Service Grants A138260, A104717, A135956, and A130230 from the National Institutes of Health. O. Liesenfeld is recipient of a Walter Marget Foundation Infectious Disease Fellowship and an Infectious Disease Research Fellowship from the German Ministry of Research and Technology (BMFT).

References

1. Johnson AM. Strain-dependent, route of challenge-dependent, murine susceptibility to toxoplasmosis. Zentralbl Parasitenk. 1984;70:303–309.
2. McLeod R, Estes, RG, Mack, D, Cohen, H. Immune response of mice to ingested *Toxoplasma gondii*: a mode of *Toxoplasma* infection acquired by ingestion. J Infect Dis. 1984;149: 234–244.
3. McLeod R, Eisenhauer P, Mack D, Brown C, Filice G, Spitalny G. Immune responses associated with early survival after peroral infection with *Toxoplasma gondii*. J Immunol. 1989;142: 3247–3255.
4. Liesenfeld O, Kosek J, Remington J, Suzuki, Y. Association of CD4[+] T cell-dependent, interferon-γ mediated necrosis of the small intestine with genetic susceptibility of mice to peroral infection with *Toxoplasma gondii*. J Exp Med. 1996;184:597–609.
5. Suzuki Y, Orellana, MA, Schreiber RD, Remington, JS. Interferon-γ: the major mediator of resistance against *Toxoplasma gondii*. Science. 1988;240:516–518.
6. Johnson L. A protective role for endogenous tumor necrosis factor in *Toxoplasma gondii* infection. Infect Immun. 1992;60:1979–1983.
7. Powrie R, Orrea-Olivera R, Mauze S, Coffman RL. Regulatory interactions between CD45RB[high] and CD45RB[low] CD4[+] T cells are important for the balance between protective and pathogenic cell-mediated immunity. J Exp Med. 1994;179:589–600.
8. Neurath F, Fuss I, Kelsall B, Stüber E, Strober W. Antibodies against interleukin 12 abrogate established experimental colitis in mice. J Exp Med. 1995;182:1281–1290.
9. Berg DJ, Davidson N, Kühn R et al. Enterocolitis and colon cancer in interleukin-10-deficient mice are associated with aberrant cytokine production and CD4[+] TH1-like responses. J Clin Invest. 1996;98:1010–1020.

Section V
Mechanisms of inflammatory disease 3: Down-regulation of inflammatory processes and disturbances in IBD

22

Physiological role of apoptotic mechanisms in the gut

M. BOIRIVANT, M. MARINI and G. DI FELICE

INTRODUCTION

Intestinal lamina propria-associated lymphoid tissues constitute a major lymphoid compartment which is continuously exposed to potentially stimulatory mucosal antigens[1]. Nevertheless, although lamina propria T cells show increased expression of surface markers of cell activation[2,3], lamina propria is normally a site of controlled chronic inflammation[1]. Maintaining homeostasis requires effective mechanisms for preventing and terminating lymphocyte responses which evolved in this area to allow fine discrimination between pathogen and resident luminal antigens. The unresponsiveness toward the latter antigens is defined as oral tolerance[4]. Some unique features of lymphocytes isolated from human lamina propria indeed suggest that regulatory mechanisms are operating in maintaining such homeostasis.

Lamina propria T cells, in comparison to peripheral blood T cells, represent a population enriched in CD45R0+ activated T cells, which express Fas antigen[5]. When stimulated via the TCR/CD3 pathway they show proliferative hyporesponsiveness, but relative normoresponsiveness when stimulated via the CD2 accessory signalling pathway, compared with peripheral blood T cells[6–9]. This pattern of hyporesponsiveness is underscored by the fact that in inflammatory bowel disease, the TCR/CD3 pathway proliferative response is further diminished whereas CD2 normoresponsiveness is maintained[10]. Among the several immunological mechanisms involved in maintaining homeostasis and T-cell tolerance (anergy, apoptosis and cytokine modulation), we have, in the last few years, investigated the role of apoptosis in maintaining homeostasis in human lamina propria.

APOPTOSIS

Cell death is an important event during the immune response, allowing the removal of cells that are no longer needed and/or are potentially autoreactive.

This naturally occurring programmed cell death is a morphologically defined process that ultimately leads to activation of endogenous nucleases and internucleosomal DNA degradation. Nuclear fragmentation and formation of apoptotic bodies follow this process. Apoptotic cells and bodies are specifically recognized by phagocytic cells which degrade them. This process prevents the release of cell constituents and therefore prevents injury to neighbouring cells[11,12].

Apoptosis of T cells is involved in both eliminating activated T cells which are no longer engaged by the antigen when growth factors decline and T cells repeatedly activated to prevent overstimulation. The second event is associated with the triggering of such designated molecules as Fas and its ligand[13,14].

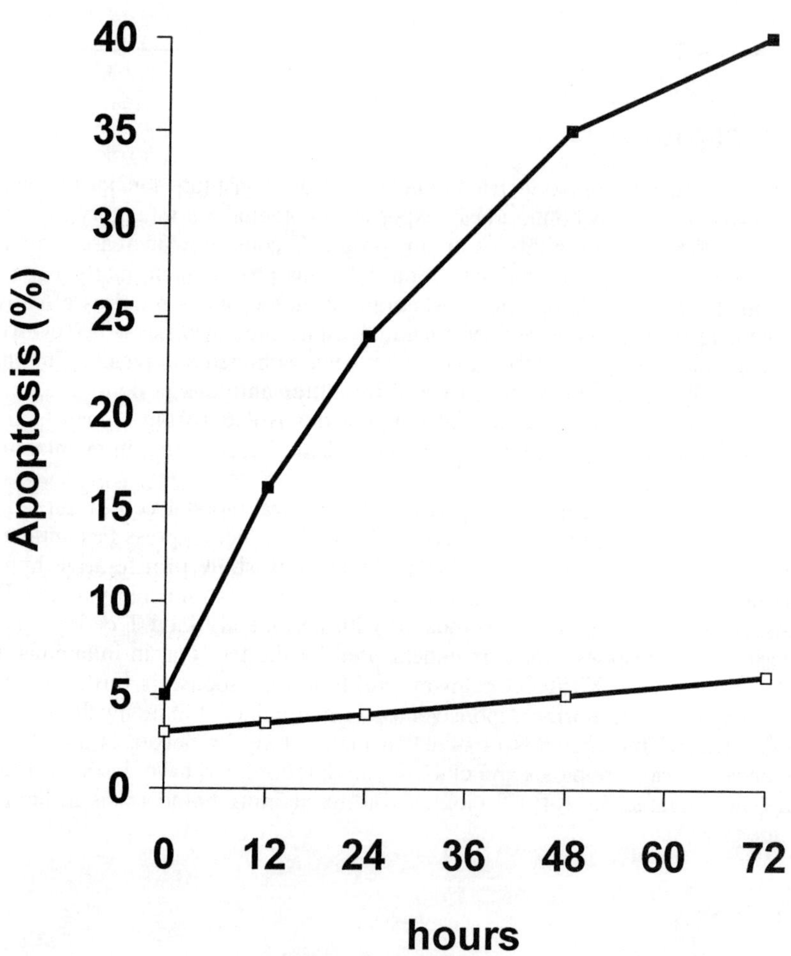

Figure 1 Relative proportion of apoptotic T lymphocytes during culture in absence of stimulation. ■ Lamina propria T cell; □ peripheral blood T cell

APOPTOSIS IN HUMAN LAMINA PROPRIA T CELLS

When we initially analysed the apoptosis of isolated lamina propria T lymphocytes, we observed an increased apoptosis in unstimulated T cells compared with autologous peripheral blood T lymphocytes (Figure 1). This apoptosis was partially rescued by incubation with cytokines which signal through the interleukin-2 (IL-2) receptor common γ-chain, IL-2, IL-7 and IL-15[15]. We previously observed that CD3/TCR hyporesponsive lamina propria T cells can recover their ability to proliferate when cultured in IL-2 in the absence of antigen stimulation[8], suggesting that these cells are partially anergic cells (if one defines the latter via TCR/CD3 responsiveness) which are more susceptible to apoptosis. From these observations we can derive that death by deprivation of growth factors contributes, at least in part, to increased levels of spontaneous apoptosis in activated, partially anergic, lamina propria T cells. Since IL-2 is not able to rescue the apoptosis of unstimulated T cells completely, some apoptotic mechanisms should be already activated *in vivo* and cannot be counteracted during culture. We observed that a discrete fraction of freshly isolated lamina propria T cells constitutively expresses Fas ligand[5] and shows an increase in the protease activity of CPP32 when compared to peripheral T lymphocytes (2.36-fold increase over the peripheral blood T lymphocyte value, preliminary data). These data strongly suggest that activation-induced cell death, mediated by Fas–Fas ligand, affects human lamina propria T cells *in vivo*.

We therefore investigated the *in vitro* susceptibility of different activation pathways to regulation by apoptosis. TCR/CD3 stimulation induced no increase in the apoptosis level over that observed in unstimulated T cells, while CD2 stimulation was associated with a significant increase in apoptosis compared with unstimulated lamina propria T cells (Table 1)[15]. CD2 stimulation was associated with increased levels of Fas ligand mRNA (Figure 2) and, more recently, we also found increased CPP32 enzymatic activity (preliminary data). In addition, we were able to block CD2 stimulation-associated apoptosis using a blocking anti-Fas monoclonal antibody. Pretreatment of LPT lymphocytes with this antibody completely prevented the observed CD2 stimulation-induced increase in apoptosis but failed to modify apoptosis in unstimulated T cells (Figure 3). Thus, the augmented apoptosis that follows CD2 pathway stimulation is mediated by Fas signalling. Intracellular events that follow Fas triggering are, in

Table 1 Relative proportion of apoptotic cells after 18 h of culture with different stimuli

	PBTC (%)	LPTC (%)
Unstimulated	4 ± 2	17 ± 5*
CD3 pathway-stimulated	3 ± 2	18 ± 5
CD2 pathway-stimulated	3.5 ± 3	31 ± 7**

Apoptosis was quantitated by propidium iodide staining, followed by FACS analysis.
PBTC = peripheral blood T cells; LPTC = lamina propria T cells.
* $p = 0.001$ unstimulated PBTC vs unstimulated LPTC.
** $p = 0.007$ CD2 pathway-stimulated LPTC vs unstimulated LPTC. Values are mean ± SD from 8 different experiments.

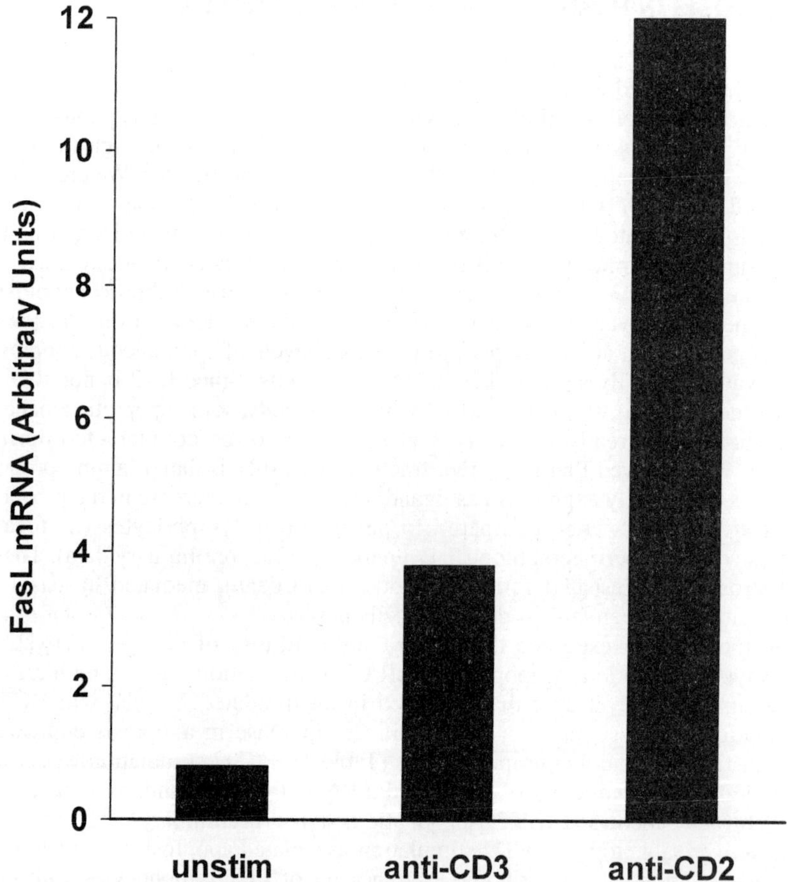

Figure 2 FasL mRNA expression after 18 h culture with different stimuli. FasL mRNA was evaluated by RT-PCR. Gel runs were photographed and the negative was scanned for the detection of optical density area by densitometry. Fas ligand values are expressed as arbitrary units after normalization with the corresponding GAPDH value (Fas ligand/GAPDH optical density area)

human lamina propria T lymphocytes, mediated by acidic sphingomyelinase pathway activation with ceramide generation[5]. Since LP T cells show an increased capacity to secrete cytokines compared with peripheral blood T cells, especially when triggered via the CD2 stimulation pathway[8,9], one would predict that the increased apoptosis cell death that follows CD2 pathway stimulation would be an important mechanism in the down-regulation of lamina propria T cell cytokine production that might otherwise induce inflammation in the lamina propria; this indeed proved to be true in that lamina propria T cells in cultures in which apoptosis was inhibited produced significantly increased amounts of IFN-γ (Figure 4).

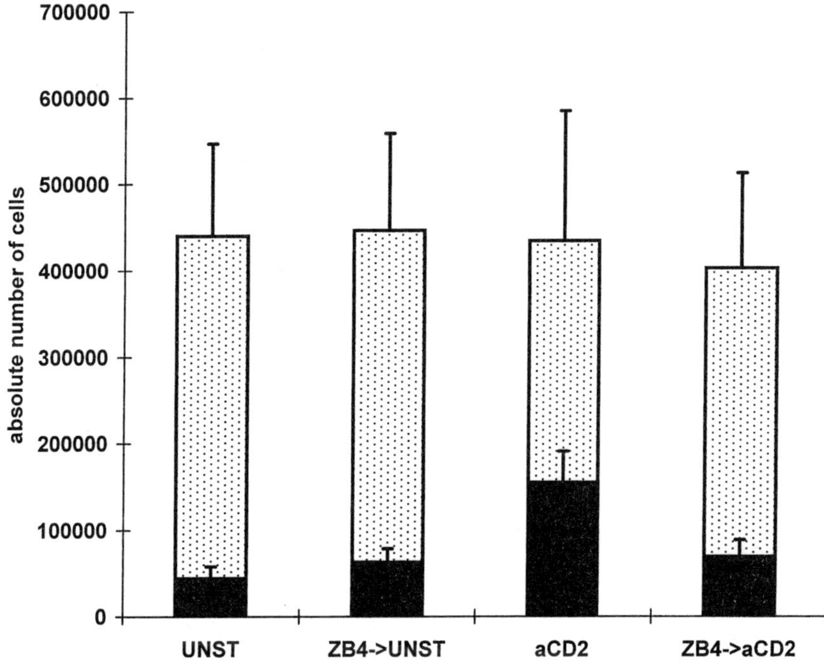

Figure 3 Effect of Fas blockade on CD2-mediated apoptosis. Assessment of apoptosis by acridine orange/ethidium bromide fluorescence staining after 24 h of culture. Cells were preincubated where indicated for 1 h at 37°C in the presence of anti-Fas blocking mAb (IgG1) ZB4. Values represent mean ± SD from 4 different experiments. Number of apoptotic cells ▉ and number of cells recovered ▨ at the end of the culture period

From the above data, we suggest that functional condition of LP T cells resembles that of a recently described human peripheral blood allogeneic T cell clone, intentionally rendered anergic and then cultured in IL-2. These cells respond to TCR/CD3 stimulation only if co-stimulated via CD2. In addition, whereas fully anergic T cells do not express a signalling CD2 epitope upon stimulation, anergic cells cultured in IL-2 do express this epitope upon stimulation, accounting for the recovered CD2-mediated proliferative capacity[16]. According to this model, activation-induced apoptosis is involved only in the CD2 activation pathway, where it is responsible for down-modulating proliferation and cytokine production. The TCR/CD3 pathway is somehow differently down-modulated and, therefore, it is not apparently regulated by activation-induced apoptosis. CD3/TCR-pathway hyporesponsiveness is strictly related to the microenvironment in the tissue since T cell lines derived from lamina propria lymphocytes and maintained with alternate CD28+CD2/IL-2 stimulation are able to proliferate under TCR/CD3 stimulation as T cell lines derived from autologous peripheral blood. In addition, after proper induction, they undergo apoptosis after TCR/CD3 stimulation as well as after CD2 stimulation (Figure 5).

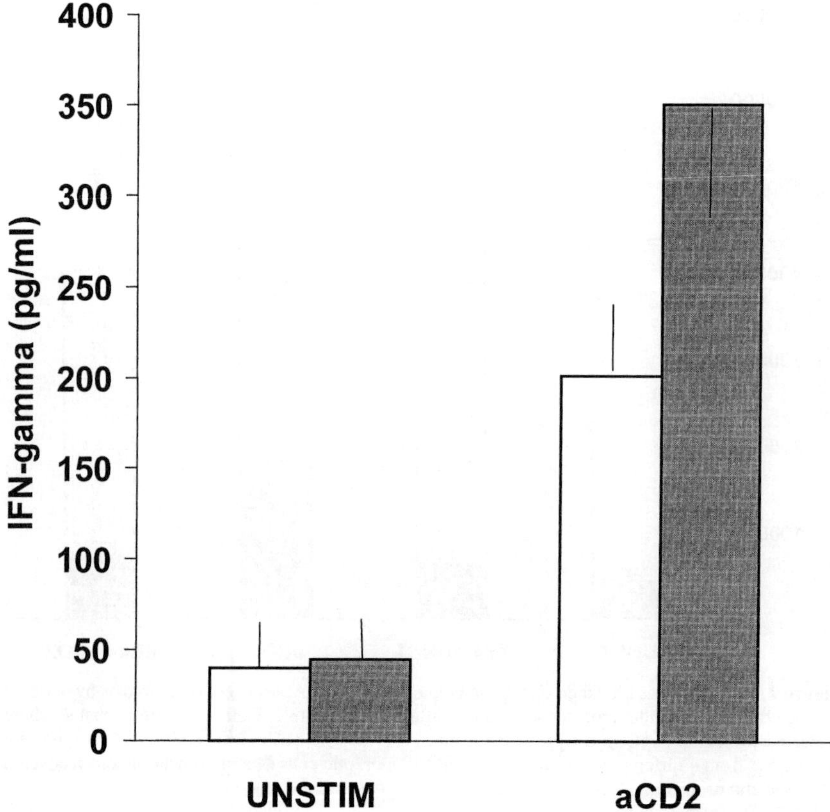

Figure 4 Effect of apoptosis bockade on CD2-induced LP T cell IFN-γ production. Cells were preincubated for 1 h at 37°C in the presence ■ or in the absence □ of anti-Fas blocking mAb (IgG1) ZB4. After preincubation cells were stimulated, where indicated, with anti-CD2 mAb. Values represent mean ± SD from 4 different experiments

APOPTOSIS IN CROHN'S DISEASE

In view of the above findings, it is of interest to determine the ability of cells in the lamina propria of patients with inflammatory bowel disease to undergo apoptosis. Preliminary results suggest that Crohn's disease-derived T cell lines are less sensitive to IL-2 deprivation-associated apoptosis than are control-derived T cell lines[17]. Our preliminary data suggest that activation-induced cell death is also defective[18].

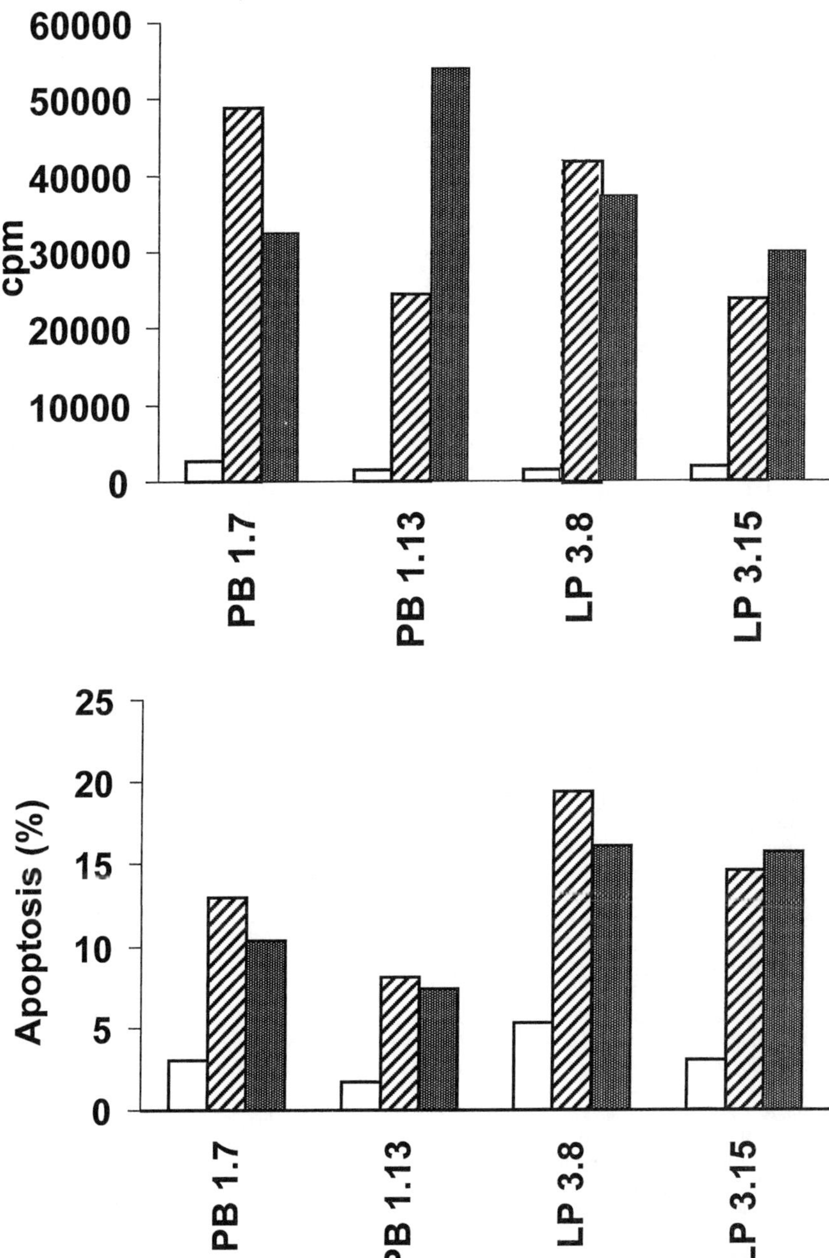

Figure 5 Upper panel: Proliferative response to different stimuli by lamina propria-derived T cell lines (LP) and autologous peripheral blood-derived T cell lines (PB). Proliferation was assessed as [³H]thymidine incorporation during the last 18 h of 48 h stimulation with the different stimuli. Unstimulated □; anti-CD3 ▨ ; anti-CD2▨ . Lower panel: Relative proportion of apoptotic T cells in T cell lines derived from LP and autologous PB. Apoptosis was quantitated by propidium iodide staining followed by FACS analysis. In order to induce apoptosis T cell lines were treated for 24 h with rIL-2 (20 U/ml) followed by TCR/CD3 or CD2 pathway stimulation. Unstimulated □; anti-CD3 ▨; anti-CD2▨ .

References

1. Brandtzaeg P, Halstesen TS, Kett K et al. Immunobiology and immunopathology of human gut mucosa: humoral immunity and intraepithelial lymphocytes. Gastroenterology. 1989;97: 1562–1586.
2. Pallone F, Fais S, Squarcia O, Biancone L, Pozzilli P, Boirivant M. Activation of peripheral and intestinal lamina propria lymphocytes in Crohn's disease. 'In vivo' state of activation and 'in vitro' response to stimulation as defined by the expression of early activation antigens. Gut. 1987;28:745–753.
3. Peters MG, Secrist H, Anders KR, Nash GS, Rich SR, MacDermott RP. Normal human intestinal lymphocytes. Increased activation compared with the peripheral blood. J Clin Invest. 1989;83:1827–1831.
4. Weiner HL, Friedman A, Miller A et al. Oral tolerance: immunologic mechanisms and treatment of animal and human organ-specific autoimmune diseases by oral administration of autoantigens. Annu Rev Immunol. 1994;12:809–837.
5. De Maria R, Boirivant M, Cifone MG et al. Functional expression of Fas and Fas ligand on human gut lamina propria T lymphocytes: a potential role for the acidic sphingomyelinase pathway in normal immunoregulation. J Clin Invest. 1996;97:316–322.
6. Pirzer UC, Schurmann G, Post S, Betzler M, Meuer SC. Differential responsiveness to CD3-Ti vs. CD2-dependent activation of human intestinal T lymphocytes. Eur J Immunol. 1990;20: 2339–2342.
7. Qiao L, Schurmann G, Betzler M, Meuer SC. Activation and signaling status of human lamina propria T lymphocytes. Gastroenterology. 1991;101:1529–1536.
8. Boirivant M, Fuss I, Fiocchi C, Klein JS, Strong SA, Strober W. Hypo-proliferative human lamina propria T cells retain the capacity to secrete lymphokines when stimulated via the CD2/CD28 accessory signaling pathways. Proc Assoc Am Phys. 1996;108:55–67.
9. Targan SR, Deem RL, Liu M, Wang S, Nel A. Definition of lamina propria T cell responsive state. Enhanced cytokine responsiveness of T cells stimulated through the CD2 pathway. J Immunol. 1995;154:664–675.
10. Fuss IJ, Neurath M, Boirivant M et al. Disparate CD4+ lamina propria (LP) lymphokine secretion profiles in inflammatory bowel disease. Crohn's disease LP cells manifest increased secretion of IFN-gamma, whereas ulcerative colitis LP cells manifest increased secretion of IL-5. J Immunol. 1996;157:1261–1270.
11. Cotter TG, Al-Rubeai M. Cell death (apoptosis) in cell culture systems. Tibtech. 1995;13: 150–155.
12. Savill J, Fadok V, Henson P, Haslett C. Phagocyte recognition of cells undergoing apoptosis. Immunol Today. 1993;14:131–136.
13. Akbar AN, Salmon M. Cellular environments and apoptosis: tissue microenvironment control activated T-cell death. Immunol Today. 1997;18:72–76.
14. Van Parijs L, Abbas AK. Homeostasis and self-tolerance in the immune system: turning lymphocytes off. Science. 1998;280:243–248.
15. Boirivant M, Pica R, DeMaria R, Testi R, Pallone F, Strober W. Stimulated human lamina propria T cells manifest enhanced Fas-mediated apoptosis. J Clin Invest. 1996;98:2616–2622.
16. Boussiotis VA, Freeman GJ, Griffin JD, Gray GS, Gribben JG, Nadler LM. CD2 is involved in maintenance and reversal of human alloantigen-specific clonal anergy. J Exp Med. 1994;180: 1665–1674.
17. Ina K, Binion DG, West GA, Dobrea GM, Fiocchi C. Crohn's disease (CD) mucosal T-cells are resistant to apoptosis. Gastroenterology. 1995;108:A841.
18. Marini M, Di Felice G, Pronio AM, Montesani C, Boirivant M. Lamina propria mononuclear cells (LPMC) from Crohn's disease (CD) patients show reduced apoptosis levels when stimulated via the CD2-activation pathway. Gastroenterology. 1997;112:A1034.

23
Shifting T_H1/T_H2 responses as therapeutic approach

P. PARRONCHI and S. ROMAGNANI

T_H1/T_H2 CELLS IN HUMANS

Convincing evidence for the existence of human T cells exhibiting polarized phenotypes similar to those first described in mice has been clearly provided in recent years[1,2]. In 1991 we showed that T cell clones specific for protein purified derivative (PPD) of *Mycobacterium tuberculosis* and excretory/secretory (TES) antigens from *Toxocara canis* showed different abilities to produce cytokine: TES-specific T cells were able to produce IL-4 and IL-5 but no interferon-γ (IFN-γ) showing a clear-cut T_H2 profile, while PPD-specific T cells produced IFN-γ but no IL-4 and IL-5 (T_H1 phenotype)[3]. Different functional properties are also exhibited by human T_H1 and T_H2 cells, as T_H1 cells show cytolytic potential, can activate macrophages and can help B cells (at low T:B ratios) to produce antibodies. They are implicated in the host defence against micro-organisms, in particular intracellular microbes, and viruses. T_H2 cells show no cytolytic potential and no ability to activate macrophage functions, but they can actively help B cells to produce antibodies, including IgE. Complex parasites (helminths) usually induce a T_H2 response which interferes with parasite physiology through the activation and recruitment of eosinophils, induction of IgE and degranulation of mast-cells and basophils[4].

Recently it has been reported that human T lymphocytes showing polarized phenotypes preferentially express different surface antigens. Expression of lymphocyte activation gene 3 (LAG-3), a member of the immunoglobulin super-family with unknown function, has been associated with IFN-γ-producing T cells. Streptokinase (SK)-specific T cell lines from normal donors which show a prevalent T_H1 phenotype are positive for LAG-3 expression, while allergen (Der p 1)-specific T cell lines obtained from atopic donors which produce high amounts of IL-4 and low IFN-γ exhibit poor expression of the molecule[5]. T cell clones with established T_H1 phenotype express LAG-3 on their surface and are able to release sLAG-3 in supernatants after stimulation. Recently we have demonstrated the naive T cells derived from cord blood after polyclonal stimulation in the presence of modulating agents such as interleukin (IL)-12 and IL-4 show different ability to express LAG-3. IL-12-conditioned T cell lines show a prevalent T_H1 phenotype and express high levels of LAG-3. The expression of LAG-3 is dependent on IFN-γ production, since a neutralizing anti-IFN-γ monoclonal antibody down-regulates the expression of the molecule in IL-12 primed T cell lines[6]. High expression of CD26 antigen, a dipeptidyl peptidase IV, correlates with a T_H1/T_H0 phenotype as IL-12 and IFN-γ modulated PBMC show increased levels of CD26 while allergen (Bet V 1)-specific T cell clones with T_H2 phenotype display low expression of this molecule[7]. Moreover, LAG-3 and CD26 are present in pathological tissues where the pathogenetic role of T_H1 cells has been demonstrated[8]. Finally, high expression of chemokine receptors such as CXCR3 and CCR5 and P and E selectins has been described recently on the surface of T_H1 cells.

Despite initial conflicting results, we and others have provided convincing evidence in favour of the expression of CD30, a member of the TNF superfamily, as a molecule preferentially associated with T_H2 phenotype. High level and long-lasting CD30 expression is seen after activation in T cell clones showing the T_H2 phenotype, while transient and low expression of the receptor is present on T_H1/T_H0 cells[9]. High numbers of CD30[+] lymphocytes are present in lymph nodes of patients affected by Omenn's syndrome, a rare immunodeficiency characterized by hypereosinophilia and increased serum levels of IgE. Sorting CD30[+] T cells from the peripheral blood of these patients allowed the generation of T cell clones with a clear-cut T_H2 phenotype[10]. CD30[+] cells and high levels of the soluble form of this receptor have been demonstrated in pathological conditions where T_H2 cells predominate, such as systemic sclerosis and atopic conditions[11]. CD30 is also expressed in medullary area of the thymus where IL-4 production is present[12]. Finally, both murine and human naive T cells polyclonally stimulated in the presence of IL-4 develop into cells able to produce IL-4 and IL-13 and express CD30[6,13]. More recently other receptors have been described as preferentially associated with the T_H2 phenotype, including L-selectin and CCR3, CCR4, CXCR4 chemokine receptors.

THE T_H1/T_H2 PARADIGM IN HUMAN DISEASES

Several studies have demonstrated the role of T_H1 and T_H2 cells in the pathogenesis of different pathological conditions in humans. T_H1 cells are implicated in organ-specific autoimmune disease such as Hashimoto's thyroiditis and Graves' disease, as demonstrated by clonal studies and reverse transcriptase-polymerase chain reaction (RT-PCR) analysis[14,15]. An homogeneous T_H1 phenotype was also observed in CD4[+] T cell clones derived from retro-orbital infiltrates of patients with Graves' ophthalmopathy[15]. Several studies suggest a role for tumour necrosis factor-α (TNF-α) and IFN-γ in the pathogenesis of multiple sclerosis (MS): high levels of TNF-α in both plasma and cerebrospinal fluid may predict relapses in MS patients[16] and T cell clones specific for myelin antigens derived from both peripheral blood and cerebrospinal fluid show a T_H1 profile[17]. Soluble LAG-3 has been found in high levels in the serum of patients with more severe forms of MS[5] and RT-PCR has demonstrated the presence of TNF-α, TNF-β and IL-12p40 in active cerebral plaques[18]. In rheumatoid and reactive arthritis subsequent to infection from *Borrelia burgdorferi* and *Yersinia enterocolitica* T$_H$1 cells have been demonstrated[4].

More recently we have demonstrated that two gastrointestinal diseases are associated with a prevalent T$_H$1 phenotype of infiltrating T lymphocytes. *Helicobacter pylori* (Hp) infection is the primary cause of chronic antral gastritis and is associated with the majority of cases of duodenal ulcer[19]. Antral mucosa specimens from patients infected by Hp show massive infiltration by CD4$^+$ lymphocytes, and mRNA for IL-12, TNF-α and IFN-γ has been demonstrated. High numbers of CD4$^+$ T cell clones have been derived from infiltrating lymphocytes and a high proportion of these (15%) show reactivity against Hp antigens. These clones have a clear-cut T$_H$1 profile and exhibit cytolytic activity against autologous B cells carrying Hp antigens[20]. Crohn's disease (CD) represents an inflammatory bowel disease in which insults from microbial agents are suspected, although not proved. Increased levels of pro-inflammatory cytokines have been demonstrated in the intestinal mucosa or in the serum of patients with CD. High numbers of LAG-3$^+$ CD26$^+$ CD4$^+$ lymphocytes can be seen in the gut of patients affected by CD, and large IL-12 expressing macrophages are scattered in the muscularis propria. T cell clones derived from the gut mucosa of CD patients are able to produce high amounts of IFN-γ showing a T$_H$1 profile. IL-12 production by activated infiltrating macrophages plays a role in the induction of IFN-γ- producing cells, as the addition of neutralizing antibodies to cultures of gut mucosa fragments determines a decrease to normal values in the percentage of IFN-γ expressing lymphocytes[8].

Atopy is a genetically determined condition characterized by an increased ability of B cells to produce IgE against a group of antigens which can activate the immune system after inhalation, penetration through the skin and ingestion (allergens). A large body of evidence has been accumulated to demonstrate the role played by T$_H$2 cells in atopic disorders. Since the beginning of the 1990s we and others have shown that allergen-specific T cells are IL-4-producing[1,2] and T$_H$2 cells accumulate at the sites of allergic reactions, such as in vernal conjunctivitis, allergic asthma and rhinitis[4]. Specific successful immunotherapy determines a shift from a prevalent T$_H$2 response to T$_H$1 with a decrease in IL-4 or increase in IFN-γ production.

Other pathological conditions are correlated with the presence of T$_H$2 cells. Systemic sclerosis (SSc) is a connective tissue disorder characterized by inflammatory, vascular and fibrotic changes of the skin leading to sclerosis with involvement of internal organs. Several soluble factors secreted by different cells may modulate fibrosis or promote vascular damage in SSc such as IL-1α and β, IL-6, TNF-β and TGF-β. In addition, IL-4 is able to induce human fibroblasts to synthesize elevated levels of extracellular matrix[21,22]. mRNA for IL-4 can be shown in the infiltrating perivascular T lymphocytes and expression for CD30 is seen in the same areas. A prevalent T$_H$2 phenotype of the T cell clones derived from the skin of patients with active SSc is also seen[11]. Finally, we have recently shown that pregnancy is a pathophysiological condition in which IL-4 is needed for preventing embryo rejection. CD30 is highly expressed in the decidua of pregnant women and higher numbers of IL-4-producing T cell clones can be derived from the decidua of pregnant women than from those affected by recurrent unexplained abortions[23]. Moreover progesterone, a hormone produced by the corpus luteum in high concentration during pregnancy, is able to shift T cells to L-4 production[24].

MODULATION OF T_H1/T_H2 RESPONSES

Increasing amounts of data indicate that T cells exhibiting established T_H1 or T_H2 phenotype can be influenced by the use of different signals both *in vitro* and *in vivo*, and antigen-specific or non-specific modulating agents have been described.

Synthetic peptides, eventually associated with particular adjuvants (CFA, liposomes) might be suitable vaccines showing advantages over traditional ones, as they are safe and pure and can be rapidly synthesized in large amounts with high reproducibility. Selected peptides with the ability to induce a prevalent T_H1 or T_H2 phenotype can be obtained from antigens. In particular a recombinant protein from *Leishmania braziliensis* and the promastigote surface antigen 2 of *Leishmania major* preferentially induce a T_H1 response[25,26]. Moreover modification of even one single amino acid in the sequence of a peptide, which varies MHC class binding affinity, can deviate T cells to produce particular cytokines. Several antigen modifications have been shown to favour a T_H1 response such as polymerization, incorporation in immune complexes, coupling with oxidized mannan, injection with components of mycobacterial cell wall, stimulating IL-12 production by macrophages[27–29]. Recombinant BCG injected together with *Leishmania major* or measles virus and live orally administered recombinant *Salmonella* can shift the T_H2 response towards a prevalent T_H1 profile[30]. Even cytokines can be used in addition to antigens in vaccines, boosting humoral and cellular responses and improving the ability of the vaccine to confer protection. In particular, recombinant IL-12 has been used in animal models in conjunction with T_H2-inducing agents such as protozoa and helminths[31]. A new approach, originally developed for gene therapy, is represented by the so called 'naked DNA vaccines' or plasmid DNA vaccination, in which the gene coding for the relevant antigen (or allergen) is inserted in plasmid DNA which remains episomally in cells close to the site of injection. In this system antigen-specific CD8+ cells are stimulated as MHC class I presentation is possible. Immunization of mice with β-galactosidase in alum or saline evokes a prevalent T_H2 response with induction of high concentrations of IgE and IL-4/IL-5 production by stimulated splenic cells, while intradermal immunization with naked plasmid DNA encoding β-gal induces a T_H1 response[32]. More recently oligonucleotides containing CpG motifs have been demonstrated to induce T_H1-type cytokines in mice but evidence that they may exert similar functions in the human system is still lacking.

In non-antigen-specific modulatory systems, cytokines or anti-cytokines or antibodies both *in vitro* and *in vivo* can shift established T_H1/T_H2 responses. Interferons (α and γ) and IL-12 can shift T_H2 responses towards the T_H1 pathway[33,34]. Administration of recombinant IL-12 to *Leishmania*-infected mice together with pentostam leads to a sensible reduction in the parasite load. IL-12 given *in vivo* can reduce pulmonary inflammation and nebulized IFN-γ normalizes airway function in animal models of allergy[35]. In specific immune responses in which T$_H$2 cells predominate, IL-4 activity can be antagonized by antibodies, soluble IL-4 receptors or IL-4 mutant protein, while humanized anti-IL-5 antibodies are able to inhibit eosinophil accumulation and normalize airway hyperactivity in animals infected by *Ascaris suis*[36,37]. In autoimmune disorders, oral tolerance, which can be defined as a specific reduction in immune response by feeding the relevant antigen, has been successfully used in both mice and humans. Modulation of experimental allergic encephalomyelitis, autoimmune uveitis, collagen-induced arthritis and myasthenia gravis can be achieved by oral administration of the relevant antigen and intranasal administration of glutamate decarboxylase is effective in preventing IDDM in NOD mice[38]. In humans, administration of myelin has been used in severe relapsing-remitting MS unresponsive to conventional therapies and good results have been achieved in a number of patients affected by rheumatoid arthritis treated with oral type II collagen[39]. The oral route is also used for specific immunotherapy in allergic patients, and peptides of Fel d I and PLA2 administered intranasally or orally have been successfully used. Finally, redirection of T$_H$1-mediated immune responses by the use of recombinant IL-4 and IL-10 has been achieved in animal models of autoimmune diseases (EAE, IDDM and collagen-induced arthritis). Both cytokines are able to down-regulate the T$_H$1 response, inflammatory cytokines and mediators such as IL-1, TNF-α and NO. In humans, clinical trials with IL-10 are under investigation in some pathological conditions, such as Crohn's disease.

CONCLUDING REMARKS

Evidence is accumulating for a central role of T cells and related cytokines in human diseases and it is now clear that under some *in vivo* and *in vitro* conditions T cell stimulation can result in the development of a restricted T$_H$1- or T$_H$2-type response.

The understanding of the fine mechanisms underlying the activation of a polarized form of response and the demonstration that memory T cells retain the ability to be further influenced by different signals may be therapeutically exploited not only in situations in which either the T$_H$1 or the T$_H$2 response is necessary for protection, but also in conditions in which harmful immune response develops against environmental antigens or autoantigens, such as allergic or autoimmune disorders.

References

1. Wierenga EA, Snoek M, de Groot C et al. J Immunol. 1990;144:4651.
2. Parronchi P, Macchia D, Piccinni M-P et al. Proc Natl Acad Sci USA. 1991;88:4538.
3. Del Prete, GF, De Carli, M, Mastromauro et al. J Clin Invest. 1991;88:346–351.
4. Romagnani S. The Th1/Th2 paradigm in disease. Heidelberg: Springer; 1997.
5. Annunziato F, Manetti R, Tomasevic L et al. FASEB J. 1996;10:767.
6. Annunziato F, Manetti R, Cosmi L et al. Eur J Immunol. 1997;27:1730.
7. Willheim M, Ebner C, Baier K et al. J Allergy Clin Immunol. 1997;100:348.
8. Parronchi P, Romagnani P, Annunziato F et al. Am J Pathol. 1997;50:823.
9. Del Prete G-F, De Carli M, Almerigogna F et al. FASEB J. 1995;9:81.
10. Chilosi M, Facchetti F, Notarangelo LD et al. Eur J. Immunol. 1996;26:329.
11. Mavilia C, Scaletti C, Romagnani P et al. Am J Pathol. 1997;151:1751.

12. Romagnani P, Annunziato F, Manetti R et al. Blood 1998;91:3223.
13. Nakamura T, Lee RK, Nam SY et al. J Immunol. 1997;158:2090.
14. Del Prete GF, Tiri A, Mariotti S et al. Clin Exp Immunol. 1987;69:323
15. De Carli M, D'Elios MM, Mariotti S et al. J Clin Endocrinol Metab. 1993;77:1120.
16. Sharief MK, Hentges R. N Engl J Med. 1991;325:467.
17. Selmaj K, Raine CS, Cannella B, Brosnan CF. J Clin Invest. 1991;87:949.
18. Windhagen A, Newcombe J, Dangond F et al. J Exp Med. 1995;182:1985.
19. D'Elios MM, Manghetti M, Almerigogna F et al. Eur J Immunol. 1997;27:1751.
20. D'Elios MM, Manghetti M, De Carli M et al. J Immunol. 1997;158:962.
21. Kovacs EJ. Immunol Today. 1991;12:17–23.
22. Gillery P, Fertin C, Nicolas JF et al. FEBS Lett. 1992;302:231.
23. Piccinni M-P, Beloni L, Scaletti C et al. Nature Med. 1998;4:1020–1024.
24. Piccinni M-P, Giudizi M-G, Biagiotti R et al. J Immunol. 1995;155:128.
25. Skeiky JAW, Gauderian JA, Benson DR et al. J Exp Med. 1995;181:1527.
26. Handman E, Symons FM, Baldwin TM et al. Infect Immunol. 1995;63:4261.
27. Gieni RS, Yang X, HayGlass KT. J Immunol. 1993;150:302.
28. Villacres-Eriksson M. Clin Exp Immunol. 1995;102:46.
29. Apostolopoulos V, Peitersz GA, Loveland BE et al. Proc Natl Acad Sci USA. 1995;92:10128.
30. VanCott JL, Staats HF, Pascual DW et al. J Immunol. 1995;156:1504.
31. Taylor CE. Infect Immun. 1995;63:3241.
32. Raz E, Tighe E, Sato Y et al. Proc Natl Acad Sci USA. 1996;93:5141
33. Parronchi P, Mohapatra S, Sampognaro S et al. Eur J Immunol. 1996;26:697.
34. Manetti R, Parronchi P, Giudizi M-G et al. J Exp Med. 1993;177:1199.
35. Lack G, Renz H, Saloga J et al. J Immunol. 1994;152:2546.
36. Renz H, Enssle K, Lauffer L et al. Int Arch Allergy Immunol. 1995;106:46.
37. Egan RW, Athwahl D, Chou C-C et al. Int Arch Allergy Immunol. 1995;107:321.
38. Tian JD, Atkinson MA, Salzler MC et al. J Exp Med. 1996;183:1561.
39. Sieper J, Kary S, Sorensen H et al. Arthritis Rheum. 1996;39:41–51.

24
TGF-β mediated oral tolerance

T. MARTH, B. KELSALL, W. STROBER and M. ZEITZ

CHARACTERISTICS OF ORAL TOLERANCE

Oral tolerance (OT) describes the antigen-specific suppression of an immune response following administration of oral antigen. Both cellular and humoral immune responses are suppressed by such orally induced tolerance, and the tolerance achieved is often associated with the generation of cytokine-producing suppressor T cells. The mechanisms and potential clinical applications of oral tolerance have been studied with increasing interest in recent years. Ferguson and Mowat studied the immune regulation and immunosuppressive mechanisms of oral tolerance following the intake of normal food protein antigens with the diet. This laid the basis for the hypothesis that allergy to dietary antigens and food sensitive enteropathies could be due to a dysregulation of oral tolerance mechanisms[1,2]. In the last decade, investigators have also studied in more detail oral tolerance as a possible option to treat antigen-specific autoimmune disease in animal models and humans[3].

Oral tolerance has been studied with a variety of antigens such as thymic-dependent antigens, heterologous cells (e.g. erythrocytes), killed bacteria and viruses, but most studies have addressed orally induced tolerance following the feeding of soluble non-adjuvanted dietary proteins which probably represent the dietary antigens of the highest immunological relevance. It has been shown by many investigators that specific systemic immunoglobulin responses (IgM, IgG and IgE) can be suppressed by oral antigen feeding. The suppression of IgE responses can be achieved with relatively low amounts of fed antigen and lasts usually for a long time, whereas reduction of other immunoglobulins either may be short-term or may require higher doses of antigen[4–6]. The application of oral antigen also leads to the suppression of cellular immune responses. Thus, it has been shown that *in vitro* parameters of cell-mediated immunity (proliferation and cytokine production by T cells) as well as *in vivo* functions of cell-mediated immunity (CMI) such as delayed type hypersensitivity (DTH) reactions and contact hypersensitivity can be suppressed by oral antigen feeding. Similar to the IgE response, cellular immune functions can be relatively easily suppressed with low amounts of fed antigens, and the suppression of CMI persists longer[4,7–10]. The suppression of cell-mediated immune functions by oral

"

antigens does not only apply to naive mice hosts but also to models where the host has been pre-immunized with the antigen[9,11].

It has long been presumed that the Peyer's patches (PP) have a central role in the generation of oral tolerance since PP have been shown to be the site of generation of suppressor cells[12–14]. Subsequently, it was found that the suppressor cells generated in the PP migrate to other lymphoid organs, i.e., to mesenteric lymph nodes and to the spleen (and then to other peripheral lymphoid tissues)[14–16]. Moreover, it has been shown that an adoptive transfer of cells from the PP will transfer oral tolerance; similar findings have been made with cells from the mesenteric lymph nodes and the spleen. The primary cytokine milieu in the intestine and in the PP following antigen feeding is not well defined. On the one hand, repeated low dose feeding of the same antigen, for example in the model of experimental autoimmune encephalomyelitis (EAE), is associated with a mucosal T helper type 2 (T_H2) cytokine response as well as a peripheral immune tolerance[14]. On the other hand, recent studies from our laboratory have demonstrated that feeding a high dose of protein antigens (ovalbumin, OVA) leads to a generation of T_H1 responses in the PP and is not associated with induction of tolerance of mucosal T cells[10]. It is therefore possible that the initial T_H1 response following high-dose antigen feeding serves as a defence and is not associated with tolerance at mucosal sites. Repeated low-dose antigen delivery or, alternatively, inhibition of a T_H1 response, may be the prerequisites for the generation of a more protective cytokine response, i.e., a T_H2 cytokine response and the generation of other suppressor cytokines[17].

IMMUNOLOGICAL MECHANISMS OF ORAL TOLERANCE

While orally induced tolerance has distinct immunological characteristics, there are some overlaps with the mechanisms underlying the occurrence of tolerance achieved by other forms of antigen delivery. One important difference between systemic and orally induced tolerance seems to be based on antigen processing by structures of the mucosal immune system. Serum of mice previously fed OVA, but not serum of mice injected systemically with OVA, when injected into naive animals, causes a reduction of antigen-specific DTH reactions and to the activation of suppressor cells in recipients. Thus, the serum of OVA-fed mice seems to contain a tolerogen which rapidly appears in the serum of the mice[18–20]. In addition, the significance of the intestinal proteolysis and the role of mucosal barrier is indicated by observations that oral tolerance cannot be induced when either inhibitors of endopeptidases are being pre-fed or when mucosal integrity is disturbed by substances such as saponin or cholera toxin[21–23].

The possibility that tolerance versus immunization following an antigen feeding may be influenced by the strength of activation of antigen-presenting cells (APC) was addressed by studies of Mowat *et al.* and others. They proposed a model in which the intestinal antigen proteolysis and antigen processing usually will not lead to a highly activated APC and thus, the development of tolerance rather than an active immunity can occur. Consistent with this notion, it has been shown that oral tolerance against OVA can be prevented by the simultaneous induction of a graft-versus-host reaction, the application of oestrogens, and the administration of muramyl-peptides, all of which will lead to an activation of the reticuloendothelial system and thus to an activation of the APC[24–26].

As mentioned above, orally induced tolerance has some common features with systemically induced tolerance and the well-studied phenomenon of suppression, anergy and deletion of systemic tolerance[27] can also be found in oral tolerance.

Active suppression and transforming growth factor-β (TGF-β)

Active suppression is now a well-characterized mechanism of oral tolerance. Lymphoid cells obtained following oral antigen feeding can adoptively transfer tolerance in other animals[28,29]. Later, it was also shown that primarily the cell-mediated immunity, and to a much lesser extent humoral immunity, could be transferred[4,11]. Moreover, it has been demonstrated that immunosuppressive agents such as cyclophosphamide can inhibit the generation of suppressor cells[5]. More recently, cytokines have been recognized as main mediators of suppression, and subsequently the term active suppression, meaning cytokine-mediated suppression of immune reactions, has been designated[3].

Active suppression has been well studied in several animal models of oral tolerance. The cytokines associated with active suppression are T_H2-like cytokines such as IL-4, IL-10 as well as TGF-β[3,30]. TGF-β seems to have a central role in mediating oral tolerance in several animal models of chronic inflammation. In EAE, for example, TGF-β mediates the immunosuppressive and therapeutic effects[14,31,32]. Studies by Weiner and others have pointed out that neutralization of anti-TGF-β may reverse orally induced tolerance in the EAE model both *in vitro* and *in vivo*[14,30,32,33]. Thus, relating to the *in vivo* studies, mice were immunized with myelin basic protein (MBP) and subsequently developed EAE unless a feed of MBP was given at the start point of the study. The injection of anti-TGF-β inhibited the occurrence of oral tolerance in this model completely[32]. Hence, the *in vivo* neutralization of TGF-β by administration of antibodies reversed the previously induced oral tolerance[32]. In the model of trinitrobenzene sulphonic acid (TNBS)-induced colitis, a murine model of Crohn's disease which is mainly mediated by T_H1-like cytokine responses, the repeated application of anti-TGF-β resulted in an abrogation of oral tolerance induced by prefeeding of haptenated colonic proteins[34]. Similarly, TGF-β possesses relevance in mediating suppression in another chemically induced tolerance model, namely the hapten-induced oral tolerance model, since anti-TGF-β reversed *in vitro* inhibition in cells from 2,4-dinitrochlorbenzene-fed mice[35]. In these models TGF-β also mediates active suppression *in vitro*, i.e. cell culture supernatants induce active suppression which can be reversed by anti-TGF-β as demonstrated in *in vitro* cell mixing studies (discussed below).

Moreover, it has been shown in the model of collagen induced arthritis that injection of recombinant TGF-β induces an immunological tolerance similar to that induced by feeding of collagen type II[36]. Finally, there are reports of increased levels of TGF-β in healing phases of autoimmune diseases in animals as well as in humans (i.e. in multiple sclerosis and myasthenia gravis)[37].

In summary, there is increasing evidence that the suppressive cytokine TGF-β plays a central role in mediating immunological tolerance following antigen feeding. In addition, TGF-β is apparently important in different stages of the induction of oral tolerance. It is therefore important to understand the mechanisms regulating the generation of TGF-β producing immune cells (such as T cells) following oral antigen feeding.

Regulation of TGF-β and influence of interleukin-12 (IL-12)

TGF-β-producing cells are generated in the intestinal mucosa following antigen feeding and migrate subsequently to systemic lymphoid tissues and inflamed target organs (such as the central nervous system in the EAE model)[3,14]. Upon activation these cells then specifically suppress immune responses of nearby T cells. This phenomenon has been termed 'bystander suppression' and, based on this principle, the therapy of autoimmune diseases should be possible even though the exact nature of the causative antigen may not be known[30,32].

The phenotype and the functional features of the TGF-β-producing cells generated at mucosal sites is still poorly defined. TGF-β mediated oral tolerance can still be generated in the absence of CD8 cells (after *in vivo* depletion of CD8 cells)[38], and other studies showed that in different models CD8 cells are capable of transferring oral tolerance[39]. Thus, in different models both CD4 and CD8 cells seem to be capable of mediating active suppression mediated by TGF-β. More recently, it has become apparent that the TGF-β-producing cells might be distinct from T_H1 and T_H2 T cell populations. Based on these observations, and although it had been observed previously that TGF-β-producing cells often occur concurrently with a T_H2 cytokine response, it was suggested that TGF-β-producing cells may be a T_H1- and T_H2-independent T_H3 population, the regulation of which remains to be defined[40–42].

Recent work from one group has shown that the generation of TGF-β-producing cells can be regulated by IL-12 and T_H1 cytokines. First, it was shown that feeding of high doses of OVA to OVA-T cell receptor (TCR) transgenic mice induced systemic tolerance and, at the same time, resulted in a mucosal cytokine response dominated by IFN-γ production. When this IFN-γ production was inhibited by systemic neutralization of IL-12 simultaneously with the OVA feeding, we observed a significant increase in the production of TGF-β but not of the T_H2 cytokine IL-4 by cells from the mucosal lymphoid tissue, i.e. from PP cells (Figure 1). A similar pattern of cytokine responses was observed when the OVA-TCR transgenic mice were exposed to a second *in vivo* antigen challenge. The increased production of TGF-β was associated with active suppression *in vitro*, as demonstrated in cell mixing studies (Figure 2). These results therefore suggest that a combination of oral tolerance induction and neutralization of IL-12 may be useful to test models of autoimmune diseases[10]. In further studies, treatment with anti-IL-12 antibodies also induced an elevated amount of apoptosis in T lymphocytes. Preliminary studies suggest that this induction of programmed cell death by anti-IL-12 may be a Fas-mediated event (Marth *et al.*, unpublished observation). In accord with these studies on the negative role of IL-12 in oral tolerance, systemic neutralization of IL-12 prevents contact hypersensitivity and induces hapten-specific tolerance *in vivo*[43,44]; in addition, mucosally delivered IL-12 reversed tolerance induced by OVA feeding in mice[45].

We have also shown recently in an *in vitro* T cell differentiation system (consisting of naive TCR transgenic cells stimulated with antigen-primed dendritic

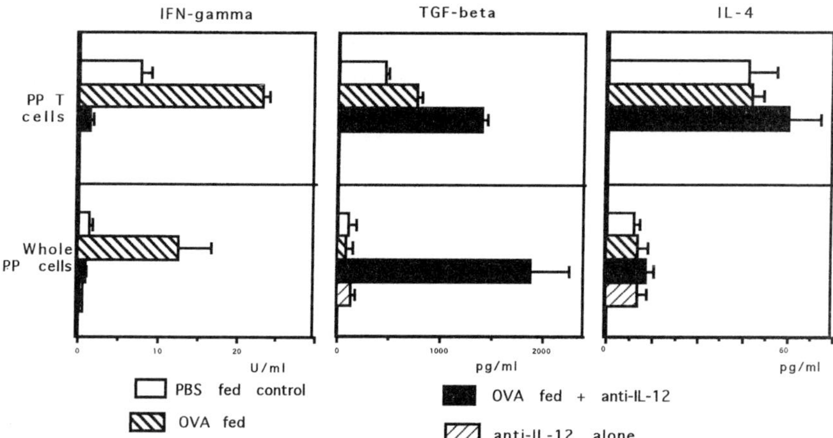

Figure 1 Reciprocal relation of IFN-γ and TGF-β responses in an oral tolerance model. OVA-TCR transgenic mice were fed high doses of OVA (3 × 250 mg), and lymphoid tissues were isolated 3 days after the last feeding. Other groups of mice served as control (untreated), or were treated with antigen feeding plus systemic anti-IL-12, or with anti-IL-12 alone. Cells from the PP were restimulated *in vitro* with OVA and cytokine responses were determined by ELISA as described elsewhere[10]

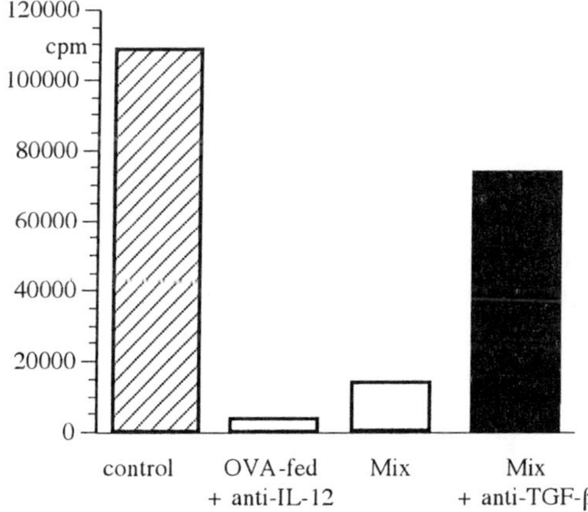

Figure 2 TGF-β mediates active suppression *in vitro*. PP cells from OVA-TCR transgenic mice treated with oral OVA plus systemic anti-IL-12 injection were isolated, restimulated *in vitro* with OVA and proliferative responses were determined by [³H]thymidine incorporation. In other assays, cells were mixed in a 1:1 ratio with cells from the untreated control groups which revealed a suppressed proliferative capacity; this phenomenon could be reversed when cells were incubated with neutralizing anti-TGF-β at 0 h of culture but not with control antibody (data not shown) arguing for the TGF-mediated active suppression

cells) that TGF-β production from T cells can be significantly increased when anti-IL-12 or anti-IFN-γ antibodies are added at the start point of the cell culture. This was a specific to anti-IL-12 and T_H1 cytokines since other antibodies to cytokines such IL-2, IL-4, or IL-10 did not result in a significant increase in TGF-β. This phenomenon was observed with a variety of stimulation methods including stimulation with dendritic cells, macrophages, and direct stimulation of the T cells with anti-CD3. The increase of TGF-β production in this system was, in contrast to some previous reports in the EAE model, not associated with a rise in T_H2 cytokines. It is important to note, however, that IL-14 had growth factor-like influences in the generation of TGF-β producing cells[46].

In another study by Seder *et al.*, using a two-phase cell culture system, a number of factors were shown to influence the development of T cells producing TGF-β[47]. In the culture system used, naive CD4/CD62L double-positive T cells from TCR transgenic mice are primed in the presence of appropriate antigen, APC, IL-2, and various other conditions, e.g., IL-4, IL-12, IFN-γ, or various anti-cytokine antibodies, and then in a second phase restimulated with anti-CD3/anti-CD28 to expand the differentiated cells. Cells from different mouse strains and cells from knock-out mice were used in the study. T_H1 cytokines had a negative effect on the differentiation of TGF-β-producing T cells, both directly and through their capacity to inhibit T_H2 differentiation and cytokines. Thus, cells from IFN-γ deficient mice displayed a high capacity to differentiate into TGF-β-producing cells. In addition, IL-4 had a marked positive effect on T cells producing TGF-β; it should be noted, however, that IL-4 was not essential for the differentiation of TGF-β-producing cells since TGF-β production was also seen in IL-4 deficient mice. Thus, while IL-4 is necessary for optimal TGF-β responses, its absence does not prevent the occurrence of TGF-β-producing cells. Further studies showed that other cytokines, such as IL-7 and IL-10, also enhanced the differentiation of TGF-β-producing T cells, mainly indirectly through their effects on IL-2 and IL-4 production, respectively. Finally, TGF-β itself had a positive effect on the differentiation of TGF-β-producing cells which operated through its ability to inhibit IFN-γ production[47].

Third and last, in the TNBS-induced colitis model in the mouse, TGF-β is a central mediator of suppression following oral antigen feeding (administration of the haptenized colonic proteins). The disease can be cured by the injection of anti-IL-12 antibodies or by injection of recombinant TGF-β, and injection of IL-12 will reinduce the disease[34,48]. Since the TNBS model is a reflection of cytokine regulation similar to Crohn's disease in the humans, these observations show the potential of targeting cytokines (e.g. TGF-β, T_H1 cytokines and IL-12) as potential treatments for human inflammatory bowel diseases.

Taken together, these studies indicate that the suppression of T_H1-like cytokines and IL-12 has a major influence on the production of TGF-β and also that the TGF-β response by T cells is independent of T_H2 cytokines. These data suggest that a microenvironment oriented toward the development of T_H2 cells (i.e. rich in IL-4 and poor in IFN-γ) is optimal for the induction of TGF-β-producing T cells[17]. In regard to recent data showing that TGF-β can suppress T_H1 and IL-12 responses[49], it is tempting to assume that TGF-β and IFN-γ/IL-12 constitute a regulatory feed-back loop.

Clonal anergy and clonal deletion

Clonal anergy is defined as a state of tolerance of clonal T cells which can be reversed *in vitro* by IL-2. Clonal anergy was found in studies of oral tolerance mainly after a single feed of a high dose of protein antigens. In these systems the anergy was defined as reduced T cell proliferation and cytokine production which could be reversed when the cells were pre-cultured with IL-2[50,51].

The availability of TCR transgenic mice, which have a high percentage of circulating antigen-specific T cells, enables one to study the clonal deletion in different lymphoid organs *in vivo* in a more suitable way than has been possible before with the use of conventional animal models. We and others have previously shown that feeding of high doses of antigen can lead to deletion of T cells in the periphery by apoptosis. It was found that feeding OVA-TCR transgenic mice leads to a higher proportion of apoptosis of antigen specific cells in the spleen and the Peyer's patches[10,52].

CONCLUDING REMARKS

The occurrence of TGF-β mediated antigen-induced oral tolerance is dependent on a complex interplay of different immunoregulatory mechanisms. It has been shown that several mechanisms including active suppression, clonal anergy and clonal deletion may lead to the development of oral tolerance. Peripheral tolerance is more likely, and occurs to a greater extent, when a T_H1 cytokine response is reduced at mucosal sites and when simultaneously suppressor cytokines such as TGF-β and IL-4 occur. The modulation of the TGF-β response following oral antigen delivery represents a particularly interesting target to enhance peripheral tolerance.

References

1. Ferguson A, Gillett H, Mahony SO. Active immunity or tolerance to foods in patients with celiac disease or inflammatory bowel disease. Ann NY Acad Sci. 1996;778:202–216.
2. Mowat AMcI. The regulation of immune responses to dietary protein antigens. Immunol Today. 1987;8:93–98.
3. Weiner HL, Friedman A, Miller A et al. Oral tolerance: immunologic mechanisms and treatment of animal and human organ-specific autoimmune diseases by oral administration of autoantigens. Annu Rev Immunol. 1994;12:809–831.
4. Strobel S, Ferguson A. Persistence of oral tolerance in mice fed ovalbumin is different for humoral and cell-mediated immune responses. Immunology. 1987;60:317–318.
5. Mowat AM, Strobel S, Drummond HE, Ferguson A. Immunological responses to fed protein antigens in mice. I. Reversal of oral tolerance to ovalbumin by cyclophosphamide. Immunology. 1982;45:105–113.
6. Challacombe SJ, Tomasi JB. Systemic tolerance and secretory immunity after oral immunisation. J Exp Med. 1980;152:1459–1472.
7. Kay R, Ferguson A. The immunological consequences of feeding cholera toxin. I. Feeding cholera toxin suppresses the induction of systemic delayed-type hypersensitivity but not humoral immunity. Immunology. 1989;66:410–415.
8. Lamont AG, Gordon M, Ferguson A. Oral tolerance in protein-deprived mice. I. Profound antibody tolerance but impaired DTH tolerance after antigen feeding. Immunology. 1987;61:333–337.
9. Lamont AG, Bruce MG, Watret KC, Ferguson A. Suppression of an established DTH response to ovalbumin in mice by feeding antigen after immunization. Immunology. 1988;64:135–140.
10. Marth T, Strober W, Kelsall BL. High dose oral tolerance in ovalbumin TCR transgenic mice: systemic neutralization of interleukin-12 augments TGFβ secretion and T cell apoptosis. J Immunol. 1996;157:2348–2357.
11. Mowat AM. Oral tolerance and regulation of immunity to dietary antigens. In: Ogra PL, Lamm ME, McGhee JR, Mestecky J, Strober W, Bienenstock J (eds). Handbook of Mucosal Immunology. San Diego: Academic Press, 1994:185–201.

12. MacDonald TT. Immunosuppression caused by antigen feeding. II. Suppressor T cells mask Peyer's patches B cell priming to orally administered antigen. Eur J Immunol. 1983;13:138–142.
13. Mattingly JA. Immunological suppression after oral antigen administration. III. Activation of suppressor-inducer cells in the Peyer's patches. Cell Immunol. 1984;86:46–52.
14. Santos LMB, Al-Sabbagh A, Londono A, Weiner HL. Oral tolerance to myelin basic protein induces regulatory TGF-β secreting cells in Peyer's patches of SJL mice. Cell Immunol. 1994;157:439–447.
15. Mattingly JA, Waksman BH. Immunologic suppression after oral administration of antigen. I. Specific suppressor cells formed in rat Peyers patches after oral administration of sheep erythrocytes and their systemic migration. J Immunol. 1978;121:1878–1883.
16. MacDonald TT. Immunosuppression caused by antigen feeding. I. Evidence for the activation of a feedback suppressor pathway in the spleens of antigen-fed mice. Eur J Immunol. 1982;12:767–773.
17. Strober W, Kelsall BL, Fuss I et al. Reciprocal IFN-gamma and TGF-beta responses regulate the occurrence of mucosal inflammation. Immunol Today. 1997;18:61–64.
18. Bruce M, Ferguson A. The influence of intestinal processing on the immunogenicity and molecular size of absorbed, circulating ovalbumin in mice. Immunology. 1986;59:295–300.
19. Peng HJ, Turner MW, Ferguson A. The generation of a tolerogen after the ingestion of ovalbumin is time dependent and unrelated to the serum level of immunoreactive protein. Clin Exp Immunol. 1990;81:510–515.
20. Strobel S, Mowat AMcI, Drummond HE, Pickering MG, Ferguson A. Immunological responses to fed protein antigens in mice. II. Oral tolerance for CMI is due to activation of cyclophosphamide sensitive cells by gut processed antigen. Immunology. 1983;49:451–456.
21. Hanson DG, Roy MJ, Green GM, Miller SD. Inhibition of orally-induced immune tolerance in mice by prefeeding an endopeptidase inhibitor. Reg Immunol. 1993;5:85–93.
22. Mowat AM, Thomas JJ, Parrott DMV. Divergent effects of bacterial lipopolysaccharide on immunity to orally administered protein and particular antigens in mice. Immunology. 1986;58:677–684.
23. Mowat AMcI, Maloy KJ, Donachie AM. Immune-stimulating complexes as adjuvants for inducing local and systemic immunity after oral immunization with protein antigens. Immunology. 1993;80:527–534.
24. Mowat AMcI, Parrott DMV. Immunological responses to fed protein antigens in mice. IV. Effects of stimulating the reticuloendothelial system on oral tolerance and intestinal immunity to ovalbumin. Immunology. 1983;50:547–554.
25. Mowat AMcI, Felstein MV, Borland A. Experimental studies of immunologically mediated enteropathy: development of cell-mediated immunity and intestinal pathology during a graft-versus-host reaction in irradiated mice. Gut. 1988;29:949–954.
26. Strobel S, Mowat AMcI, Ferguson A. Prevention of oral tolerance induction to ovalbumin and enhanced antigen presentation during graft-versus-host reaction in mice. Immunology. 1985;56:57–64.
27. Schwartz R. Immunological tolerance. In: Paul WE (ed.). Fundamental Immunology. New York: Raven Press, 1993:677–731.
28. Thomas HC, Ryan CJ, Benjamin IS, Blumgart LH, MacSween RN. The immune response in cirrhotic rats. The induction of tolerance to orally administered protein antigens. Gastroenterology. 1976;71:114–117.
29. Chase MW, Battisto JR. The duration of dermal sensitization following cellular transfer in guinea pigs. J Allergy. 1955;26:83.
30. Miller A, Lider O, Weiner HL. Antigen-driven bystander suppression after oral administration of antigens. J Exp Med. 1991;174:791–798.
31. Khoury SJ, Hancock WW, Weiner HL. Oral tolerance to myelin basic protein and natural recovery from experimental autoimmune encephalomyelitis are associated with downregulation of inflammatory cytokines and differential upregulation of transforming growth factor beta, interleukin 4, and prostaglandin E expression in the brain. J Exp Med. 1992;176:1355–1364.
32. Miller A, Lider O, Roberts AB, Sporn MB, Weiner HL. Suppressor T cells generated by oral tolerization to myelin basic protein suppress both in vitro and in vivo immune responses by the release of transforming growth factor beta after antigen-specific triggering. Proc Natl Acad Sci USA. 1992;89:421–425.

33. Karpus WJ, Swanborg RH. CD4[+] suppressor cells inhibit the function of effector cells of experimental autoimmune encephalomyelitis through a mechanism involving transforming growth factor β. J Immunol. 1991;146:1163–1169.

34. Neurath MF, Fuss I, Kelsall BL, Presky DH, Waegell W, Strober W. Experimental granulomatous colitis in mice is abrogated by induction of TGFβ-mediated oral tolerance. J Exp Med. 1996;183:2605–2616.

35. Galliaerde V, Desvignes C, Peyron E, Kaiserlian D. Oral tolerance to haptens: intestinal epithelial cells from 2,4-dinitrochlorbenzene-fed mice inhibit hapten-specific T cell activation in vitro. Eur J Immunol. 1995;25:1385–1390.

36. Thorbecke GJ, Shah R, Leu CH, Kuruvilla AP, Hardison AM, Palladino MA. Involvement of endogenous tumor necrosis factor α and transforming growth factor β during induction of collagen type II arthritis in mice. Proc Natl Acad Sci USA. 1992;89:7375–7379.

37. Link J, He B, Navikas V et al. Transforming growth factor beta I suppresses autoantigen-induced expression of pro-inflammatory cytokines but not of interleukin 10 in multiple sclerosis and myasthenia gravis. J Neuroimmunol. 1995;58:21–35.

38. Chen Y, Inobe JI, Weiner HL. Induction of oral tolerance to myelin basic protein in CD8-depleted mice: Both CD4[+] and CD8[+] cells mediate active suppression. J Immunol. 1995;155:910–916.

39. Lider O, Santos LMB, Lee CSY, Higgins PJ, Weiner HL. Suppression of experimental autoimmune encephalomyelitis by oral administration of myelin basic protein. II. Suppression of disease and in vitro responses is mediated by antigen-specific CD8[+] T lymphocytes. J Immunol. 1989;142:748–752.

40. Fukaura H, Kent SC, Pietrusewic MJ, Khoury SJ, Weiner HL, Hafler DA. Induction of circulating myelin basic protein and proteolipid protein-specific transforming growth factor-beta 1-secreting Th3 T cells by oral administration of myelin in multiple sclerosis patients. J Clin Invest. 1996;98:70–77.

41. Chen Y, Kuchroo VK, Inobe JI, Hafler DA, Weiner HL. Regulatory T cell clones induced by oral tolerance: Suppression of autoimmune encephalitis. Science. 1994;265:1237–1240.

42. Chen Y, Inobe JI, Kuchroo VK, Baron JL, Chaneway CA, Weiner HL. Oral tolerance in myelin basic protein T-cell receptor transgenic mice: Suppression of autoimmune encephalomyelitis and dose-dependent induction of regulatory cells. Proc Natl Acad Sci USA. 1996;93:388–391.

43. Muller G, Saloga J, Germann T, Schuler G, Knop J, Enk AH. IL-12 as mediator and adjuvant for the induction of contact sensitivity in vivo. J Immunol. 1995;155:4661–4668.

44. Riemann H, Schwarz A, Grabbe S et al. Neutralization of IL-12 in vivo prevents induction of contact hypersensitivity and induces hapten-specific tolerance. J Immunol. 1996;156:1799–1803.

45. Claessen AM, von Blomberg BM, De Groot J, Wolvers DA, Kraal G, Scheper RJ. Reversal of mucosal tolerance by subcutaneous administration of interleukin-12 at the site of attempted sensitization. Immunology. 1996;88:363–367.

46. Marth T, Strober W, Seder RA, Kelsall BL. Regulation of transforming growth factor-beta production by interleukin-12. Eur J Immunol. 1997;27:1213–1220.

47. Seder RA, Marth T, Sieve MC et al. Factors involved in the differentiation of TGF-beta-producing cells from naive CD4+ T cells: IL-4 and IFN-gamma have opposing effects, while TGF-beta positively regulates its own production. J Immunol. 1998;160:5719–5728.

48. Neurath MF, Fuss I, Kelsall BL, Stuber E, Strober W. Antibodies to interleukin 12 abrogate established experimental colitis in mice. J Exp Med. 1995;182:1281–1290.

49. Schmitt E, Hoehn P, Huels C et al. T helper type 1 development of naive CD4+ T cells requires the coordinate action of interleukin-12 and interferon-gamma and is inhibited by transforming growth factor-β. Eur J Immunol. 1994;24:793–798.

50. Whitacre CC, Gienapp IE, Orosz CG, Bitar DM. Oral tolerance in experimental autoimmune encephalomyelitis. III. Evidence for clonal anergy. J Immunol. 1991;147:2155–2163.

51. Friedman A, Weiner HL. Induction of anergy or active suppression in oral tolerance is determined by frequency of feeding and antigen dosage. Proc Natl Acad Sci USA. 1994;91:6688–6692.

52. Chen Y, Inobe JI, Marks R, Gonella P, Kuchroo VK, Weiner HL. Peripheral deletion of antigen-reactive T cells in oral tolerance. Nature. 1995;376:177–180.

25
Induction of immunological tolerance by antigen delivery via the colon

F. SEIBOLD, C. WEAVER, M. SCHEURLEN and C. O. ELSON

Immunological tolerance induced by antigen delivery via the mucosa is often called oral tolerance. This term is, however, something of a misnomer in that such tolerance can ensue after the application of antigen to mucosal surfaces other than the upper gastrointestinal tract (e.g. nasal mucosa). Immunological tolerance is a very important homeostatic mechanism which maintains health despite the multitude of food and bacterial antigens in the intestine. At the same time the mucosal immune system must be able to resist infectious organisms and pathogens. Oral tolerance thus represents one end of the spectrum of the mucosal response to antigens, and it is increasingly being recognized to be an active process, i.e. not simply the absence of an immune response.

PROPERTIES OF THE COLONIC AND SMALL INTESTINAL IMMUNE SYSTEM

Colon and small intestine have different anatomy and functions. The mucosa-associated immune system is also different in small intestine and colon. Most investigations of the intestinal immune system have been performed on the murine small intestine and only recently has it been recognized that the composition of the mucosal immune system of the colon differs from that of the small intestine. The numbers of lymphocytes are much higher in small intestine than in colon, and, in contrast to the intraepithelial lymphocytes (IEL) and lamina propria lymphocytes (LPL) of the small intestine which are mainly CD8[+], colonic IEL and LPL have significantly more CD4[+] cells[1]. Likewise, small intestinal IEL contain a major proportion of $\gamma\delta$ TCR-expressing cells, whereas colonic IEL are mainly $\alpha\beta$ TCR. Other markers, including CD2, CD5, and L-selectin, have a much lower expression in small intestinal IEL than in the colon IEL[1,2].

INDUCTION OF TOLERANCE BY ANTIGEN ADMINISTRATION VIA THE COLON?

The classical way to induce mucosal tolerance is done by feeding the antigen prior to a systemic immunization. As mentioned above it is known that tolerance induction occurs after antigen application to other mucosal surfaces. Because of the differences in cell numbers and cell populations in the colon in comparison to small intestine we asked whether tolerance could be induced by antigen delivery into the colon. To answer this question we used a transgenic mouse model (DO11.10) which allows the identification and specific stimulation of T cells specific for ovalbumin (OVA). Transgenic T cells (5×10^6) were adoptively transferred into BALB/c mice and the animals were then treated with three consecutive enemas containing 10 mg of OVA. Treated and control animals were immunized parenterally with 100 μg OVA in multiple emulsion at day 14 and 28. Mice were bled day 42 and their antibody production was determined by ELISA. Mice treated with three consecutive enemas had a one log lower antibody response (0.3 mg/ml versus 3.2 mg/ml) than control animals. This indicates that colonic delivery of this antigen did induce immunological tolerance.

MECHANISMS OF TOLERANCE

T cells appear to be the major target of tolerance and the reductions in antibody responses after antigen feeding are due to the reductions in helper activity of T cells rather than to a tolerization of B cells directly. Several mechanisms leading to tolerance have been identified and probably more than one of them are operative simultaneously after antigen feeding. The most common mechanisms appear to be clonal deletion[3], clonal anergy[4], and the induction of suppressor cells[5]. The mode of feeding (repetitive, dosage) seems to influence the mechanism of tolerance. Thus, multiple feedings of 1 mg doses have been shown to generate cells producing inhibitory cytokines, whereas large doses (20 mg or more) appear to preferentially induce clonal anergy[6]. Anergy can be reversed by culturing cells with recombinant interleukin-2 (IL-2)[6]. Active cellular suppression seems to be mediated by suppressive cytokines such as transforming growth factor-β (TGF-β), IL-4 and IL-10[7]. There is little known about the early cytokine response during tolerance induction.

EARLY CYTOKINE RESPONSE

To investigate the early cytokine response the above animal model with transgenic T cells was used. To detect how many transgenic cells were activated after a single enema or after i.p. immunization the frequency of IL-2R-and CD69-positive TCR transgenic T cells was determined by fluorescence activated cell sorting (FACS) at different time points. A high frequency of transgenic T cells from spleen or lymph nodes expressed IL-2R (67%) after enema, which was similar to the frequency after parenteral immunization (76%) in adjuvans. The frequency of IL-2, IL-4, IL-10 and IFN-γ mRNA-producing cells was determined at 3, 6, 12, 24 and 48 h on lymphocytes from spleen, mesenteric lymph nodes and caudal lymph node by *in situ* hybridization with cytokine-specific riboprobes. The maximal cytokine response was found 12 h after antigen application in all tested organs. IL-2 mRNA was found in a high percentage of transgenic T cells in tolerized and in immunized animals (42% versus 37%). However, in contrast to parenterally immunized animals, the IL-2 response was of shorter duration in animals given enemas. The frequency of IL-10 mRNA producing transgenic T cells was higher in animals given OVA via the colon than in those which were parenterally immunized (7.5 versus 2.2%). Conversely, parenterally immunized animals had more IFN-γ-producing T cells than animals given OVA by enema (4.2 versus 2.3%). An important question was whether early IL-2 production had an influence on the proliferation of specific T cells. Therefore the frequency of transgenic T cells was determined by FACS at different times after immunization or enema application. Interestingly, there was no significant increase of transgenic T cells after antigen application via enema, whereas there was a significant increase in transgenic T cells after parenteral immunization. This indicates that despite the early IL-2 mRNA secretion there was no cell proliferation after OVA delivery by enema. Because the duration of IL-2 mRNA expression was very short, there might be not enough IL-2 protein to induce a proliferatory effect. Alternatively functional anergy may be due to the increased IL-10 mRNA production.

CONCLUSION

Repetitive antigen application into the colon is a very efficient way to induce tolerance. The function of the specific T cells in the colonic epithelium and lamina propria is not clear, but only a few hours after antigen application into the colon there is a strong systemic response with a short peak of IL-2 mRNA production. Despite this, specific T cells do not expand, which may be due to the short duration of IL-2 production, to the secretion of inhibitory cytokines such as IL-10, or both.

References

1. Beagley KW, Fujihashi K, Lagoo AS et al. Differences in intraepithelial T cell subsets isolated from murine small versus large intestine. J Immunol. 1995;154:5611–5619.
2. Seibold F, Seibold-Schmid B, Cong Y et al. Regional differences in intestinal lymphocytes: Regulation of L-selectin. Gastroenterology. 1998;114:965–974.
3. Chen Y, Inobe J, Marks R, Gonella P, Kuchroo VK, Weiner HL. Peripheral deletion of antigen-reactive T cells in oral tolerance. Nature. 1995;376:177–180.
4. Melamed D, Friedman A. Direct evidence for anergy in T lymphocytes tolerized by oral administration of ovalbumin. Eur J Immunol. 1993;24:78–80.
5. Richman LK, Chiller JM, Brown WR, Hanson DG, Vaz NM. Enterically induced immunologic tolerance. J Immunol. 1978;121:2429–2434.
6. Friedman A, Weiner HL. Induction of anergy and/or active suppression following oral tolerance is determined by antigen dosage. Proc Natl Acad Sci USA. 1994;140:6688–6692.
7. Chen Y, Kuchroo VK, Inobe JI, Hafler DA, Weiner HL. Regulatory T cell clones induced by oral tolerance: suppression of autoimmune encephalomyelitis. Science. 1994;265:1237–1240.

26
Immunological findings in inflammatory bowel disease

M. F. NEURATH

Ulcerative colitis (UC) and Crohn's disease (CD) are the two major forms of inflammatory bowel disease (IBD) in humans. Although the precise aetiology of both diseases remains unknown, there is increasing evidence for an alteration of mucosal immunoregulation in patients with IBD. This review focuses on the role of different components of the mucosal immune system in IBD. In particular, the role of epithelial cells, lamina propria (LP) macrophages and lymphocytes is discussed.

ROLE OF THE INTESTINAL FLORA

Recent data suggest that hyper-responsiveness to otherwise less immunogenic or harmless products of the intestinal flora is a key phenomenon in the pathogenesis of IBD (Figure 1)[1,2]. These data are in agreement with the clinical observations that IBD manifests itself most frequently at intestinal sites with the highest bacterial concentrations, and that increases in gut permeability precede acute flares in CD. Finally, it was shown that development of chronic intestinal inflammation in various animal models is abrogated when mice are kept under germfree conditions[3,4]. Based on these results, loss of tolerance and hyper-responsiveness to mucosal antigens appear to be key events in the pathogenesis of IBD.

EPITHELIAL CELLS

Recent data suggest that intestinal epithelial cells (IEC) may play an important role in the pathogenesis of IBD (Figure 2). For instance, it has been recently found that normal IEC express high levels of gp180, a novel ligand for CD8 T cells. Decreased expression of gp180 in CD may cause loss of CD8[+] suppressor cell activity in CD thereby favouring activation of CD4[+] T cells in this disease[5]. Furthermore, various groups have shown that IEC have a different

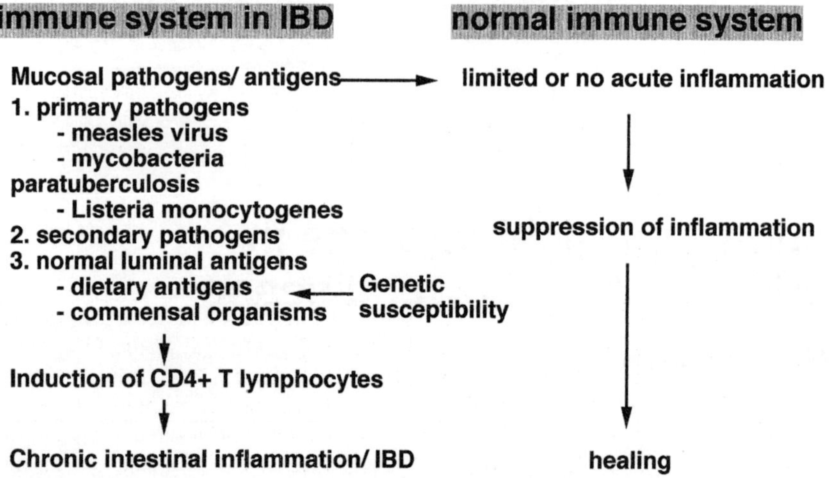

Figure 1 Hypothetical model of IBD pathogenesis. Whereas mucosal antigens normally cause no or limited acute inflammation with consequent healing, antigens in IBD cause a dysregulated mucosal immune response that leads to chronic intestinal inflammation. Although several pathogens have been suggested to be the primary cause of IBD, there are currently no unequivocal data that support this hypothesis

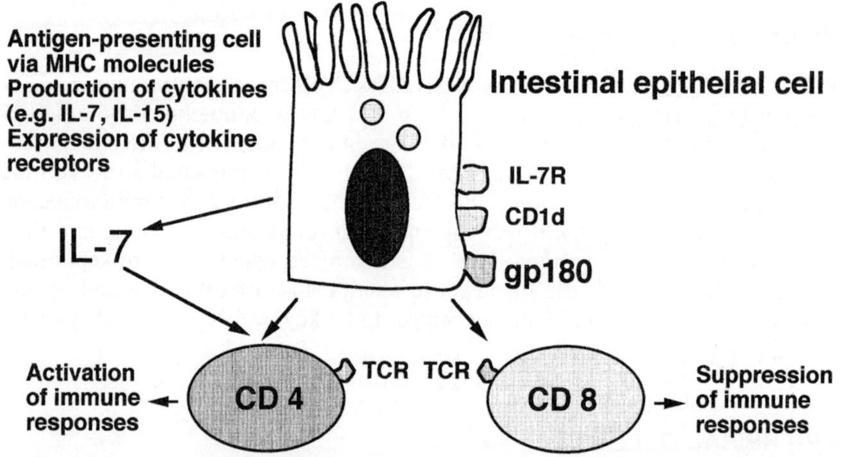

Figure 2 Role of intestinal epithelial cells (IEC) in the pathogenesis of IBD. Normal IEC express high levels of gp180, a novel ligand for CD8 T cells. A decreased expression of gp180 in CD may cause loss of CD8+ suppressor cell activity thereby favouring activation of CD4+ T cells in this disease. Furthermore, recent evidence suggests that production of IL-7 by IEC may be a key phenomenon in inducing acute flares of UC

cytokine profile in IBD. Recent evidence suggests that interleukin-7 (IL-7) produced by IEC could be a key cytokine in the pathogenesis of IBD[6]. IL-7 is normally produced by IEC at low levels and is known to activate T lymphocytes. Whereas production of IL-7 by IEC is increased in acute flares of UC, its production is decreased during chronic phases of disease. Thus, increased IL-7 production by IEC could be a more proximal event in the pathogenesis of IBD that may result in T cell activation.

LAMINA PROPRIA MACROPHAGES

Several recent studies have shown changes in the activation status of LP macrophages in patients with IBD (Figure 3). Several groups described increased levels of various proinflammatory cytokines (IL-1, IL-6, IL-8) in inflamed CD and UC tissue samples compared with control patients[7,8]. Increased levels of IL-1 and IL-6 have also been described in uninvolved CD tissue compared with control tissue. These data support the hypothesis that CD is a panenteritis that manifests itself only in some defined areas of the gut.

Various groups found an increased production of tumour necrosis factor-α (TNF-α) by LP mononuclear cells in patients with IBD[9]. The functional importance of this cytokine in IBD is supported by several studies that showed that antibodies to TNF can be successfully used to treat intestinal inflammation in

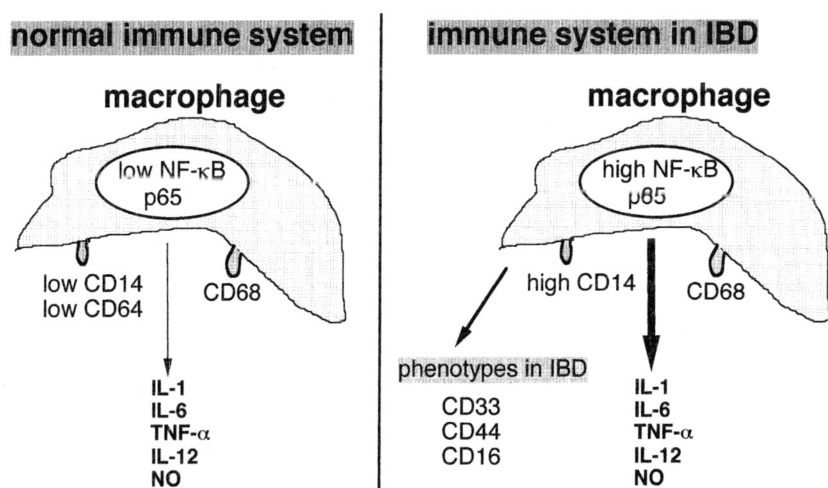

Figure 3 Role of intestinal macrophages in the pathogenesis of IBD. Normal lamina propria macrophages express CD68 but only low levels of CD14. Furthermore, they express only low levels of nuclear NF-κB p65 and produce small amounts of proinflammatory cytokines such as IL-1, IL-6 and TNF. In contrast, LP macrophages in IBD express higher levels of CD14 and CD16. Furthermore, they express high levels of nuclear NF-κB p65 and produce high amounts of proinflammatory cytokines such as IL-1, IL-6 and TNF

CD[10]. However, another cytokine central to the pathogenesis of IBD could be IL-12, a cytokine produced by dendritic cells and macrophages mainly in response to bacterial products[11,12]. Levels of the functionally active IL-12 (p35/p40) hetero-dimer are increased in the LP of patients with CD but not UC (M. Neurath *et al.*, unpublished data). Since IL-12 is potent inducer of T_H1 T cell differentiation, these data suggest that IL-12 could be a key cytokine for T_H1 T cell differentiation in CD, whereas lower IL-12 levels in UC favour T_H2 T cell differentiation. The fundamental importance of IL-12 in chronic intestinal inflammation is further underlined by studies in murine models for IBD that showed amelioration or abrogation of established disease after administration of antibodies to IL-12[11].

B LYMPHOCYTES

B lymphocytes are cells of the mucosal immune system that play a key role in mediating the humoral immunity in the gut (reviewed in Ref. 13). Various studies have found increased numbers of mucosal B lymphocytes/plasma cells and an altered production of immunoglobulins in patients with IBD. Interestingly, B lymphocytes in IBD are known to produce various auto-antibodies mainly directed against components of epithelial cells (e.g. ECAC) and antineutrophilic cytoplasmic antibodies (ANCA). It has been suggested that these autoantibodies may contribute to the pathogenesis of IBD.

LAMINA PROPRIA T LYMPHOCYTES

The intestinal immune system comprises specialized lymphocyte populations localized in Peyer's patches, the epithelium (IEL) and the LP[13]. Various studies have shown that normal LP lymphocytes exhibit changes in their proliferative capacities and cytokine production[14]. For instance, LP T cells are significantly more responsive to CD2 ligation than peripheral blood lymphocytes, as deter-mined by release of interferon-γ (IFN-γ), IL-2, IL-4 and TNF-α. In addition, LP T cells proliferate poorly and produce less cytokines in response to TCR/CD3 receptor stimulation. In CD and UC, however, LP T cells showed even lower proliferative responses than control LP T cells when stimulated via the TCR/CD3 signalling pathway. In contrast, proliferative responses of IBD LP T cells stimulated via the CD2/CD28 pathway were relatively preserved or increased[15].

Fuss *et al.*[15] found a different cytokine profile of LP T lymphocytes in IBD compared with control LP T cells. For instance, a decreased IL-2 production of LP CD4+ T cells in patients with CD but not UC was shown after accessory pathway stimulation. The production of IFN-γ, another T_H1 cytokine, in IBD has also been analysed by several groups. Breese *et al.*[16] and Autschbach *et al.*[17] found an increase of IFN-γ producing cells in CD but not UC. Conversely, Fuss *et al.*[15] showed an increased production of IFN-γ by LP CD4+ T cells in CD but not UC when cells were stimulated via accessory signalling pathways.

In further studies designed to analyse production of T_H2 cytokines in IBD, decreased production of IL-4 by LP CD4+ T cells was found in both CD and

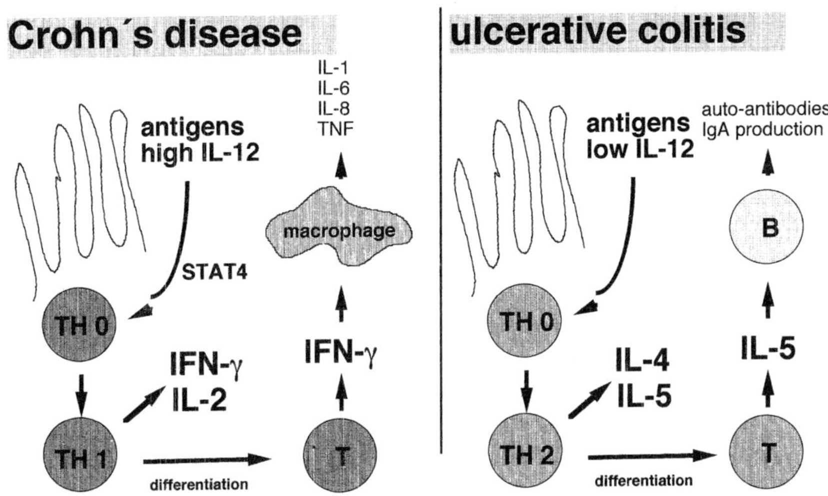

Figure 4   Hypothetical pathogenesis of IBD. Mucosal antigens are presented by antigen-presenting cells to CD4+ T lymphocytes. Activation of the CD40/CD40L interaction causes production of large amounts of IL-12 in CD but not UC. IL-12 in CD in turn promotes IFN-γ production by LP CD4+ T lymphocytes. IFN-γ then again activates macrophages with the consecutive production of proinflammatory cytokines such as TNF. In contrast, low levels of IL-12 in UC favour the generation of T cells with a different cytokine profile

UC[15]. This decrease of IL-4 production was associated with reduced numbers of IL-4 producing cells, as shown by ELISPOT analysis. Further studies focused on production of the T_H2 type cytokine IL-5 in patients with IBD. IL-5 production by LP CD4+ T cells in CD was normal or decreased, whereas strikingly increased IL-5 production was observed in UC[15]. In summary, these data provide reason to believe that mucosal T cell responses in CD are associated with an IFN-γ-like cytokine response, whereas UC is associated with an IL-5-like response[15].

In summary, the data suggest that changes of the mucosal immune system play a key role in the pathogenesis of IBD (Figure 4). A better understanding of the pathogenic mechanisms in IBD may finally lead to the design of rational immunotherapeutic strategies in IBD patients.

References

1. Duchmann R, Kaiser I, Hermann E, Mayet W, Ewe K, Meyer zum Büschenfelde KH. Tolerance exists towards resident intestinal flora but is broken in active inflammatory bowel disease (IBD). Clin Exp Immunol. 1995;102:448–455.
2. Mowat AM. The regulation of immune responses to dietary protein antigens. Immunol Today. 1987;8:93–98.
3. Sadlack B, Merz H, Schorle H, Schimpl A, Feller AC, Horvak I. Ulcerative colitis-like disease in mice with a disrupted interleukin-2 gene. Cell. 1993;75:253–261.
4. Kühn R, Löhler J, Rennick D, Rajewsky K, Müller W. Interleukin-10-deficient mice develop chronic enterocolitis. Cell. 1993;75:263–274.
5. Toy C, Mayer L. Defective expression of gp180, a ligand for CD8 T cells, on epithelial cells in IBD. J Clin Invest. 1997;78:256–269.

6. Watanabe Y, Hibi T. Chronic intestinal inflammation in IL-7 transgenic mice. J Exp Med. 1998;144:413–422.
7. Isaaks KL, Sartor RB, Haskill S. Cytokine mRNA profiles in inflammatory bowel disease mucosa detected by PCR amplification. Gastroenterology. 1992;103:1587–1595.
8. Mahida YR, Wu K, Jewell DP. Enhanced production of interleukin1-β by mononuclear cells isolated from mucosa with active ulcerative colitis and Crohn's disease. Gut. 1989;30:835–838.
9. Reinecker HC, Steffen M, Witthoeft T et al. Enhanced secretion of tumour necrosis factor-alpha, IL-6 and IL-1 beta by isolated lamina propria mononuclear cells from patients with ulcerative colitis and Crohn's disease. Clin Exp Immunol. 1993;94:174–181.
10. van Dullemen HM, van Deventer SJH, Hommes DW et al. Treatment of Crohn's disease with anti-tumor necrosis factor chimeric monoclonal antibody. Gastroenterology. 1995;109:129–135.
11. Neurath MF, Fuss I, Kelsall BL, Stüber E, Strober W. Antibodies to IL-12 abrogate established experimental colitis in mice. J Exp Med. 1995;182:1281–1290.
12. Stüber E, Strober W, Neurath MF. Blocking the CD40L-CD40 interaction in vivo specifically prevents the priming of Th1-T cells through the inhibition of IL-12 secretion. J Exp Med. 1996;183:183–189.
13. Strober W, Neurath MF. Immunological diseases of the gastrointestinal tract. In: Rich RR (ed) Clinical Immunology. St. Louis: Mosby, 1995:1401–1428.
14. Targan SR, Deem RL, Liu M, Wang S, Nel A. Definition of a lamina propria T cell responsive state. Enhanced cytokine responsiveness of T cells stimulated through the CD2 pathway. J Immunol. 1995;154:664–675.
15. Fuss I, Neurath MF, Boirivant M et al. The lymphokine production of lamina propria CD4+ T cells in Crohn's disease exhibits a TH1-like (IFN-γ) profile whereas ulcerative colitis manifests a TH2-like (IL-5) profile. J Immunol. 1996;171:1228–1238.
16. Breese E, Braegger CP, Corrigan CJ, Walker-Smith JA, MacDonald TT. IL-2 and IFN-γ-secreting T cells in normal and diseased human intestinal mucosa. Immunology. 1993;78:127–131.
17. Autschbach F, Schürmann G, Qiao L, Merz H, Wallich R, Meuer SC. Cytokine mRNA expression and proliferation status of intestinal mononuclear cells in noninflamed gut and Crohn's disease. Virchows Arch. 1995;426:51–60.

Section VI
Immunomodulatory strategies in IBD

27
Conventional drug therapy and immunomodulatory strategies in IBD

M. ZEITZ

INTRODUCTION

Standard medical therapy of patients with inflammatory bowel diseases (IBD) consists of aminosalicylates, corticosteroids and immunosuppressive agents such as azathioprine/6-mercaptopurine. The role and efficacy of these drugs in different clinical situations has been established by several controlled clinical trials. Progress in medical therapy over recent decades has been more an evolutionary rather than a revolutionary process. Only in very recent years, based on our understanding of the pathogenesis of IBD, have new immunomodulatory and anti-inflammatory strategies been developed: these are the topics of several contributions in this volume. In this chapter, several aspects of the medical therapy of IBD, especially Crohn's disease (CD), will be discussed which are important in determining how many and which groups of patients may benefit. In addition, the clinical and pathophysiological rationale for the introduction of these new agents will be covered.

EFFICACY OF ESTABLISHED ANTI-INFLAMMATORY AND IMMUNOSUPPRESSIVE AGENTS IN INFLAMMATORY BOWEL DISEASES

The basis of the current concept of medical therapy of patients with Crohn's disease was given by two major placebo-controlled randomized studies, the North American (NCCDS)[1] and European (ECCDS)[2] trials. These studies clearly have shown superiority of corticosteroids over aminosalicylates and azathioprine in treating patients with active CD. None of the drugs was effective in maintaining remission. In later trials these results were basically confirmed; however, higher doses of aminosalicylates in the form of different preparations of mesalamine (5-ASA) were shown to be effective in both active disease and remission maintenance[3]. These effects were only moderate. The important role of immunosuppressive agents especially in subgroups of patients with IBD has been increasingly recognized. The benefits of azathioprine/6-mercaptopurine have been clearly shown for steroid-dependent Crohn's disease and for complicated and severe disease[4,5]. Even in active disease azathioprine was superior to placebo in addition to high dose corticosteroids. Thus, immunosuppressive therapy with azathioprine/6-mercaptopurine has its established role in the treatment of complicated CD and there are indications that increasing the dose up to the development of mild leukopenia might be even more effective than a fixed dose schedule (2–2.5 mg/kg body weight).

It is thought by most investigators that T cell abnormalities, especially hyperresponsiveness and increased activation of mucosal T cells, play a central role in the pathogenesis of IBD. Therefore agents which suppress T cell function, such as cyclosporin, were tested with much hope in IBD. However, in spite of an initial successful trial[6], later controlled treatment studies were not able to confirm a beneficial effect of cyclosporin in CD[7–9]. This unexpected finding may be due to differential effects of cyclosporin on mucosal T cells and circulating T cells[10].

If one tries to combine the results of the different controlled trials with conventional drug therapy in patients with CD with regard to their effectiveness in either active disease or remission maintenance the following picture emerges. Of 1000 patients with active disease, 800 will respond to corticosteroid therapy. Of the remaining 200 patients about 66 will either not respond or will have an early relapse after increasing steroid doses and introducing azathioprine/6-mercaptopurine (Figure 1). Thus, about 6.6% of patients with active disease might be candidates for new treatment strategies due to insufficient treatment response. A more severe problem in treating CD is maintenance of remission: about 13% will have early relapses in spite of using 5-ASA and/or azathioprine/6-mercaptopurine (Figure 2).

In conclusion, from these theoretical calculations, one in five patients with CD will not have a satisfying response to conventional established therapy and will be a candidate for other treatment modalities.

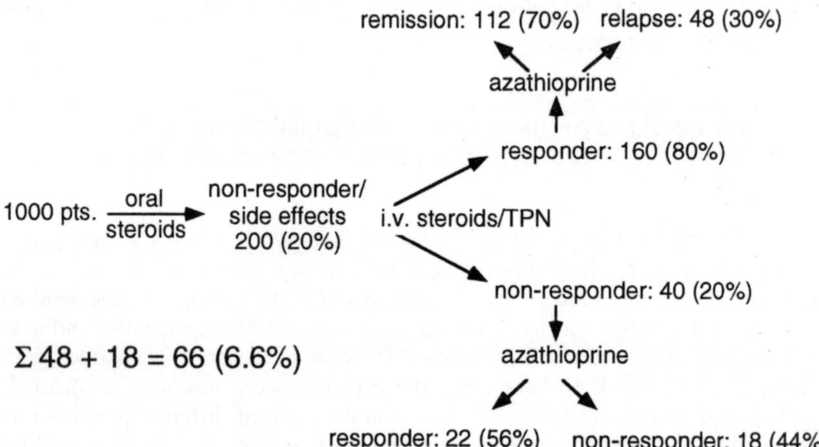

Figure 1 Theoretical calculation of the number of patients not responding to standard treatment regimens[1]

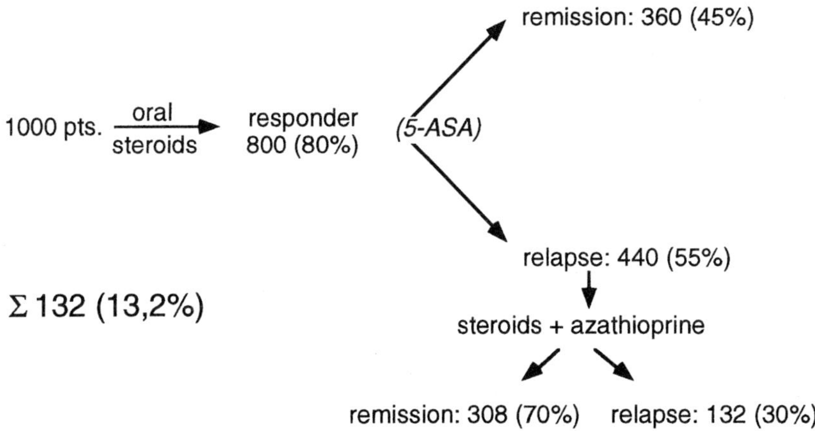

Figure 2 Theoretical calculation of the number of patients not responding to standard treatment regimens[2]

SIDE EFFECTS OF 'CONVENTIONAL' IMMUNOSUPPRESSIVE AGENTS

In addition to the ineffectiveness of established agents, the presence of side effects may be another motivation for the development of new treatment strategies. Side effects of corticosteroids are well known and arise from their endocrine activity (Table 1). Risks of treatment with the immunosuppressive agents azathioprine/6-mercaptopurine are also well characterized[11] (see Table 1). If patients are carefully followed up by experienced physicians, untoward effects of conventional agents are tolerable and it is rarely necessary to change the therapeutic approach. One attempt to reduce the side effects of corticosteroids is the use of locally active steroids with high anti-inflammatory activity and low systemic availability, such as budesonide. This compound, when given orally in distal (ileal) release formulations, is effective in low to moderately active CD with manifestations in the terminal ileum and right-sided colon[12]. Thus, this approach is limited in its clinical application.

Table 1 Undesired effects of anti-inflammatory and immunosuppressive agents in IBD

Azathioprine/6-Mercaptopurine:				
Pancreatitis	Bone marrow depression	Allergic reactions	Drug hepatitis	Infections (severe)
3.3%	2%	2%	0.3%	7.4%(1.8%)
396 patients, mean follow-up 5 yrs[11]				

Corticosteroids:
Short-term treatment: severe side effects uncommon
Long-term treatment: side effects up to 60%
Infectious complications: 12.7% (control group 8.0%)

The side effects of treating patients with IBD using recent alternative approaches such as cytokines, anti-cytokine or anti-lymphocyte receptor antibodies and anti-sense oligonucleotides are poorly characterized for obvious reasons. Several problems are associated with these agents. The risk of developing an immune response to antibodies from non-human species can be minimized by the use of humanized antibodies. A more severe and, so far unpredictable risk, arises from the consequences of immunomodulation by cytokines and anti-cytokines/anti-receptors with regard to the development of immunodeficiency and immune dysregulation and pathological immunoproliferation with the development of malignancy. Although there are no published reports in this regard so far, such consequences of immunomodulation may be possible and have to be kept in mind.

TARGET STRUCTURES OF ANTI-INFLAMMATORY AGENTS IN IBD

Intestinal mucosal immune responses are usually characterized by down-regulation of T cell responses to luminal antigens. In IBD patients this tolerance towards antigens of the own luminal flora seems to be broken and hyper-responsiveness of intestinal T cells, especially CD4[+] T cells, is observed which might explain the ongoing inflammatory response in the gut mucosa[13]. Therefore strategies to down-regulate the overshooting CD4[+] T cell-dominated immune response might be particularly helpful (Figure 3). As mentioned above, cyclosporin has been disappointing in this regard in clinical trials. One explanation might be the finding that cyclosporin is less effective in suppressing mucosal compared with systemic immune responses in an animal model of mucosal immunization[10] (Figure 4). At the moment it is not clear whether tacrolimus, a drug with similar mode of action on T cell responses, has similar shortcomings since initial pilot studies in IBD patients indicate a beneficial effect.

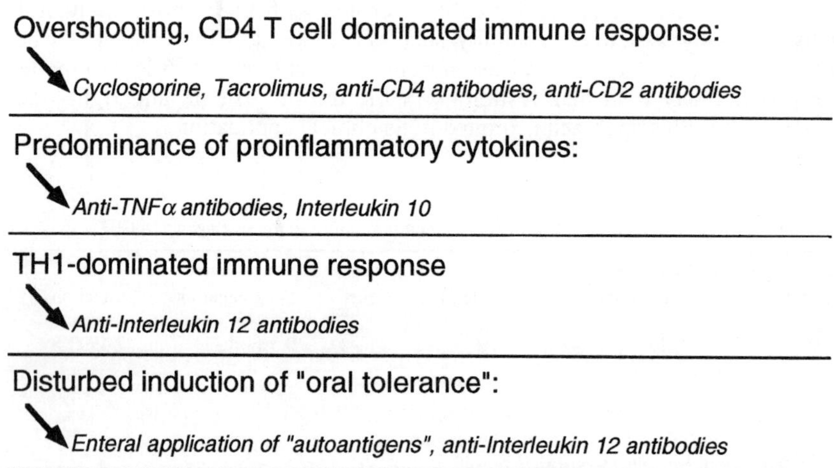

Figure 3 Immunomodulating therapy in IBD

In Vivo Treatment with Cyclosporin A

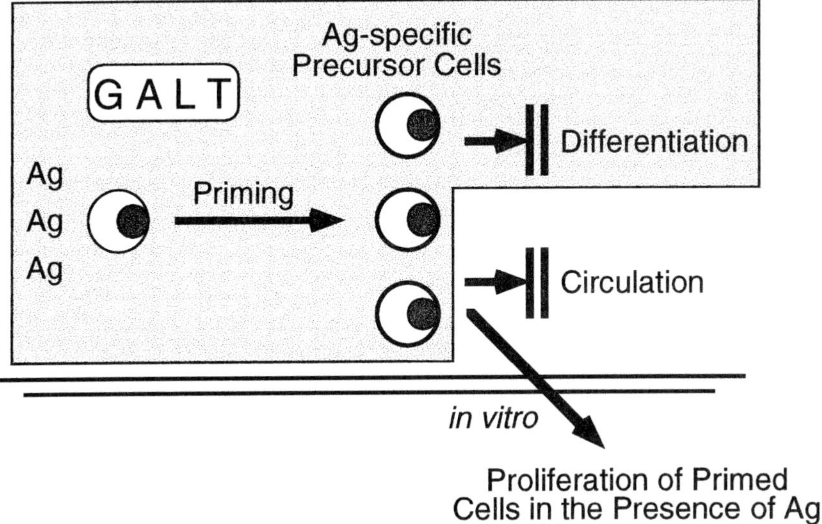

Figure 4 Schematic summary of a study in which non-human primates were treated for 2 weeks with cyclosporin, then rectally infected with *Chlamydia trachomatis*[10]. This investigation has shown that cyclosporin was unable to prevent the induction of antigen-specific T cells in the mucosal immune system (mesenteric lymph nodes). However, reactive T cells were not found in the circulation and specific antibodies did not appear compared with untreated infected control animals. These results implicate that cyclopsorin might have different effects on the mucosal immune system versus the systemic compartment

Other strategies for down-regulation of CD4+ T cell responses include the administration of antibodies to the CD4 receptor. This has been tried in small numbers of patients with severe inflammatory bowel disease. Again, some activity has been documented. However, long-term risks of this form of inducing immunodeficiency are unpredictable so far. Many groups have documented an increase of the proinflammatory cytokine TNF-α in the mucosa of CD patients and have shown its pathophysiological role. Based on these findings, clinical trials have been initiated using antibodies to this cytokine, such as the humanized chimeric antibody cA2. These studies clearly documented clinical efficacy in severe disease and even have shown beneficial effects in fistulating disease[14–16]. At the moment there is concern about this treatment since long-term trials in rheumatoid arthritis showed the development of malignant lymphomas in some patients. It is important to notice that these findings are so far unpublished and there is no convincing evidence proving the relationship to the treatment with anti-TNF-α antibodies. Based on our knowledge on mucosal immunoregulation, the application of the down-regulating cytokine interleukin-10 (IL-10) has also been tested. IL-10 is produced by T cells, B cells and macrophages, and inhibits a wide variety of macrophage functions, including the production of proinflammatory cytokines. Recently, the results of a controlled trial have been presented in preliminary form[17]. Limited efficacy and no significant side effects were documented in active disease; however, more studies are necessary to define the role of this promising approach.

There is increasing evidence that at least in CD there is dominance of a T_H1 T cell response in the mucosa characterized by high levels of IFN-γ production[18]. In the induction of T_H1 T cells IL-12 plays a pivotal role[19]. In an established animal model of Crohn's disease, TNBS colitis in mice, administration of anti-IL-12 antibodies was highly effective in healing mucosal inflammation[20,21]. Therefore the blockade of IL-12 in patients might be a highly specific therapeutic approach in CD. So far, clinical studies are completely missing.

CONCLUSIONS

Conventional drug therapy in IBD patients is clinically effective in the vast majority of patients. The main clinical problems in treating IBD patients are (1) remission maintenance, (2) decreasing disease activity in the small subgroup of patients with highly active disease refractory to conventional drugs, and (3) decreasing side effects of conventional anti-inflammatory and immuno-suppressive agents by the use of more specific approaches. The most potent agents in IBD are corticosteroids. Glucocorticosteroids induce their effect mainly via cytosolic glucocorticosteroid receptors, which finally results in an increase or decrease of gene transcription. This mechanism of action explains both their multiple anti-inflammatory actions (via down-regulation of transcription factor AP-1) (Table 2) and also their untoward side effects (via induction of glucocorticoid responsive gene transcription). Immunosuppressive agents such as azathioprine/6-mercaptopurine act mainly by their anti-proliferative properties which also explain the main side effects. Therefore, based on our current knowledge on the pathogenesis of mucosal inflammation, more specific approaches to down-regulate mucosal inflammation have been developed recently. These approaches include antibodies to various cytokines or surface

Table 2   Anti-inflammatory and immunosuppressive effects of glucocorticoids

---

Suppression of cytokine synthesis:
  IL-1 through 6, IL-8
  TNF-α
  GMCSF

Inhibition of the induction of proinflammatory enzymes
  Phospholipase A2
  Cyclooxygenase 2
  iNOS

Inhibition of the expression of adhesion molecules
  Selectins
  ICAM-1

Suppression of T_H1 cells, stimulation of apoptosis of eosinophils
  and others ...

---

molecules on T cells as well as direct administration of contra-inflammatory cytokines (see Figure 3). The main problem with these agents is that their efficacy also seems to be limited. Probably more important is the fact that long-term toxicity is poorly characterized. In particular, the consequences of immunodeficiency induced by these agents, including the development of lymphoproliferative diseases, are unpredictable. Therefore, carefully performed preclinical investigations, exact patient selection, and intense long-term follow-up of treated patients are prerequisites of these new approaches. However, the major goal for future investigations is the development of treatment modalities to specifically inhibit the underlying immunoregulatory disturbance in inflammatory bowel disease in a safe way. This goal clearly can only be achieved by the collaboration of basic scientists and clinical investigators.

References

1. Summers RW, Switz DM, Sessions JT et al. National cooperative Crohn's disease study: results of drug therapy. Gastroenterology. 1979;77:870–882.
2. Malchow H, Ewe K, Brandes J et al. European Cooperative Crohn's Disease Study (ECCDS): results of drug treatment. Gastroenterology. 1984;86:249–266.
3. Messori A, Brignola C, Trallori G et al. Effectiveness of 5-aminosalicylic acid for maintaining remission in patients with Crohn's disease: a meta-analysis. Am J Gastroenterol. 1994;89: 592–598.
4. Stange EF. Immunosuppression in inflammatory bowel disease. In: Campieri M, Bianchi-Porro G, Fiocchi C, Schölmerich J (eds). Clinical Challenges in Inflammatory Bowel Diseases: Diagnosis, Prognosis and Treatment. Dordrecht: Kluwer Academic Publishers, 1998: 146–152.
5. Pearson DC, May GR, Fick GH, Sutherland LR. Azathioprine and 6-mercaptopurine in Crohn's disease. A meta-analysis. Ann Intern Med. 1995;122:132–142.
6. Brynskov J, Freund L, Rasmussen SN et al. A placebo-controlled, double-blind, randomized trial of cyclosporine therapy in active chronic Crohn's disease. N Engl J Med. 1989;321: 845–850.
7. Feagan BG, McDonald JWD, Rochon J et al. Low-dose cyclosporin for the treatment of Crohn's disease. N Engl J Med. 1994;330:1846–1851.
8. Jewell DP, Lennard-Jones JE. Oral cyclosporin for chronic active Crohn's disease: a multicentre controlled trial. Eur J Gastroenterol Hepatol. 1994;6:499–505.
9. Stange EF, Modigliani R, Pena AS et al. European trial of cyclosporin in chronic active Crohn's disease: a 12-month study. Gastroenterology. 1995;109:774–782.
10. Zeitz M, Quinn TC, Graeff AS, James SP. Oral administration of cyclosporine does not prevent the expansion of antigen-specific gut-associated and spleen lymphocytes during *Chlamydia trachomatis* proctitis in non-human primates. Dig Dis Sci. 1989;34:585–595.
11. Present DH, Meltzer STJ, Krummholz MP, Wolke A, Korelitz BI. 6-Mercaptopurine in the management of inflammatory bowel disease: short- and long-term toxicity. Ann Intern Med. 1989;111:641–649.
12. Rutgeerts P, Lofberg R, Malchow H et al. A comparison of budesonide with prednisolone for active Crohn's disease [see comments]. N Engl J Med. 1994;331:842–845.
13. Zeitz M. Pathogenesis of inflammatory bowel disease. Digestion. 1997;58(S1):59–61.
14. van Dullemen HM, van Deventer SJ, Hommes DW et al. Treatment of Crohn's disease with anti-tumor necrosis factor chimeric monoclonal antibody (cA2). Gastroenterology. 1997;109: 129–135.
15. van Dullemen HM, de Jong E, Slors F, Tytgat GN, van Deventer SJ. Treatment of therapy-resistant perineal metastatic Crohn's disease after proctectomy using anti-tumor necrosis factor chimeric monoclonal antibody, cA2: report of two cases. Dis Colon Rectum. 1998;41: 98–102.
16. Targan SR, Hanauer SB, van Deventer SJ et al. A short-term study of chimeric monoclonal antibody cA2 to tumor necrosis factor alpha for Crohn's disease. Crohn's Disease cA2 Study Group. N Engl J Med. 1997;337:1029–1035.

17. Schreiber S, Fedorak RN, Nielson OH et al. A safety and efficacy study of recombinant human interleukin-10 (rHuIL-10) treatment in 329 patients with chronic active Crohn's disease (CACD). Gastroenterology. 1998;114:A1080.
18. Fuss IJ, Neurath M, Boirivant M et al. Disparate CD4+ lamina propria (LP) lymphokine secretion profiles in inflammatory bowel disease. Crohn's disease LP cells manifest increased secretion of IFN-gamma, whereas ulcerative colitis LP cells manifest increased secretion of IL-5. J Immunol. 1996;157:1261–1270.
19. Strober W, Kelsall B, Fuss I et al. Reciprocal IFN-gamma and TGF-beta responses regulate the occurrence of mucosal inflammation. Immunol Today. 1997;18:61–64.
20. Neurath MF, Fuss I, Kelsall B, Meyer zum Buschenfelde KH, Strober W. Effect of IL-12 and antibodies to IL-12 on established granulomatous colitis in mice. Ann NY Acad Sci. 1996;795: 368–370.
21. Stuber E, Strober W, Neurath M. Blocking the CD40L-CD40 interaction in vivo specifically prevents the priming of T helper 1 cells through the inhibition of interleukin 12 secretion. J Exp Med. 1996;183:693–698.

28
Antagonists of pro-inflammatory cytokines

T. ANDUS and G. ROGLER

INTRODUCTION

The surface of the intestinal mucosa represents the largest part of our barrier against the environment (Figure 1)[1,2]. Large quantities of fluids, electrolytes, nutrients and secretions must cross this border every day in order to maintain the physiological homeostasis of the body. However, the colon is a location with one of the highest concentrations of potential pathogenic microorganisms, which can cause severe harm if they cross the epithelium and invade the circulation. Evolution has solved this conflict by the development of the intestinal immune system.

The intestinal immune system is a complex network consisting of different inflammatory cells, including intraepithelial lymphocytes, intestinal

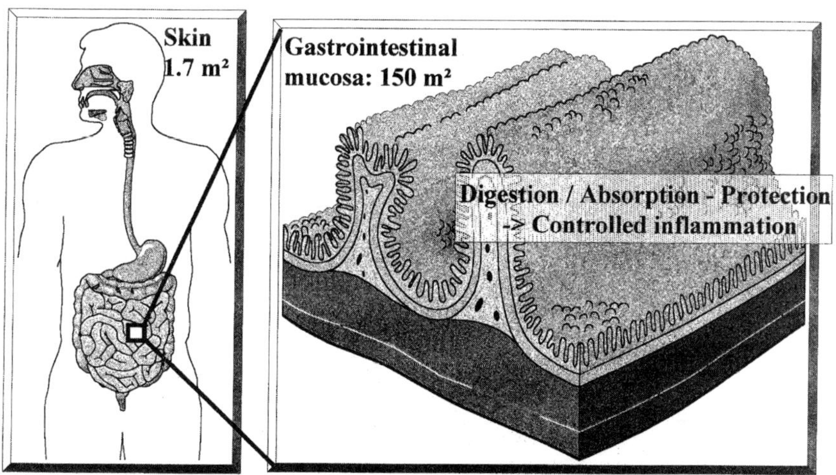

Figure 1   Scheme of the proportions of the surfaces of the gastrointestinal mucosa and the skin

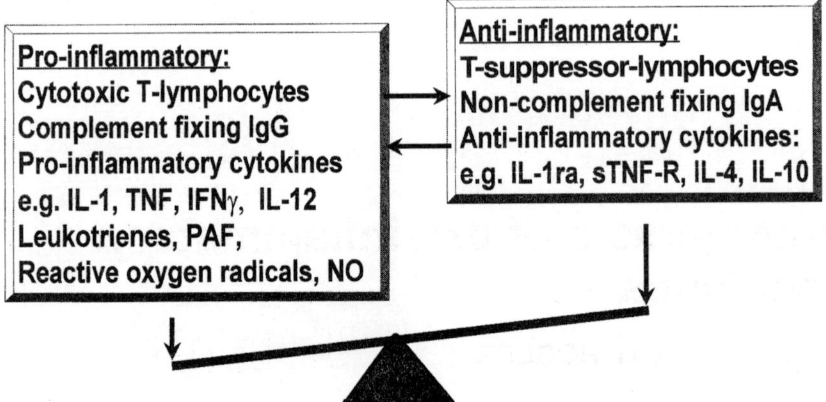

Figure 2 Balance of pro- and anti-inflammatory mediators and cytokines. IL-1 = interleukin-1, TNF = tumour necrosis factor, IFNγ = interferon γ, IL-12 = interleukin-12, PAF = platelet activating factor, NO = nitric oxide, IL-1ra = interleukin-1 receptor antagonist, sTNF-R = soluble tumour necrosis factor receptors, IL-4 = interleukin-4, IL-10 = interleukin-10

macrophages, polymorphonuclear phagocytes, eosinophils, mast cells and other non-primary immune cells such as fibroblasts, endothelial cells and, not least, the intestinal epithelial cells[3–10]. These cells communicate with each other by direct cell–cell contact and by soluble inflammatory mediators acting in paracrine and endocrine ways[11–13]. Cytokines play a key role in this complex network[14–20]. The intestinal immune system must be tightly controlled to prevent the immune reaction being either too weak, resulting in a systemic infection of the host, or too strong resulting in major damage of the intestine by the 'friendly fire' of overreacting inflammatory cells[21–23] (Figure 2). Some pro-inflammatory cytokines, such as interleukin-1 (IL-1) and tumour necrosis factor (TNF) even have specific antagonists and/or soluble receptors antagonizing their action[24–27].

RESULTS AND DISCUSSION

We measured the mucosal concentrations of IL-1α and β, and of IL-1 receptor antagonist (IL-1ra) in colonic biopsies from patients with active or inactive Crohn's disease (CD) or ulcerative colitis (UC), and from inflammatory and non-inflammatory controls[28]. All three cytokines were significantly increased in the inflamed mucosa of patients with CD and UC and in patients with infectious colitis (Figure 3a–c). However, the increase of the pro-inflammatory cytokines IL-1α and β was much greater than the increase of the anti-inflammatory IL-1ra, leading to a significant decrease of the IL-1:IL-1ra ratio (Figure 3d). In the inflamed colonic mucosa there was no difference between IBD and infectious colitis. However, in the non-inflamed mucosa a significant increase of IL-1α and β was found[28].

Genetic polymorphisms have been found for IL-1α, β and IL-1ra[29–32]. Interestingly, genotype 2 of the IL-1ra has been found to be more frequent in

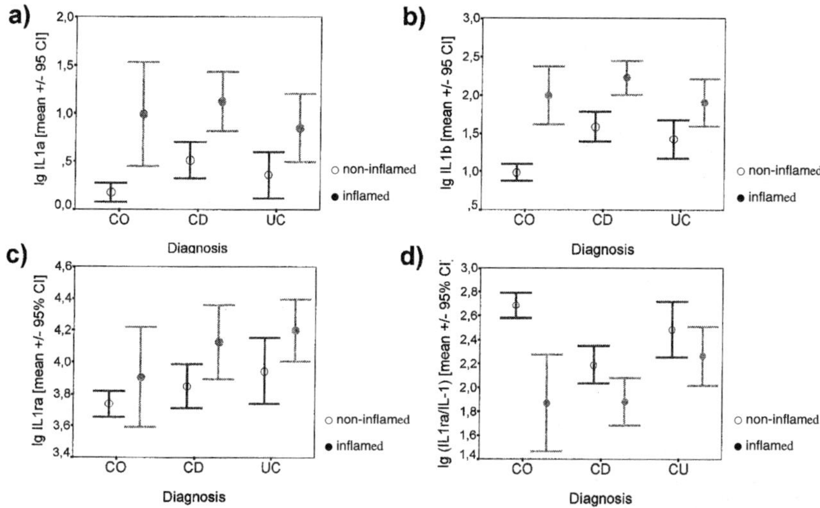

Figure 3 Determination of interleukin-1α (IL-1a), interleukin-1β (IL-1b), interleukin-1 receptor antagonist (IL-1ra), and the ratios between IL-1ra/(IL-1a + IL-1b) in colonic biopsies. Data are given as means of natural logarithms with 95% confidence intervals. CO = controls, CD = Crohn's disease, UC = ulcerative colitis

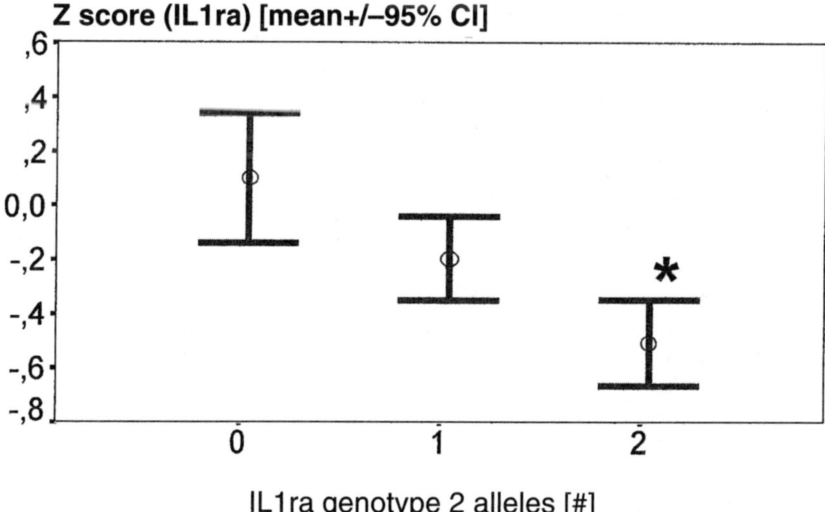

Figure 4 Association between mucosal concentrations of interleukin-1 receptor antagonist and the genotype of interleukin-1 receptor antagonist. Data are given as Z score (patient's value − mean/ standard deviation) and 95% confidence intervals. *Significantly different from patients with no genotype 2 alleles

some groups of patients with UC than in controls and patients with CD[28,33–37]. We therefore looked for an association between this genetic polymorphism and the concentrations of IL-1ra in the colonic mucosa. Interestingly, we found that persons with genotype 2 of the IL-1ra had a significantly decreased concentration of IL-1ra in their colonic mucosa. This effect of the IL-1ra alleles was dose dependent[28] (Figure 4).

In order to determine the sites of synthesis of the IL-1ra in the colonic mucosa we isolated and cultured intestinal lamina propria mononuclear cells and

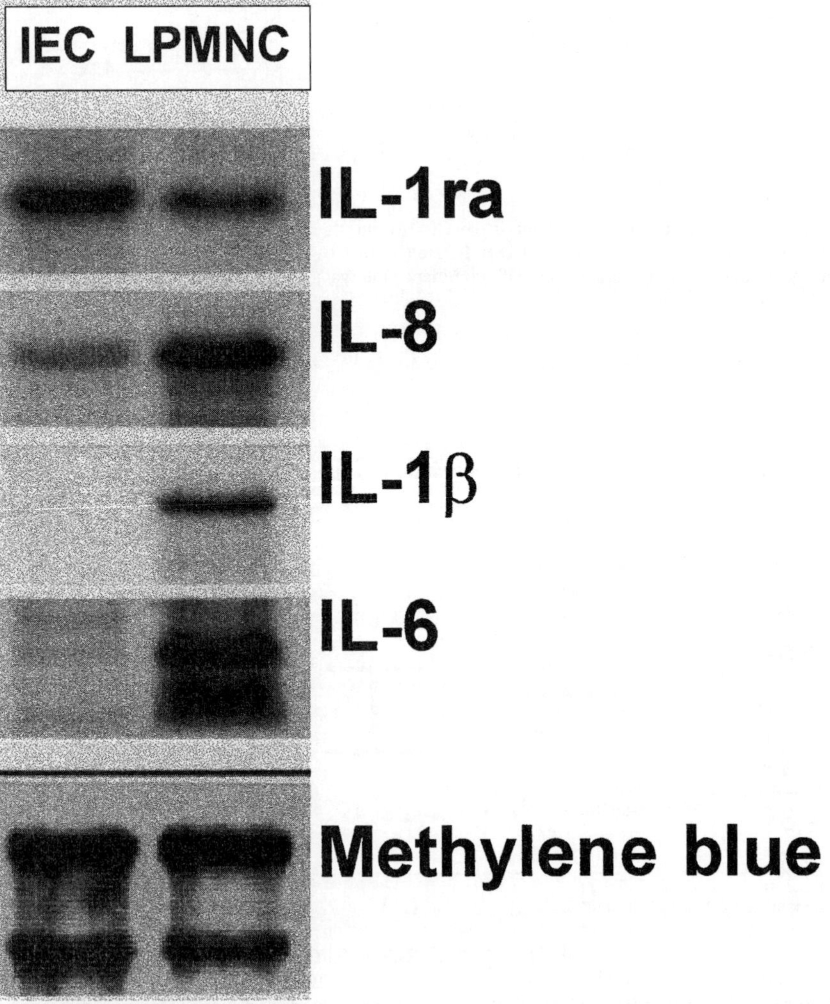

Figure 5 Northern blot analysis of intestinal epithelial cells (IEC) and lamina propria mononuclear cells (LPMNC). IL-1ra = interleukin-1 receptor antagonist, IL-8 = interleukin-8, IL-1β = interleukin-1β, IL-6 = interleukin-6

intestinal epithelial cells. Interestingly, we found that intestinal epithelial cells produced higher amounts of IL-1ra than the intestinal macrophages[38], whereas the pro-inflammatory cytokine was produced significantly more in the intestinal lamina propria mononuclear cells, as shown by Northern blot analysis (Figure 5). IL-1β and IL-6 mRNA were only found in the lamina propria mononuclear cells but not in the intestinal epithelial cells. Production of IL-1ra was significantly increased in intestinal epithelial cells and in lamina propria mononuclear cells from patients with inflammatory bowel disease. In all patients the amount of IL-1ra produced was higher in the intestinal epithelial cells than in the lamina propria mononuclear cells on a cellular basis.

These data suggest that colonic intestinal epithelial cells exert an anti-inflammatory function by producing IL-1ra, so shifting the balance between IL-1 and IL-1ra to the anti-inflammatory site. In patients with the genotype 2 of the IL-1ra this shift may be disturbed in the colonic mucosa, which may lead to chronic inflammation under some circumstances. However, this seems not to be an effect specific for inflammatory bowel disease, since the genotype 2 of the IL-1ra has also been found in many patients without inflammatory bowel disease.

ACKNOWLEDGEMENTS

This work was supported by the Deutsche Forschungsgemeinschaft An168/3-2 and the Wilhelm-Sander Stiftung.

References

1. Wilson JP. Surface area of the small intestine in man. Gut. 1967;8:618–621.
2. Liptschenko VJ, Spiridonova LI. The crypt surface, free and total surface of human large intestine. Verh Anat Ges. 1977;303–305.
3. Brandtzaeg P. The human intestinal immune system: basic cellular and humoral mechanisms. Baillieres Clin Rheumatol. 1996;10:1–24.
4. Otto HF, Gebbers JO, Laissue JA. The functional importance of the intestinal immune system. A review. 1. Orthology. Z Gastroenterol. 1982;20:125–138.
5. Otto HF, Gebbers JO, Laissue JA. The functional importance of the intestinal immune system. A review. 2. Pathology. Z Gastroenterol. 1982;20:245–256.
6. Ruchti C, Luscieti P, Laissue J, Schaffner T, Hess MW, Cottier H. Functional morphology of the intestinal immune system. Z Gastroenterol Verh. 1978;16–24.
7. Liptschenko VJ, Spiridonova LI. The crypt surface, free and total surface of human large intestine. Verh Anat Ges. 1977;303–305.
8. Doe WF. The intestinal immune system. Gut. 1989;30:1679–1685.
9. Dancygier H. Bacteria and the intestinal immune system. Internist Berl. 1989;30:370–381.
10. Laissue JA, Chappuis BB, Muller C. Reubi JC, Gebbers JO. The intestinal immune system and its relation to disease. Dig Dis. 1993;11:298–312.
11. Fitz G. Paracrine regulation of intestinal secretion. Gastroenterology. 1994;107:1206–1208.
12. Kandil HM, Berschneider HM, Argenzio RA. Tumour necrosis factor alpha changes porcine intestinal ion transport through a paracrine mechanism involving prostaglandins. Gut. 1994;35:934–940.
13. Madara JL, Patapoff TW, Gillece CB et al. 5′-Adenosine monophosphate is the neutrophil-derived paracrine factor that elicits chloride secretion from T84 intestinal epithelial cell monolayers. J Clin Invest. 1993;91:2320–2325.
14. Henderson B, Poole S, Wilson M. Microbial/host interactions in health and disease: who controls the cytokine network? Immunopharmacology. 1996;35:1–21.

15. Harrison LC, Campbell IL. Cytokines: an expanding network of immunoinflammatory hormones. Mol Endocrinol. 1988;2:1151–1156.
16. Castell JV, Andus T, Kunz D, Heinrich PC. Interleukin-6. The major regulator of acute-phase protein synthesis in man and rat. Ann NY Acad Sci. 1989;557:87–99.
17. Andus T, Heinrich PC, Castell JC, Gerok W. Interleukin-6: a key hormone of the acute phase reaction. Dtsch Med Wochenschr. 1989;114:1710–1716.
18. Andus T, Holstege A. Cytokines and the liver in health and disease. Effects on liver metabolism and fibrogenesis. Acta Gastroenterol Belg. 1994;57:236–244.
19. Andus T, Palitzsch KD, Gross V, Schölmerich J. The metabolic and endocrine functions of the cytokines. Dtsch Med Wochenschr. 1993;118:306–313.
20. Gross V, Andus T, Leser HGA, Schölmerich J. Inflammatory mediators in chronic inflammatory bowel diseases. Klin Wochenschr. 1991;69:981–987.
21. MacDermott RP. Alterations of the mucosal immune system in inflammatory bowel disease. J Gastroenterol. 1996;31:907–916.
22. Miossec P. Pro- and antiinflammatory cytokine balance in rheumatoid arthritis. Clin Exp Rheumatol. 1995;13(Suppl 12):S13–S16.
23. Miossec P. Acting on the cytokine balance to control auto-immunity and chronic inflammation. Eur Cytokine Netw. 1993;4:245–251.
24. Brockhaus M. Soluble TNF receptor: what is the significance? Intensive Care Med. 1997;23:808–809.
25. Cominelli F, Pizarro TT. Interleukin-1 and interleukin-1 receptor antagonist in inflammatory bowel disease. Aliment Pharmacol Ther. 1996;10(Suppl 2):49–53.
26. Lennard AC. Interleukin-1 receptor antagonist. Crit Rev Immunol. 1995;15:77–105.
27. Olsson I, Gatanaga T, Gullberg U, Lantz M, Granger GA. Tumour necrosis factor (TNF) binding proteins (soluble TNF receptor forms) with possible roles in inflammation and malignancy. Eur Cytokine Netw. 1993;4:169–180.
28. Andus T, Daig R, Vogl D et al. Imbalance of the interleukin 1 system in colonic mucosa – association with intestinal inflammation and interleukin 1 receptor antagonist genotype 2. Gut. 1997;41:651–657.
29. Tarnow L, Pociot F, Hansen PM et al. Polymorphisms in the interleukin-1 gene cluster do not contribute to the genetic susceptibility of diabetic nephropathy in Caucasian patients with IDDM. Diabetes. 1997;46:1075–1076.
30. Louis E, Satsangi J, Roussomoustakaki M et al. Cytokine gene polymorphisms in inflammatory bowel disease. Gut. 1996;39:705–710.
31. Bioque G, Crusius JB, Koutroubakis et al. Allelic polymorphism in IL-1 beta and IL-1 receptor antagonist (IL-1Ra) genes in inflammatory bowel disease. Clin Exp Immunol. 1995;102:379–383.
32. Pociot F, Molvig J, Wogensen L, Worsaae H, Nerup J. A *Taq*I polymorphism in the human interleukin-1 beta (IL-1 beta) gene correlates with IL-1 beta secretion in vitro. Eur J Clin Invest. 1992;22:396–402.
33. Hacker UT, Gomolka M, Keller E et al. Lack of association between an interleukin-1 receptor antagonist gene polymorphism and ulcerative colitis. Gut. 1997;40:623–627.
34. Louis E, Satsangi J, Roussomoustakaki M et al. Cytokine gene polymorphisms in inflammatory bowel disease. Gut. 1996;39:705–710.
35. Bioque G, Bouma G, Crusius JB et al. Evidence of genetic heterogeneity in IBD: 1. The interleukin-1 receptor antagonist in the predisposition to suffer from ulcerative colitis. Eur J Gastroenterol Hepatol. 1996;8:105–110.
36. Bioque G, Crusius JB, Koutroubakis et al. Allelic polymorphism in IL-1 beta and IL-1 receptor antagonist (IL-1Ra) genes in inflammatory bowel disease. Clin Exp Immunol. 1995;102:379–383.
37. Mansfield JC, Holden H, Tarlow JK et al. Novel genetic association between ulcerative colitis and the anti-inflammatory cytokine interleukin-1 receptor antagonist. Gastroenterology. 1994;106:637–642.
38. Rogler G, Daig R, Aschenbrenner E et al. Establishment of long term primary cultures of human intestinal epithelial cells. Lab Invest. 1998;78:879–890.

29
Mechanisms and clinical efficacy of interleukin-10

A. J. G. SCHOTTELIUS and A. S. BALDWIN

INTRODUCTION

Human interleukin-10 (hIL-10) is a 17–20 kDa glycoprotein that exhibits a high degree of homology with mouse IL-10 (73%) and with an open reading frame of the Epstein–Barr virus (84%): BCRF1 or viral IL-10 (vIL-10)[1]. It is a true pleiotropic cytokine produced in the mouse mainly by T_H2 cells and activated macrophages, and in humans by activated monocytes, macrophages and lamina propria mononuclear cells as well as T_H0, T_H1 and T_H2 T cell clones, some CD8[+] T cells, activated B cells and B cell lymphomas[1].

BIOLOGICAL ACTIVITIES OF IL-10

Table 1 summarizes the important suppressive and stimulatory biological activities of IL-10. IL-10 has been called a cytokine synthesis inhibitory factor as one of its most prominent effects is its inhibiting function on cytokine

Table 1 IL-10: biological activities

Suppressive activities	*Stimulatory activities*
Cytokine production of macrophages, neutrophils, T cells	B cell viability, proliferation and class II MHC expression
Autoregulation of macrophages – NO production in macrophages	B cell differentiation and Ig secretion Growth of mast cell and megakaryocyte progenitors
Antigen-specific proliferation of T cell clones – class II MHC expression in macrophages – ICAM-1 expression on monocytes	Growth of thymocytes Development of cytotoxic T cells
Direct inhibition of T cell proliferation/anergy of CD4[+] cells – IL-2 production/secretion of T cells	

expression in various cell types. In activated macrophages/monocytes IL-10 inhibits the production of the pro-inflammatory cytokines IL-1, IL-6, IL-8 and tumour necrosis factor-α (TNF-α) and granulocyte-macrophage colony-stimulating factor (GM-CSF) and granulocyte colony-stimulating factor (G-CSF)[2]. It also exerts its cytokine synthesis inhibitory function on other cell types, inhibiting the synthesis of IL-1, IL-8, and TNF-α in neutrophils[3], of IL-2, TNF-β, interferon-γ (IFN-γ), and GM-CSF in T cells[4], and IFN-γ and TNF-α, GM-CSF and G-CSF in NK cells. These results collectively indicate that IL-10 exerts strong anti-inflammatory activities and it has thus been termed a 'macrophage deactivating factor'[5].

IL-10 was originally identified as a murine T_H2 product[6]. Depending on the cytokine milieu in the microenvironment, $CD4^+$ T_H0 cells differentiate along either or both of the two pathways of T cell differentiation, that is into T_H1 cells that mediate cellular immune responses or into T_H2 cells that mediate humoral immunity[7]. T_H1 and T_H2 cells are distinguished by their production of certain cytokines. These two subsets regulate one another and in this interplay IL-10 has emerged as a hinge cytokine, suppressing, on the one hand, cell-mediated immunity and inflammatory responses characteristic of T_H1 responses, while promoting, on the other hand, humoral immunity and mast cell development characteristic of T_H2 responses. In the presence of monocyte/macrophage antigen-presenting cells, IL-10 inhibits the antigen-specific activation and proliferation of T cell clones belonging to the T_H0, T_H1 or T_H2 subsets[8–10]. The suppressive activity of IL-10 does not directly affect T cell clones, but interferes with the ability of macrophages to act as antigen presenting cells. Indeed, endogenously produced IL-10 down-regulates constitutive class II major histocompatibility complex (MHC) expression on monocytes, which impairs their ability to effectively present antigen to reactive T cell clones[6,8]. A recent study showed the mechanism of MHC class II down-regulation to be not on the level of transcription but to be on the level of MHC exocytosis and recycling[11]. In addition, the expression of intercellular adhesion molecule-1, and the up-regulation of the B7 molecule, which both function as important costimulatory molecules for T cell activation, are suppressed by IL-10[12–14]. IL-10 also has autoregulatory effects since it not only suppressed the production of pro-inflammatory monokines, but also suppressed its own production in activated monocytes, indicating that expression of IL-10 may be regulated by negative feedback in these cells. Moreover, it suppresses the production of reactive oxygen intermediates such as nitric oxide in macrophages[5,15].

In addition to its indirect effects on T cell activation, IL-10 possesses direct effects on T cell proliferation and causes a state of anergy in $CD4^+$ cells by specifically interfering with activation processes leading to IL-2 production and secretion[16,17]. The observation that high levels of IL-10 are associated with transplantation tolerance, and that this cytokine has been shown to inhibit both the antigen-presenting and accessory function of monocytes and IL-2 production by T cells, suggested that IL-10 could be involved in the induction of anergy in $CD4^+$ T cells and it was only recently that IL-10 was actually demonstrated to induce a long-lasting antigen-specific unresponsiveness against allogeneic antigens that cannot be reversed by IL-2 or CD28 stimulation[18].

Looking at the stimulatory activities of IL-10, this cytokine sustains viability and proliferation of activated B lymphocytes and allows them to differentiate into high-rate immunoglobulin-secreting B cells[4]. In addition, IL-10 induces CD-40-activated B lymphocytes to undergo an isotype switch toward IgA[19] IgG1, and IgG3[20]. Moreover, IL-10 co-stimulates growth and differentiation of mast cells and megakaryocyte progenitors as well as thymocytes[3] and enhances cytotoxic T cell development[21]. A wide variety of human tumours express IL-10, for reasons which are poorly understood. New evidence supports the hypothesis that IL-10 is produced by tumours because of its immunosuppressive activities, and that this may be due either to inhibition of recognition by immune cells or inhibition of destruction of tumour cells by effector cells[22].

MOLECULAR MECHANISMS

Some molecular mechanisms of monocyte deactivation by IL-10 have been described. IL-10 inhibits protein tyrosine kinase (PTK) activation induced by LPS binding to the CD14 receptor, and consequently blocks the down-stream Ras signalling pathway[23]. Interestingly, in monocytes and T cells IL-10 induces tyrosine phosphorylation of the Janus kinases Jak1 and tyk2, which then phosphorylate the signal transducers and activators of transcription, STAT1, STAT3 and STAT5 in a differential manner, enabling them to translocate to the nucleus where they transactivate target genes[24,25].

As the inhibition of proinflammatory cytokine production by IL-10 is mainly at the level of gene transcription the possibility was raised that IL-10 affects the activities of transcription factors involved in proinflammatory cytokine gene expression. Indeed, IL-10 has been shown to inhibit the activation of the transcription factor NF-κB in monocytes and T-cells, indicating that inhibition of NF-κB activation may be an important mechanism for IL-10 suppression of cytokine gene transcription. NF-κB has been clearly shown to be critical for the induction of the cytokine genes of for example IL-1β, IL-6, IL-8 and TNF-α. NF-κB is constitutively present in the cytoplasm as an inactive dimer bound to its inhibitory molecule IκBα. Various stimuli including TNF-α and lipopolysaccharide lead to a rapid degradation of IκBα, releasing the NF-κB complex and enabling its nuclear translocation and activation of gene transcription[26]. Studies have produced conflicting results on the ability of IL-10 to inhibit LPS-induced NF-κB DNA-binding activity and the exact mechanisms of this action have not been established[27,28].

Preliminary results obtained in our laboratory in human monocytic THP-1 and U937 cells suggest an IL-10 induced rapid and strong, dose-dependent inhibition of NF-κB DNA binding in gel shift analysis. In contrast to other studies, inhibition of NF-κB by IL-10 in our cell system was caused by two distinct mechanisms. IL-10 treatment preserved IκBα degradation upon short treatment with TNFα and was able to block nuclear translocation of NF-κB. Whereas under conditions of longer TNF-α treatment, IL-10 inhibited NF-κB DNA-binding without affecting NF-κB nuclear translocation.

IMPORTANCE OF IL-10 FOR IBD

A potential role of IL-10 in maintaining normal intestinal homeostatis and net immunosuppression was raised by the observation that IL-10 knock-out mice develop enterocolitis with similarities to IBD[29]. It is well established that pro-inflammatory cytokines are increased in IBD and that IL-10 can down-regulate the enhanced secretion as well as RNA levels of pro-inflammatory cytokines in IBD peripheral monocytes and isolated lamina propria mononuclear cells in a dose-dependent manner[30]. In addition, the *in vivo* topical application of IL-10 down-regulated IL-1 and TNF-α secretion *in vitro*, both systemically and locally[30].

More evidence for a role of IL-10 as a potent immunoregulator in intestinal inflammation comes from animal models with induced colitis. In the SCID mouse model with severe combined immunodeficiency syndrome, transfer of the CD45 Rb[hi] subpopulation of CD4[+] cells from normal mice induces an IBD-like colitis[31]. IL-10 administration significantly protected these SCID mice from developing severe colitis. The protection from colitis was dependent on continuous treatment: the disease developed when treatment was stopped and mice were sacrificed to assess colitis 4 weeks after the last IL-10 treatment[32].

In a recent study performed in a rat model with chronic, granulomatous inflammation induced by bacterial cell wall polymers (PG-APS) IL-10 treatment significantly reduced grossly detectable intestinal inflammation in the chronic granulomatous phase of PG-APS induced enterocolitis in a preventive protocol[33], but had no ability to reverse established inflammation[41].

CLINICAL EFFICACY

In the past few years IL-10 has been tested for the treatment of IBD in clinical trials. A multicentre, randomized, double blind, placebo-controlled and dose-rising study to evaluate the safety and tolerance of multiple doses of recombinant human IL-10 (rhu-IL-10; SCH52000) given i.v. in steroid-refractory Crohn's disease ([CDAI] Crohn's disease activity index 200–350) showed that IL-10 administered at a dose of 0.5–25 μg/kg daily i.v. by bolus for 7 consecutive days in 32 patients was safe and well tolerated with no significant toxicity and only mild adverse events, consisting of headache and nausea[34]. Remission, defined as a CDAI of 150 and a decrease in baseline CDAI of >100, was achieved in 50% of patients in the treatment group versus 23% of patients in the placebo group. In contrast, no significant changes in CDAI (decrease in baseline CDAI of < 100) occurred in 52% of the treatment and in 19% of the placebo group.

A more recent multicentre, randomized, double blind, placebo-controlled, rising dose and placebo-controlled study was conducted in 95 patients with mild to moderately active Crohn's disease (CDAI > 200 ≤ 350), not on steroids or 5-ASA[35]. IL-10 was administered subcutaneously in five dose groups ranging from 1 to 20 μg/kg/day over a treatment period of 28 consecutive days, or placebo was given. Efficacy was measured using clinical (CDAI) and endoscopic outcome and quality of life measurements. Complete remission at the end of the treatment phase was defined as a CDAI < 150 with a decrease in baseline CDAI of >100 points and the improvement or resolution of endoscopic appearance. Complete remission of disease after 28 days of treatment with 1, 5, 10 and

20 μg/kg/day was achieved in 13, 29, 14 and 6% of patients, respectively versus 0% in the placebo group.

In a parallel study in mild to moderately active ulcerative colitis safety and tolerance of multiple subcutaneous doses of IL-10 was evaluated in 94 patients[36]. Mild to moderate disease was defined by an ulcerative colitis severity score (UCSS) ranging from 3 to 10. Patients requiring i.v. steroids were excluded. During the 28 days treatment phase IL-10 treatment was safe and well tolerated, and most adverse events were mild to moderate in severity. The mean percentage change in total UCSS at treatment endpoint was higher for the 5, 10 and 20 μg/kg/day dose levels (–28.9, –26.2 and –34.1 respectively) than the placebo group (–13.4). There was, however, no significant difference in the IL-10 treated groups and placebo for patients achieving complete remission (UCSS of 0).

A large, placebo-controlled trial evaluated the safety and efficacy of subcutaneously administered IL-10 in steroid-unresponsive chronic active Crohn's disease in 329 patients (CDAI 200–400, steroids 10–40 mg/day for 3 months prior to study given alone or in combination with 6-MP or AZA and kept stable throughout the study)[37]. Adverse events were mild to moderate and a transient, reversible asymptomatic decrease in platelet counts and haemoglobin concentration was observed in the two highest dose groups. A clinical response that was measured using baseline haematocrit adjusted CDAI was observed in 27%, 34%, 46% and 40% of patients in the 1, 4, 8 and 20 μg/kg/day dose groups respectively, compared with 27% in the placebo group. In conclusion IL-10 therapy in this study was well tolerated and associated with clinical benefit.

SUMMARY AND DISCUSSION

In vitro and *in vivo* studies in animal models of IBD and in IBD patients have demonstrated IL-10 to be an important intestinal immunoregulator with potent anti-inflammatory and immunosuppressive activities. One of the most prominent effects of IL-10 is its down-regulation of pro-inflammatory cytokines in activated monocytes and macrophages[2,8]. IL-10 also has autoregulatory effects and suppresses its own production in activated monocytes. This contra-inflammatory cytokine interferes with the ability of macrophages to act as antigen-presenting cells by down-regulating MHC class II expression[6,8] and thereby inhibiting antigen-specific activation and proliferation of T cell clones[9,10,38].

Conflicting results exist on the ability of IL-10 to inhibit the transcription factor NF-κB[27,28], which is critical for the induction of pro-inflammatory cytokines and has been found to be activated in IBD[39,40]. The mechanisms by which IL-10 suppresses NF-κB have not been established. Preliminary results from our laboratory suggest a rapid and strong, dose-dependent inhibition of NF-κB activity in monocytic cells. Inhibition of NF-κB by IL-10 in our monocytic cell system is mediated by preservation of IκBα degradation and direct inhibition of NF-κB DNA-binding.

Intravenous IL-10 therapy in steroid-refractory Crohn's disease is safe and associated with clinical improvement and when given subcutaneously in mild to moderate active Crohn's disease was safe, well tolerated and associated with modest but significant rates of clinical and endoscopic remission. A relatively low remission rate in some dose groups could reflect certain patient sub-populations that do not respond to IL-10 treatment as well as other patient populations. IL-10 therapy was also well tolerated and associated with clinical benefits in a large, placebo-controlled trial in chronic active Crohn's disease. In a first trial assessing the safety of IL-10 therapy in ulcerative colitis, IL-10 treatment was safe and well tolerated but the percentage of patients achieving remission was not significantly different in the treated versus the placebo group.

Future studies could test for the contra-inflammatory synergism between IL-10 and other immune-modulators such as IL-4 or corticosteroids, possibly improving clinical efficacy of IL-10 treatment in IBD.

References

1. Moore K, O'Garra A, de Waal Malefyt R, Vieira P, Mosmann T. Interleukin-10. Annu Rev Immunol. 1993;11:165–190.
2. Fiorentino D, Zlotnik A, Mosmann T, Howard M, O'Garra A. IL-10 inhibits cytokine production by activated macrophages. J Immunol. 1991;147:3815–3822.
3. Thompson-Snipes L, Dhar V, Bond M, Mosmann T, Moore K, Rennick D. Interleukin-10: a novel stimulatory factor for mast cells and their progenitors. J Exp Med. 1991;173: 507–510.
4. Rousset F, Garcia E, Defrance T et al. IL-10 is a potent growth and differentiation factor for activated human B lymphocytes. Proc Natl Acad Sci USA. 1992;89:1890–1893.
5. Bogdan C, Vodovotz Y, Nathan C. Macrophage deactivation by interleukin-10. J Exp Med. 1991;174:1549–1555.
6. Fiorentino D, Bond M, Mosman T. Th2 clones secrete a factor that inhibits cytokine production by Th1 clones. J Exp Med. 1989;170:2081–2095.
7. Mosmann T, Coffman R. Th1 and Th2 cells: different patterns of lymphokine secretion lead to different functional properties. Annu Rev Immunol. 1989;7:145–174.
8. de Waal Malefyt R, Abrams J, Bennett B, Figdor CG, de Vries JE. IL-10 inhibits cytokine synthesis by human monocytes: an autoregulatory role of IL-10 produced by monocytes. J Exp Med. 1991;174:1209–1220.
9. Taga K, Tosato G. IL-10 inhibits T cell proliferation and IL-2 production. J Immunol. 1992;148:1143–1148.
10. Ding L, Shevach E. T cell proliferation by selectively inhibiting macrophage costimulatory function. J Immunol. 1992;148:3133–3139.
11. Koppelman B, Neefjes JJ, de Vries JE, de Waal Malefyt R. Interleukin-10 down-regulates MHC Class II $\alpha\beta$ peptide complexes at the plasma membrane of monocytes by affecting arrival and recycling. Immunity. 1997;7:861–871.
12. Ding L, Linsley P, Huang L-Y, Germain R, Shevach E. IL-10 inhibits macrophage costimulatory activity by selectively inhibiting the up-regulation of B7 expression. J Immunol. 1993;151: 1224–1234.
13. Willems F, Marchant A, Delville J-P et al. Interleukin-10 inhibits B7 and intercellular adhesion molecule-1 expression on human monocytes. Eur J Immunol. 1994;24:1007.
14. Chang C, Furue M, Tamaki K. b7-1 expression of Langerhans cells is up-regulated by proinflammatory cytokines, and is down-regulated by interferon-gamma or by interleukin-10. Eur J Immunol. 1995;25:394–398.
15. Gazzinelli R, Oswald I, James S, Sher A. IL-10 inhibits parasite killing and nitric oxide production by IFN-γ activated macrophages. J Immunol. 1992;148:1792–1796.
16. de Waal Malefyt R, Yssel H, de Vries JE. Direct effects of IL-10 on subsets of human CD4[+] T cell clones and resting T cells. J Immunol. 1993;150:4754–4765.
17. Taga K, Mostowski H, Tosato G. Human interleukin-10 can directly inhibit T-cell growth. Blood. 1993;81:2964–2971.
18. Groux H, Bigler M, de Vries JE, Roncarolo MG. Interleukin-10 induces a long-term antigen-specific anergic state in human CD4[+] T cells. J Exp Med. 1996;184:19–29.

19. Defrance T, Vanberliet B, Briere F, Durand I, Rousset F, Banchereau J. Interleukin 10 and transforming growth factor β co-operate to induce anti-CD40-activated naive human B cells to secrete immunoglobulin A. J Exp Med. 1992;175:671–682.
20. Briere F, Servet-Delprat C, Bridon J-M, Saint-Remy J-M, Banchereau J. Human interleukin 10 induces naive sIgD-B cells to secrete IgG1 and IgG3. J Exp Med. 1994;179:757–762.
21. Chen W-F, Zlotnik A. Interleukin-10: a novel cytotoxic T cell differentiation factor. J Immunol. 1991;147:528–534.
22. Qin Z, Noffz G, Mohaupt M, Blankenstein T. Interleukin-10 prevents dendritic cell accumulation and vaccination with granulocyte-macrophage colony-stimulating factor gene-modified tumor cells. J Immunol. 1997;159:770–776.
23. Geng Y, Gulbins E, Altman A, Lotz M. Monocyte deactivation by interleukin-10 via inhibition of tyrosine kinase activity and the Ras signaling pathway. Proc Natl Acad Sci USA. 1994;91: 8602–8606.
24. Finbloom D, Winestock K. IL-10 induces the tyrosine phosphorylation of tyk2 and Jak1 and the differential assembly of STAT1a and STAT3 complexes in human T cells and monocytes. J Immunol. 1995;155:1079–1090.
25. O'Farrell A-M, Liu Y, Moore K, Mui AL-F. IL-10 inhibits macrophage activation and proliferation by distinct signaling mechanisms: evidence for STAT2 dependent and -independent pathways. EMBO J. 1998;17:1006–1018.
26. Baldwin A. The NF-κB and IκB proteins: new discoveries and insights. Annu Rev Immunol. 1996;14:649–681.
27. Wang P, Wu P, Siegel M, Egan R, Billah M. IL-10 inhibits NF-κB activation in human monocytes. J Biol Chem. 1995;270:9558–9563.
28. Dokter W, Koopmans S, Vellenga E. Effects of IL-10 and IL-4 on LPS-induced transcription factors which are involved in IL-6 regulation. Leukemia. 1996;10:1308–1316.
29. Kühn R, Löhler J, Rennick D, Rajewski K, Müller W. Interleukin-10-deficient mice develop enterocolitis. Cell. 1993;75:263–274.
30. Schreiber S, Heinig T, Thiele H-G, Raedler A. Immunoregulatory role of interleukin-10 in patients with inflammatory bowel disease. Gastroenterology. 1995;108:1434–1444.
31. Powrie F, Leach M, Mauze S, Caddle L, Coffman R. Phenotypically distinct subsets of CD4$^+$ T cells induce protection from chronic intestinal inflammation in C.B-17 scid mice. Int Immunol. 1993;5:1461–1471.
32. Powrie F, Leach M, Mauze S, Menon S, Caddle L, Coffman R. Inhibition of Th1 responses prevents inflammatory bowel disease in scid mice reconstituted with CD45RB^{hi} CD4$^+$ T cells. Immunity. 1994;1:553–562.
33. Herfarth H, Mohanty S, Rath H, Tonkonogy S, Sartor R. Interleukin-10 suppresses experimental chronic, granulomatous inflammation induced by bacterial cell wall polymers. Gut. 1996;39: 836–845.
34. van Deventer S, Elson C, Fedorak R. Multiple doses of intravenous interleukin-10 in steroid-refractory Crohn's disease. Gastroenterology. 1997;113:383–389.
35. Fedorak R, Gangl A, Elson C et al. Safety, tolerance and efficacy of multiple doses of subcutaneous interleukin-10 in mild to moderate active Crohn's disease. Gastroenterology. 1998;114:A974.
36. Schreiber S, Fedorak R, Wild G et al. Safety, tolerance of rHuIL-10 treatment in patients with mild/moderate active ulcerative colitis. Gastroenterology. 1998;114:A1080.
37. Schreiber S, Fedorak R, Nielson O et al. A safety and efficacy study of recombinant human interleukin-10 (rHuIL-10) treatment in 329 patients with chronic active Crohn's disease (CACD). Gastroenterology. 1998;114:A1080.
38. de Waal-Malefyt R, Haanen J, Spits H et al. IL-10 and viral IL-10 strongly reduce antigen-specific human T cell proliferation by diminishing the antigen-presenting capacity of monocytes via downregulation of class II MHC expression. J Exp Med. 1991;174:915–924.
39. Schreiber S, Nikolaus S, Hampe J. Activation of nuclear factor κB in inflammatory bowel disease. Gut. 1998;42:477–484.
40. Neurath M, Pettersson S, Meyer zum Büscherfelde K. Local administration of antisense phosphorothioate oligonucleotides to the p65 subunit of NF-κB abrogates experimental colitis in mice. Nature Med. 1996;2:998–1004.
41. Herfarth H, Böcker U, Janardhanam R, Sartor B. Subtherapeutic corticosteroids potentiate the ability of interleukin-10 to prevent chronic inflammation in rats. Gastroenterology. 1998;115:856–865.

30
Interleukin-10 induces apoptosis of activated neutrophils via the nuclear factor kappa-B

T. KÜHBACHER, R. D. LOHMANN and S. SCHREIBER

INTRODUCTION

Mature human neutrophils die rapidly *in vitro* and *in vivo* because they constitutively undergo apoptosis[1–3]. Life span and functional activity can be expanded significantly by immunological activation[2,4]. The aim was to investigate the regulation of neutrophil apoptosis by interleukin-10 (IL-10).

METHODS

The apoptotic DNA fragmentation was measured by diphenylamine reaction, flow cytometry and gel electrophoresis.

RESULTS

LPS stimulation of neutrophils results in an increased concentration of activated nuclear factor kappa-B (NFκ-B) (p65) in the nucleus and reduced apoptosis as previously shown. The contrainflammatory cytokine IL-10 promoted apoptosis in LPS (1 μg/ml)-stimulated human neutrophils in a dose-dependent manner (70% inhibition at 50 U IL-10/ml). There was no significant influence of the cytokine on the spontaneous apoptosis rate of non-activated neutrophils *in vitro* after 24 h incubation. The apoptosis-inducing effect of IL-10 was associated with a decreased level of transcription factor NFκ-B (p65) in the nucleus of stimulated neutrophils and stabilization of NFκ-B inhibitor α (IκBα) in the cytosol (western blot).

Direct inhibitors of NFκ-B activation also induced apoptosis in neutrophils.

CONCLUSIONS

Activation of NFκ-B involving p65 is directly linked to inhibition of spontaneous apoptosis in neutrophils. The antagonizing effect of interleukin 10 versus LPS may be an important principle in the regulation of the neutrophil apoptosis in host defence.

References

1. Svill JS, Henson PM, Haslett C. Phagocytosis of aged human neutrophils by macrophages is mediated by a novel charge-sensitive recognition mechanism. J Clin Invest. 1989;84:1518–1527.
2. Colotta F, Re F, Polentarutti N, Sozzani S, Mantovani A. Modulation of granulocyte survival and programmed cell death by cytokines and bacterial products. Blood. 1992;80:2012–2020.
3. Whyte MKB, Meagher LC, Macdermot J, Haslett C. Impairment of function in aging neutrophils is associated with apoptosis. J Immunol. 1993;150:5124–5134.
4. Weiss SJ. Tissue destruction by neutrophils. N Engl J Med. 1989;320:365–375.

31
Additive and synergistic effects of T$_H$2-cytokines in inflammatory bowel disease: balance of proinflammatory and immunosuppressive mediators

N. LÜGERING, T. KUCHARZIK, R. STOLL, C. SORG and W. DOMSCHKE

MONOCYTE/MACROPHAGE ACTIVATION IN IBD

Macrophages are important in providing the first line of intestinal defence against microorganisms or toxins that break the epithelial barrier, by presenting antigen to sensitized T cells and releasing a variety of cytokines[1-7]. Since mucosal macrophages are probably derived from circulating monocytes, several studies have investigated circulating monocyte function in inflammatory bowel disease[8,9]. There is an increase in monocyte turnover due to increased demand from the inflamed bowel. Circulating monocytes in inflammatory bowel disease (IBD) are activated, as assessed by a variety of functional measures, but the cause is unclear. The binding of phagocytes to blood vessel endothelial cells followed by migration into the diseased bowel is facilitated by interactions between molecules on the leukocyte cell surface and their counterparts on the endothelial cell. The process of homing into areas of disease involves adhesion molecules expressed on both leukocytes and endothelial cells[10,11]. Studies by several groups show that the expression of nearly all adhesion molecules (ELAM-1, ICAM-1, E-, P- and L-selectin as well as different integrins) is highly increased in active IBD[10-12].

Differentiation of monocytes is associated with changes in morphological, biochemical and functional properties[1-7]. Progress in the development of monoclonal antibodies has provided further information by showing the appearance of macrophage subpopulations with a changed phenotype in IBD. Mahida *et al.* identified unique subsets of macrophages in active inflammatory bowel disease, staining with the monoclonal antibodies RFD9 and 3G8[5]. 3G8-positive cells were distributed throughout the inflamed lamina propria while RFD9-positive cells were mainly located at the bases of disrupted crypts and adjacent to and within mucosal fissures. In some cases, there was a complete replacement of crypts by RFD9[+] cells. Though Selby *et al.*[2,3] encountered a distribution of scavenger macrophages in the normal gut similar to that found by Seldenrijk *et al.*[7], they reported decreased numbers of such cells in both Crohn's disease and ulcerative colitis, which contrasts to the findings of Seldenrijk *et al.* An explanation of this discrepancy might be the use of biopsy material, which necessarily only includes analysis of the infiltrate of the superficial mucosal layer. Seldenrijk *et al.* used surgical specimens and, therefore, were able to analyse deeper infiltrates, surrounding the ulcers and fissures[7].

Rugtveit *et al.* found an increased number of RFD7-positive scavenger macrophages with strong acid phosphatase activity but with no reactivity for mAb RFD1 in IBD mucosa[13]. They reported that lamina propria macrophages recruited recently in IBD preferentially express the CD14 molecule and represent the majority of those lamina propria macrophages which are activated. In addition, they observed that many newly recruited macrophages positive for the myelomonocytic L1 antigen accumulate in both Crohn's disease and ulcerative colitis, depending on the histological degree of inflammation[13,14]. L1 is a member of the S100 family, which have been named also MRP8/14 (27E10 antigen). This heterodimer, which is formed by noncovalent association of MRP8 and MRP14 (Figure 1), is expressed on the surface of infiltrating monocytes in acute inflammation, whereas no heterodimer formation occurs in chronic inflammatory lesions or in normal tissues[15–27]. MRP8/14[+] cells are either adherent to the vascular endothelium or constitute the perivascular infiltrate[16]. Interestingly, we found that epithelial cells of the terminal ileum strongly express the heterodimer 27E10 in the acute phase of Crohn's disease (Figure 2), whereas no 27E10 immunoreactivity was found in epithelial cells of the large

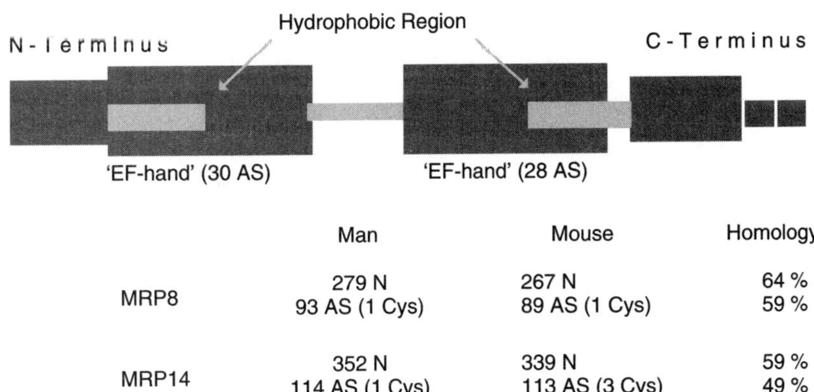

	Man	Mouse	Homology
MRP8	279 N 93 AS (1 Cys)	267 N 89 AS (1 Cys)	64 % 59 %
MRP14	352 N 114 AS (1 Cys)	339 N 113 AS (3 Cys)	59 % 49 %

Figure 1 Molecular structure of the Ca^{2+}-binding proteins MRP8 and MRP14. The sequence of MRP8 cDNA has an open reading frame (ORF) of 279 nucleotides (n), predicting a protein of 93 amino acids (aa). MRP14 cDNA contains an ORF of 352 nucleotides predicting a protein of 114 amino acids. MRP8 and MRP14 both have two Ca^{2+}-binding domains and contain a single cysteine residue, have no signal or membrane-anchor sequences, and lack consensus sequences for N-linked glycosylation

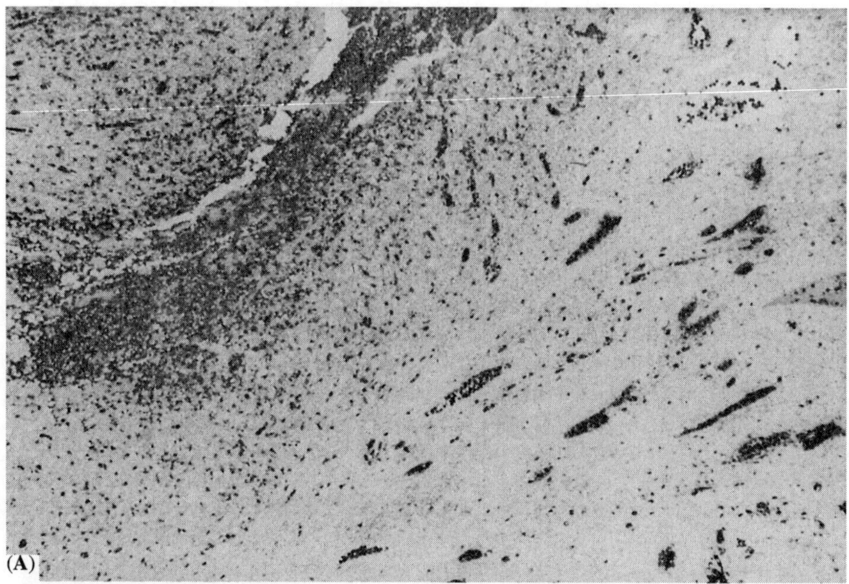

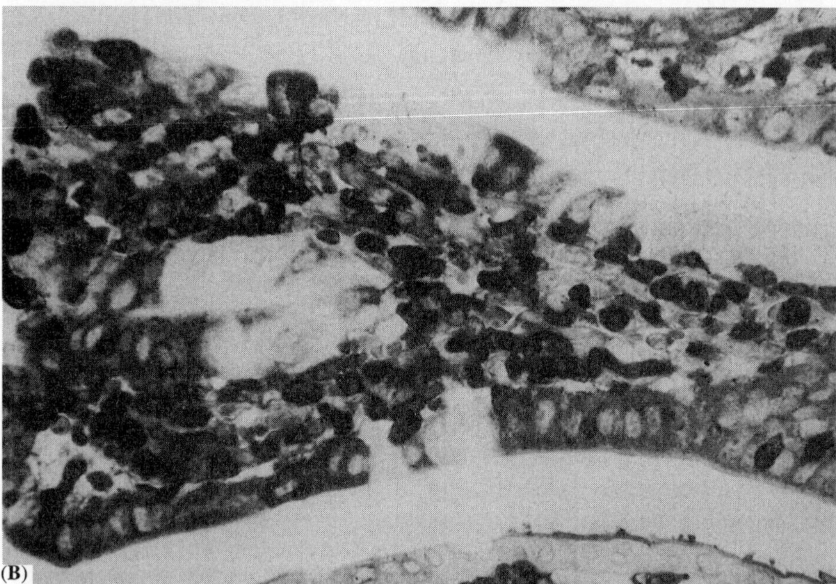

Figure 2 (A) Immunohistochemical staining for the 27E10 antigen (MRP8/14) in fissuring ulceration of the small bowel of a patient with Crohn's disease. (B) MRP8/14 (27E10 antigen) could be immunolocalized in the majority of macrophages, granulocytes and epithelial cells. APAAP technique. ×39

bowel[16]. This probably reflects a different biological behaviour between small and large bowel epithelial cells under inflammatory conditions. Accordingly, epithelial cells may serve as a (second) source responsible for the serum MRP8/14 increase observed in active Crohn's disease. It has been shown recently in an *in vitro* study that keratinocytes produce substantial amounts of MRP8/14[27]. Thus, it seems unlikely that our immunohistochemical demonstration of MRP8 and MRP14 as well as MRP8/14 complexes in small bowel epithelial cells is simply attributable to absorption of these proteins.

The functional role of the Ca^{2+}-binding proteins MRP8 and MRP14 and, in particular, their heterodimer MRP8/14 in patients with IBD is not clear at present. MRP8 and MRP14 represent a major proportion of the total cellular protein content in neutrophils and monocytes[13,15,18,26]. This distribution of MRPs may hint at an innate defence function. It was, therefore, of considerable interest when Steinbakk *et al.* described *in vitro* an antimicrobial action of the MRP8 and MRP14 containing L1-protein complex[22]. On the other hand, recombinant monomers of MRP8 and MRP14 did not exhibit antimicrobial activity at all, indicating that the biological function of these proteins is dependent on the complexed form[15]. According to the high serum levels of the heterodimer MRP8/14 without enhancement of the single monomers MRP8 and MRP14 in patients with active IBD complexes of these proteins rather than their single components may be the carriers of biological functions[17,19]. MRP8/14 (27E10 antigen) has also been claimed to act in an anti-proliferative manner on various tumour cell lines apparently because of inhibition of casein kinase II[23]. This might be of significance in controlling the development of epithelial dysplasia to neoplasia in IBD.

Up-regulation and down-regulation of the inflammatory response in IBD are both controlled by a balance of soluble mediators released by immune cells in the gastrointestinal tract. The identification of subsets of CD4$^+$ helper cells producing a distinct pattern of cytokines has provided a valuable framework for understanding how different effector populations of immune cells can be recruited *in vivo* during inflammation. Indeed, T$_H$1 cells secreting interferon-γ (IFN-γ) are involved in monocyte/ macrophage-mediated inflammatory responses, while T$_H$2-derived cytokines (IL-4, IL-5, IL-10) encourage antibody production (including IgE responses) and promote mast cell and eosinophil proliferation and function. Clinical studies and animal models suggest that human IBD can be characterized as a T$_H$1 or, alternatively, as a T$_H$2 T cell defect[28,29] providing further evidence that alterations of the cytokine balance can improve or worsen IBD. As yet, however, only equivocal or incomplete data on T$_H$1 or T$_H$2 lymphokine production in IBD are available.

PROINFLAMMATORY CYTOKINES

The proinflammatory cytokines IL-1β, tumour necrosis factor-α (TNF-α), IL-6, IL-8 and IL-12 play key roles, as they are produced early during inflammation and induce production of many other cytokines, amplifying their proinflammatory action. In IBD, increased concentrations of TNF-α in serum[30], as well as raised faecal concentrations[31] and increased TNF-α production by peripheral blood mononuclear cells[32], lamina propria mononuclear cells[33,34], and organ cultures of biopsy specimens from inflamed[34] or morphologically normal intestinal mucosa[35] have been reported. Our studies demonstrated increased levels of TNF-α and IL-6 in stimulated monocytes from Crohn's disease (CD) patients and elevated levels of IL-1β in patients with ulcerative colitis (UC)[36]. Isaacs *et al.*[37], using the polymerase chain reaction, showed a stronger mRNA-expression of IL-1β, TNF-α and IL-6 in CD and a subgroup of UC patients than in normal intestinal mucosa. MacDonald *et al.*[38] investigated the secretion of TNF-α in IBD by using a spot ELISA technique. In CD specimens, TNF-α-secreting cells were increased in frequency in comparison with normal controls. TNF-α activates endothelial cells and can induce IL-1. Both IL-1 and TNF-α stimulate PGI_2, PGE_2 and platelet activating factor secretion by cultured endothelial cells. Therefore, sustained acute inflammation leading to tissue destruction in IBD could be in large part due to the potent biological activities of IL-1 and TNF-α. Neutralization of TNF-α by anti-TNF-α antibodies has recently been suggested to be of therapeutic benefit in CD in both open[39,40] and controlled therapeutic trials[41].

Cominelli *et al.*[42,43] found that increased IL-1 concentrations play a key role in the pathogenesis of rabbit immune complex colitis and that tissue levels of IL-1 correlate with the severity of inflammation. IL-1 mRNA was detectable as early as 4 h after induction of colitis, indicating that IL-1 gene expression occurs as a very early event in experimental immune complex colitis[31]. The rise in IL-1 preceded the increase of prostaglandin B_2 (PGE_2) and leukotriene B_4 (LTB_4). Moreover, treatment with IL-1 receptor antagonist (IL-1-ra) dose-dependently inhibited the extent and severity of the inflammatory response associated with immune complex colitis in rabbits[31]. Neutralization of endogenous IL-1-ra by specific neutralizing antibodies against IL-1-ra exacerbated and prolonged inflammation in rabbit immune colitis. Therefore, modulation of the IL-l/IL-1-ra system may be a target for future treatment approaches.

The ability of macrophages to respond to external signals with secretion of lysosomal enzymes may contribute to the initiation and perpetuation of the inflammatory process in IBD[44–48]. In our experiments, the spontaneous secretion of β-hexosaminidase, β-glucuronidase and α-mannosidase was higher in involved than in non-involved IBD mucosa[48]. These data demonstrate a correlation between lysosomal enzyme secretion and the intensity and severity of local mucosal inflammation. Thus, release of these enzymes from tissue macrophages may be an important factor in the pathogenesis of the mucosal inflammation, and several non-specific stimulants may perpetuate tissue damage in this disorder[45–47]. This is especially the case when a large number of monocytes is attracted, immobilized and activated at the site of the lesion[45–48]. As no altered β-galactosidase activities could be observed in either IBD and control monocytes during treatment with LPS, differential response of the individual lysosomal enzymes towards the secretion stimuli is compatible with the existence of alternative targeting pathways being used to different extents, as well as individual regulation of the gene expression[48]. Alternatively, this might reflect functional heterogeneity of monocytes, with selective cells being less active in release of this lysosomal enzyme. Previous observations have suggested that in IBD macrophage activation is associated with increased heterogeneity and the appearance of specialized subpopulations of cells[1-7]. In contrast to published data we found no enhanced activities of β-hexosaminidase (N-acetyl-glucosaminidase) or β-glucuronidase in supernatants of unstimulated IBD monocytes compared with controls[48]. This may be due to the different techniques used for isolation of peripheral blood monocytes[9-11] and to the fact that in previous studies fetal calf serum was used for culturing monocytes[45-47]. As in

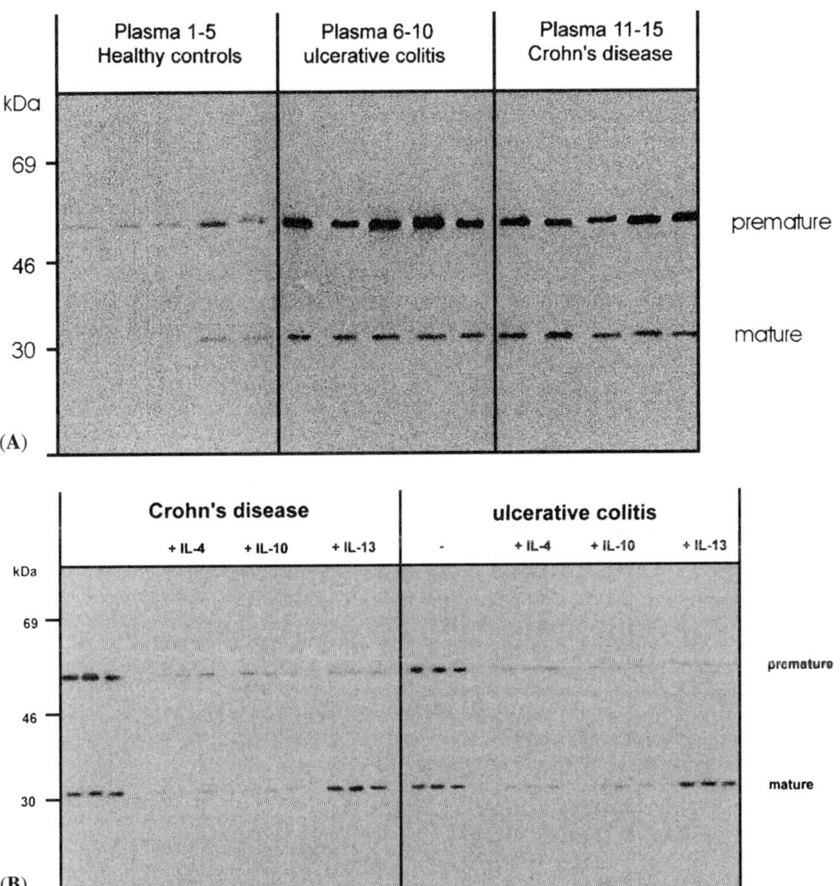

Figure 3 (A) Migration and molecular mass of major cathepsin D polypeptides in plasma of 10 patients (5 with CD and five with UC) representative of 15 patients with highly active CD and 14 patients with active UC. Venous blood samples were obtained by antecubital venipuncture and stored at $-70°C$ until analysed. Cathepsin D was separated by PAGE in the presence of SDS, electroblotted onto nitrocellulose filters and detected immunochemically. (B) Peripheral monocytes (10^6) were isolated from the same patients and cultured in the presence of either IL-13, IL-4 or IL-10 (100 U/ml) under stimulation with lipopolysaccharide. After 48 h the supernatants were harvested, centrifuged, aliquoted and examined for the production of the lysosomal enzyme cathepsin D. LPS-stimulated monocytes from healthy controls ($n \neq 2$) secreted significantly lower amounts of both the premature and mature form of cathepsin D compared with those from patients with active IBD (data not shown)

our experiments fetal calf serum, even in low concentrations, caused a strong enhancement of lysosomal enzyme activities, we used AB serum in our study[48].

Both the precursor and the mature form of the lysosomal enzyme cathepsin D are elevated in plasma and monocytic-conditioned media in patients with UC and CD (Figure 3). We assume that the precursor forms represent a fraction of newly synthesized lysosomal enzymes that escapes segregation to the lysosomes. The origin of the mature form is less clear. Possible explanations include stimuli such as viral endotoxins, antigen–antibody complexes, complement activation products, phagocytosis of organisms, lymphokines from activated lymphocytes and macrophages, as well as induction by toxic metabolites, which rupture lysosomal membranes thus liberating acid hydrolase activity through the cell. Many of these possible 'activating' factors can be presumed, or are known, to occur in patients with IBD[45–47]. This may lead to intracellular digestion and ultimately to cell death[46,47]. Whether this holds true for IBD still has to be established.

Recent studies have shown that the capacity for O_2 anion generation by peripheral monocytes and intestinal macrophages is increased in IBD[49]. The greater proportion of intestinal macrophages from IBD mucosa that are able to undergo a respiratory burst may be either the result of an up-regulation of respiratory burst capacity of the resident population of cells or may reflect an elicited population of macrophages. Rugtveit *et al.* showed that the CD14[+]L1 (MRP8/14)[+] subset was responsible for most of the increased respiratory burst activity of isolated macrophages from inflamed IBD mucosa, and that this activity could not be up-regulated in resident macrophages by IFN-γ and lipopolysaccharide (LPS), in contrast to *in vitro* matured macrophages[13,14]. MRP8/14[+] monocytes spontaneously released substantial amounts of IL-1β and TNF-α in contrast to the 27E10 population[15].

CONTRA-INFLAMMATORY CYTOKINES

Based on the suppressive actions ascribed to T_H2 cytokines in various *in vitro* assays, it has been predicted that they may negatively regulate inflammatory and cell-mediated responses *in vivo*. Previous work by our laboratory and others has demonstrated that there is a complexity of partially different actions of IL-4, IL-10 and IL-13 on human monocytes and macrophages[36,50–55]. *In vitro* experiments have shown that the effects of these cytokines in terms of both activation and deactivation are strongly influenced by the stimulatory agent, cytokine concentrations, time of cytokine addition, the source of monocytes (blood, intestinal mucosa) and the state of differentiation and activation[36]. Given its functional properties, IL-10 in particular might contribute to the specialized state of the intestinal immune system. First, IL-10 is known to suppress T cell proliferation either by acting directly on T lymphocytes or by interfering with T cell–antigen-presenting cell interactions[50,51]. Second, IL-10 down-regulates gene expression and synthesis of inflammatory cytokines/chemokines such as TNF-α, IL-1, IL-6, IL-8, and MIP-1α by activated monocytes and macrophages; decreases surface expression of accessory molecules like CD80, CD86, and CD54 on human antigen-presenting cells (monocytes, macrophages, dendritic cells); and induces antibody production by activated B lymphocytes[52–54]. IL-10 is capable of inducing IL-1-ra secretion in both peripheral monocytes and intestinal lamina propria mononuclear cells (LPMNC) and can restore the decreased IL-1-ra/IL-1β ratio in IBD to normal levels[55]. IL-10 serum levels are increased in IBD patients and significantly correlate with disease activity[56]. Recombinant IL-10 treatment affects mononuclear cell infiltration (lymphocytes and macrophages) to a greater extent than neutrophils[57]. Spontaneous intestinal inflammation occurs in IL-10 deficient (knockout) mice and continuous administration of IL-10 attenuates experimental colitis in a lymphocyte transfer model[58]. IL-10 also down-regulates the proinflammatory cytokine IL-12, which is involved in the pathogenesis of intestinal inflammation, as recently shown by the successful treatment of experimental colitis by IL-12 antibodies[28,58].

Although recent data have shown that IL-4 is decreased in IBD[29], there are also reports of increased IL-4 tissue levels in IBD[37,60]. Schreiber *et al.* presented data showing that IL-4 down-regulates the production of IL-1β and TNF-α as well as of superoxide secretion by peripheral blood monocytes from normal individuals, but not from patients with IBD[59]. They found that in peripheral blood monocytes from IBD patients the dose–response curves for IL-4-induced decreases in IL-1β and TNF-α production were shifted two logs to the right; it took 100 times more IL-4 to induce the same decreases in IL-1β and TNF-α production in IBD monocytes compared with normal monocytes[59]. In contrast, our group did not find an impaired monocyte inhibition of IL-1β by IL-4 (Figure 4). In disease controls (acute pancreatitis, diverticulitis and bacterial pneumonia) we also observed a diminished down-regulation of TNF-α during treatment with IL-13 and IL-4 and, with regard to IL-13, also for the secretion of IL-6 and IL-1β[36]. Impaired immunosuppressive activity by IL-13 and IL-4 does not, therefore, seem to be a disease-specific phenomenon, as it is also seen in other diseases with acute monocyte activation.

Many of the effects of IL-13 on cell surface phenotype, morphology, function, and cytokine production are shared with IL-4[61,62]. The amino acid sequence of IL-4 has 20–25% identity with that of IL-13, and IL-13 and IL-4 share a common receptor component that is involved in signal transduction. However, because the activities of IL-13 could not be blocked by a neutralizing anti-IL-4 mAb, and human monocytes activated with phytohaemagglutinin (PHA) and certain cloned cell lines derived from human T cells proliferate in response to IL-4, but not to IL-13, it is also true that IL-13 acts independently of IL-4[61,62]. Our studies on lysosomal enzyme protein levels by Western blot analysis revealed that, while IL-13 down-regulates the LPS-induced cathepsin D synthesis mainly by reducing the induction of the precursor form, IL-4 and IL-10 affect both the precursor and mature form of this lysosomal enzyme (Figure 3). The implication of this phenomenon in the activation of IBD monocytes is presently unknown. Whether this observation is, at least in part, responsible for the diminished monocyte response to IL-13 in IBD[36], has yet to be established. We did not observe any hyporesponsiveness of monocytes from patients with active IBD when we used a combination of IL-10/IL-4 or IL-10/IL-13[48].

Although we found a significant suppression of α-mannosidase secretion by IL-13 in IBD patients, much higher cytokine concentrations were necessary to yield the same inhibition as for β-hexosaminidase and β-glucuronidase (Figure

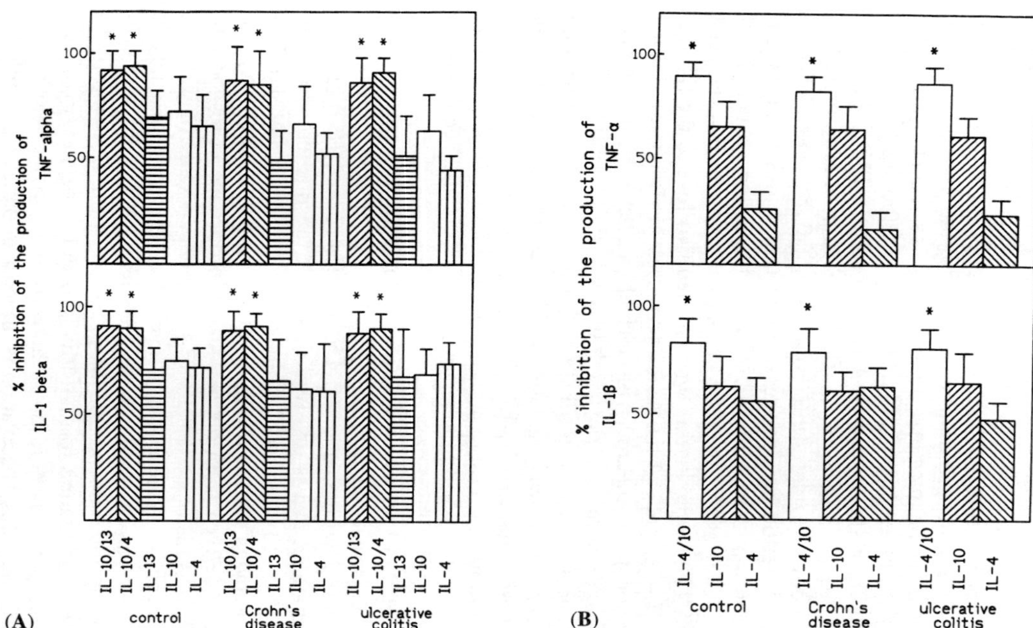

Figure 4 **(A)** Combination treatment of peripheral monocytes with immunoregulatory cytokines in patients with IBD. Peripheral monocytes from 18 patients with active CD, 16 patients with active UC and 13 controls were tested with a combination of IL-10/IL-13 and IL-10/IL-4 (100 U/ml of each cytokine) and with IL-4, IL-10 and IL-13 alone (200 U/ml of each cytokine). Results are expressed as percentage inhibition compared with controls receiving no immunosuppressive cytokine (means ± SD). In all groups, there is a significantly higher down-regulation of TNF-α and IL-1β when using a cytokine combination than when using the immunosuppressive cytokines alone. **(B)** Inhibitory effects of a combination of immunoregulatory cytokines on the production of TNF-α and IL-1β by differenti-ated macrophages in IBD patients. 7-day cultured monocytes (treated with 10 ng/ml GM-CSF) from 9 patients with ulcerative colitis, 10 patients with Crohn's disease and 8 controls were incubated with a combination of IL-4/IL-10 and with IL-4 and IL-10 alone. Results are presented as percentage inhibition compared with controls receiving no immunosuppressive cytokine. Comparable to peripheral monocytes, the use of a combination of immunoregulatory cytokines in all groups is much more effective in down-regulating. TNF-α ($p < 0.01$) and IL-β ($p < 0.01$) than using the immunosuppressive cytokine alone

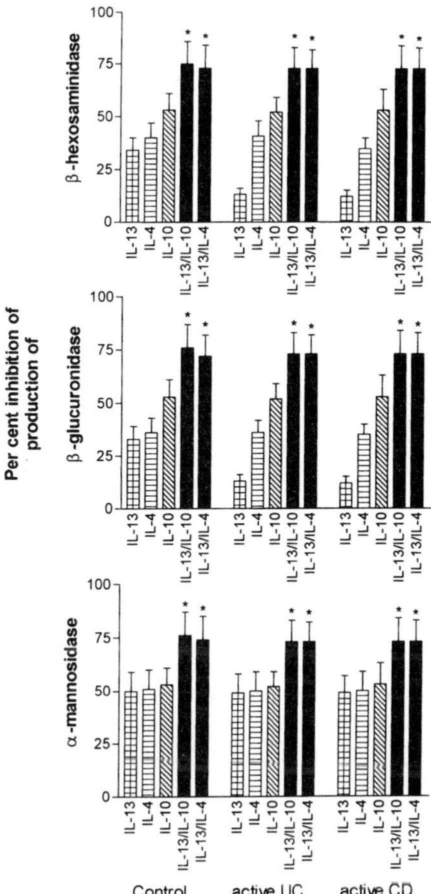

Figure 5 Combination treatment of peripheral monocytes with immunoregulatory cytokines in patients with IBD. Peripheral monocytes from 22 patients with CD, 20 patients with UC and 20 controls were tested with a combination of IL-10/IL-13 and IL-10/IL-4 (50 U/ml of each cytokine) and with IL-4, IL-10 and IL-13 alone (100 U/ml of each cytokine). Results are expressed as percentage inhibition compared with controls receiving no immunosuppressive cytokine (means ± SD). In all groups there is a significantly higher down-regulation of α-mannosidase, β-glucuronidase and β-hexosaminidase when using a cytokine combination than using the immunosuppressive cytokines alone ($p < 0.001$)

5), two lysosomal enzymes which have been shown to play a major part in the inflammatory process in IBD[45–47]. Thus, certain enzymes in UC and CD patients are apparently secreted coordinately after monocyte stimulation *in vitro* but are, in fact, not coordinately regulated by the same cytokines or other factors. These data support classification of lysosomal enzymes into separate regulatory groups sharing a few common pathways[63,64]. We found a poor response to either IL-4 or IL-10 alone for lysosomal enzyme secretion from IBD LPMNC, suggesting that the responses to anti-inflammatory cytokines detected for peripheral blood monocytes are altered by differentiation despite varied levels of monocyte/macrophage activation. On the other hand, combined cytokine treatment with IL-10 and IL-4 or IL-13 strongly suppressed LPS-induced secretion of β-hexosaminidase and α-mannosidase from intestinal IBD LPMNC. It has to be noted that the poor response to anti-inflammatory cytokines observed in the present study is not a general phenomenon but may reflect an intrinsic property of these cells; similar conditions in our test system[36] and that of others[59] resulted in significant down-regulation of production of proinflammatory cytokines. Thus, the regulation of lysosomal enzymes seems to be closely co-ordinated in the macrophage[45–47]. As a class, these products can be readily differentiated from other secretory products, e.g. pro-inflammatory cytokines.

Significant suppression by IL-10, IL-13 and IL-4 was seen only when cytokines were given prior to or simultaneously with the stimulatory agent, i.e. in the early phase of monocyte/macrophage activation. This observation indicates that these anti-inflammatory cytokines do not function as deactivation factors but interfere with some critical early step in the activation cascade of monocytic mediators.

POTENTIAL TARGETS OF PHARMACOLOGICAL INTERVENTION IN IBD

Tissue injury and inflammation in IBD have been shown to be associated with enhanced monocytic release of specific and non-specific inflammatory effector molecules. Therefore, down-regulation of protein secretion would be an important therapeutic strategy for the control of this inflammatory disease. If general immunosuppression of proinflammatory agents is necessary to achieve therapeutic effects, diminished down-regulation of these mediators does not support a therapeutic benefit of immunoregulatory cytokines in IBD patients. With respect to IL-13 and IL-4, the missing down-regulation of IL-6 as well as the reduced suppression of TNF-α in patients with active IBD argues against a therapeutic approach of these mediators in IBD[36]. The sole use of IL-13 in regulating chronic inflammation is also limited by its inability to down-regulate T lymphocyte activity. In addition, recent results of stimulatory effects on the production of TNF-α and IL-12 after 20 h pretreatment with IL-13 and IL-4 suggest an unexpected complexity in the regulatory role of these cytokines in immune responses[62].

Studies by our group and others demonstrate that combined treatment with IL-13, IL-4 and IL-10 will be of great interest as potentially novel therapeutic strategies in inflammatory bowel disease and other chronic diseases[48,65,66]. The effects of these cytokines, if combined at their optimal concentrations, are cumulative for down-regulation of production of proinflammatory cytokines[66], lysosomal enzymes[48] and other monocytic mediators, such as the Ca^{2+}-binding proteins MRP8 and MRP14[65]. In addition, a combination of IL-10 and IL-4 acts synergistically even at suboptimal concentrations (Figures 4, 5), while the immunoregulatory cytokines alone have only little effect[48,66]. Importantly, no impaired monocyte response to IL-4 and IL-13 in patients with active IBD can be observed when using combined treatment. These data speak in favour of potentially useful combined treatment which may improve chances of developing effective treatments for human IBD. Combined treatment with different immunosuppressive cytokines may result in a reduction of cytokine concentrations to be employed and incidence of potential side-effects. Future investigations must focus on cytokine profiles (proinflammatory versus anti-inflammatory; T$_H$1 versus T$_H$2), modulation of bioactivity, synergy with other soluble inflammatory mediators, and regulation of endogenous immunosuppression. Efforts to control the release and activation of proinflammatory cytokines and other potentially destructive proteins in IBD must be based on a clear understanding of their basic biosynthesis. More complete comprehension of these factors should provide clinically relevant means to more effectively diagnose, monitor and treat intestinal inflammation.

References

1. Allison MC, Poulter LW. Changes in phenotypically distinct mucosal macrophage populations may be a prerequisite for the development of inflammatory bowel disease. Clin Exp Immunol. 1991;85:504–509.
2. Selby WS, Janossy G, Mason DY, Jewell DP. Expression of HLA-DR antigens by colonic epithelium in inflammatory bowel disease. Clin Exp Immunol. 1983;53:614–618.
3. Selby WS, Poulter LW, Hobbs S, Jewell DP, Janossy G. Heterogeneity of HLA-DR-positive histiocytes in human intestinal lamina propria: a combined histochemical and immunohistological analysis. J Clin Pathol. 1983;36:379–384.
4. Hume DA, Allan W, Hogan PG, Doe WE. Immunohistochemical characterization of macrophages in human liver and gastrointestinal tract: Expression of CD4, HLA-DR, OKM1, and the mature macrophage marker 25F9 in normal and diseased tissue. J Leukocyte Biol. 1987;42:474–484.
5. Mahida YR, Patel S, Gionchetti P, Vaux D, Jewell DP. Macrophage subpopulations in lamina propria of normal and inflamed colon and terminal ileum Gut. 1989;30:826–834.
6. Choy MY, Walker-Smith JA, Williams CB, MacDonald TT. Differential expression of CD25 (interleukin-2 receptor) on lamina propria T cells and macrophages in the intestinal lesions in Crohn's disease and ulcerative colitis. Gut. 1990:31:1365–1370.
7. Seldemirijk CA, Drexhage HA, Meuwissen SCM, Pals ST, Meijer CJ. Dendritic cells and scavenger macrophages in chronic inflammatory bowel disease. Gut. 1989;30:484–491.
8. Saverymuttu SH, Peters AM, Lavender JP, Pepys MB, Hodgson NJ, Chadwick VS. Quantitative fecal indium 111-labeled leucocyte excretion in the assessment of disease activity in Crohn's disease. Gastroenterology. 1983;85:1333–1339.
9. Saverymuttu SH, Peters AM, Lavender JP, Chadwick VS, Lavender JP. In vivo assessment of granulocyte migration to diseased bowel in Crohn's disease. Gut. 1985;26:378–383.
10. Lügering N, Stoll R, Holzgreve A, Winde G, Sorg C, Domschke W. Monoclonal antibody 1F10 immunoreactivity in inflammatory bowel disease: a new marker specific only for continuous endothelial cells. Eur J Gastroenterol Hepatol. 1995;7:777–781.
11. Malizia G, Calabrese A, Cottone M et al. Expression of leukocyte adhesion molecules by mucosal mononuclear phagocytes in inflammatory bowel disease. Gastroenterology. 1991;100:150–159.
12. Koizumi M, King N, Lobb R, Benjamin C, Podolsky DK. Expression of vascular adhesion molecules in inflammatory bowel disease. Gastroenterology. 1992;103:840–847.
13. Rugtveit J, Brandtzaeg P, Halstensen T, Fausa O, Scott H. Increased macrophage subset in inflammatory bowel disease: apparent recruitment from peripheral blood monocytes. Gut. 1994;35:669–674.
14. Rugtveit J, Haraldsen G, Hogasen AK, Bakka A, Brandtzaeg P, Scott H. Respiratory burst of intestinal macrophages in inflammatory bowel disease is mainly caused by CD14$^+$L1$^+$ monocyte derived cells. Gut. 1995;37:367–373.
15. Bhardwaj RS, Zotz C, Zwadlo-Klarwasser C et al. The calcium-binding proteins MRP8 and MRP14 form a membrane associated heterodimer in a subset of monocytes/macrophages present in acute but absent in chronic inflammatory lesions. Eur J Immunol. 1992;22:1891–1897.

16. Schmid KW, Lügering N, Stoll R et al. Immunohistochemical demonstration or the calcium-binding proteins MRP8 and MRP14 and their heterodimer (27E10 antigen) in Crohn's disease. Hum Pathol. 1995;26:334–337.

17. Lügering N, Stoll R, Schmid KW et al. The myeloic related protein MRP8/14 (27E 10 antigen) – usefulness as a potential marker for disease activity in ulcerative colitis and putative biological function. Eur J Clin Invest. 1995;25:659–664.

18. Odink K, Cerletti N, Brüggen J et al. Two calcium-binding proteins in infiltrating macrophages of rheumatoid arthritis. Nature. 1987;330:80–82.

19. Lügering N, Stoll R, Kucharzik T et al. Immunohistochemical distribution and serum levels of the Ca^{2+}-binding proteins MRP8, MRP14 and their heterodimeric form MRP8/14 in Crohn's disease. Digestion. 1995;56:406–414.

20. Roth J, Burwinkel F, van dean Bos C, Goebeler M, Vollmer E, Sorg C. MRP8 and MRP14, S-100-like proteins associated with myeloid differentiation, are translocated to plasma membrane and intermediate filaments in a calcium-dependent manner. Blood. 1993;82:1875–1883.

21. Roth J, Goebeler M, Wrocklage V, van den Bos C, Sorg C. Expression of the calcium-binding proteins MRP8 and MRP14 in monocytes is regulated by a calcium-induced suppressor mechanism. Biochem J. 1994;301:655–660.

22. Steinbakk M, Naess-Andersen CE, Lingaas E, Dale I, Brandtzaeg P, Fagerhol MK. Antimicrobial actions of calcium binding leukocyte L1 protein, calprotectin. Lancet. 1990:336: 763–765.

23. Murao S, Collart FR, Huberman E. A protein containing the cystic fibrosis antigen is an inhibitor of protein kinases. J Biol Chem. 1989;264:8356–8360.

24. Zwadlo G, Sehlegel R, Sorg C. A monoclonal antibody to a subset of human monocytes found only in the peripheral blood and inflammatory tissues. J Immunol. 1986;137:512–518.

25. Zwadlo G, Brüggen J, Gerhards G, Schlegel R, Sorg C. Two calcium-binding proteins associated with specific stages of myeloid cell differentiation are expressed by subsets of macrophages in inflammatory tissues. Clin Exp Immunol. 1988;72:510–515.

26. Roth J, Teigelkamp St, Wilke M, Grün L, Tümmler B, Sorg C. Complex pattern of the myelomonocytic differentiation antigens MRP8 and MRP14 during chronic airway inflammation. Immunobiology. 1992;186:304–314.

27. Goebeler M, Roth J, van den Bos C, Ader G, Sorg C. Increase of calcium levels in epithelial cells induces translocation of calcium-binding proteins migration inhibitory factor-related protein 8 (MRP8) and MRP14 to keratin intermediate filaments. Biochem J. 1995;309:419–424.

28. Fuss IJ, Neurath M, Boirivant M et al. Disparate CD4+ lamina propria (LP) lymphokine secretion profiles in inflammatory bowel disease. J Immunol. 1996;157:1261–1270.

29. Sartor RB. Cytokines in intestinal inflammation: pathophysiological and clinical considerations. Gastroenterology. 1994;106:533–539.

30. Reimund JM, Duclos B, Sapin R, Derlon A, Chamourard P, Baumann R. Systemic tumour necrosis factor in Crohn's disease: relationship to disease activity and circulating acute phase reactants. Eur J Gastroenterol Hepatol. 1992;4:919–923.

31. Braegger CP, Nicholls S, Murch SH, Stephens S, MacDonald TT. Tumour necrosis factor alpha in stool as a marker of intestinal inflammation. Lancet. 1992;339:89–91.

32. Mazlam MZ, Hodgson HJF. Peripheral blood monocyte cytokine production and acute phase response in inflammatory bowel. disease. Gut. 1992;33:773–778.

33. Reinecker HC, Steffen M, Witthoeft T et al. Enhanced secretion of tumor necrosis factor-alpha, IL-6, and IL-1 beta by isolated lamina propria mononuclear cells from patients with ulcerative colitis and Crohn's disease. Clin Exp Immunol. 1993;94:174–181.

34. Reimund JM, Wittersheim C, Dumont S et al. Mucosal inflammatory cytokine production by intestinal biopsies in patients with ulcerative colitis and Crohn's disease. J Clin Immunol. 1996;16:144–150.

35. Reimund JM, Wittersheim C, Dumont S et al. Increased production of tumour necrosis factor-α, interleukin-β, and interleukin-6 by morphologically normal intestinal biopsies from patients with Crohn's disease. Gut. 1996;39:684–689.

36. Kucharzik T, Lügering N, Weigelt H, Adolf M, Domschke W, Stoll R. Immunoregulatory properties of interleukin-13 in patients with inflammatory bowel disease. Comparison with interleukin-4 and interleukin-10. Clin Exp Immunol. 1996;104:483–490.

37. Isaacs KL, Sartor RB, Haeskil JS. Cytokine messenger RNA profiles in inflammatory bowel disease mucosa detected by polymerase chain reaction amplification. Gastroenterology. 1992;103:1587–1595.

38. MacDonald TT, Hutchings P, Choy MY et al. Tumour-necrosis factor-alpha and interferon-gamma production measured at the single-cell level in normal and inflamed human intestine. Clin Exp Immunol. 1990;81:301–305.
39. Derkx B, Taminiau J, Radema S et al. Tumour-necrosis-factor antibody treatment in Crohn's disease. Lancet. 1993;342:173–174.
40. Van Dullemen HM, van Deventer SJH, Hommes DW et al. Treatment of Crohn's disease with anti-tumor necrosis factor chimeric monoclonal antibody (cA2). Gastroenterology. 1995;109:129–135.
41. Targan S, Rutgeerts P, Hanauer SB et al. A multicenter trial of anti-tumor necrosis factor (TNF) antibody (cA2) for treatment of patients with active Crohn's disease. Gastroenterology. 1996;110:A1026.
42. Cominelli F, Dinarello CA. Interleukin-1 in the pathogenesis of and protection from inflammatory bowel disease. Biotherapy. 1989;1:369–375.
43. Cominelli F, Nast CC, Clark BD et al. Interleukin-1 (IL-1) gene expression, synthesis and effect of specific IL-1 receptor blockade in rabbit immune complex colitis. J Clin Invest. 1990;86:972–980.
44. Mahida YR, Wu K, Jewell DP. Respiratory burst activity of intestinal macrophages in normal and inflammatory bowel diseases. Gut. 1989;30:1362–1370.
45. Ganguly NK, Kingham JGC, Lloyd B et al. Acid hydrolases in monocytes from patients with inflammatory bowel disease, chronic liver disease and rheumatoid arthritis. Lancet. 1978;i:1073–1075.
46. Mee AS, Szawatakowski M, Jewell DP. Monocytes in inflammatory bowel disease: phagocytosis and intracellular killing. J Clin Pathol. 1980;33:921–925.
47. Mee AS, Jewell DP. Monocytes in inflammatory bowel disease: monocyte and serum lysosomal enzyme activity. Clin Sci. 1980;58:295–300.
48. Lügering N, Kucharzik T, Stein H et al. IL-10 synergizes with IL-4 and IL-13 in inhibiting lysosomal enzyme secretion by human monocytes and lamina propria mononuclear cells from patients with inflammatory bowel disease. Dig Dis Sci. 1998;43:706–714.
49. Baldassano RN, Schreiber S, Johnston RB, Muraki T, McDermott RP. Monocytes of patients with Crohn's disease are primed for accentuated release of toxic oxygen metabolites: possible role for endotoxin. Gastroenterology. 1993;105:60–66.
50. Fiorentino DE, Zlotnik A, Vieira P et al. IL-10 acts on the antigen presenting cells to inhibit cytokine production by Th1 cells. J Immunol. 1991;146:3444–3451.
51. Ding L, Shevach EM. IL-10 inhibits mitogen-induced T cell proliferation by selectively inhibiting macrophage costimulatory function. J Immunol. 1992;148:3133–3139.
52. Casatella MA, Meda L, Gasperini S, Calzetti F, Bonora S. Interleukin-10 (IL-10) upregulates IL-1 receptor antagonist production from lipopolysaccharide-stimulated human polymorphonuclear leukocytes by delaying mRNA degradation. J Exp Med. 1994;179:1695–1699.
53. Hart PH, Jones CA, Finlay-Jones JJ. Monocytes cultured in cytokine-defined environments differ from freshly isolated monocytes in their responses to IL-4 and IL-10. J Leukocyte Biol. 1995;57:909–918.
54. Buelens C, Willems F, Delvaux A et al. Interleukin-10 differentially regulates B7-1 (CD80) and B7-2 (CD86) expression on human peripheral blood dendritic cells. Eur J Immunol. 1995;25:2688–2672.
55. Schreiber S, Heinig T, Thiele HG, Raedler A. Immunoregulatory role of interleukin 10 in patients with inflammatory bowel disease. Gastroenterology. 1995;108:1434–1444.
56. Kucharzik T, Stoll R, Lügering N, Domschke W. Circulating antiinflammatory cytokine IL-10 in patients with inflammatory bowel disease (IBD). Clin Exp Immunol. 1995;100:452–456.
57. Herfarth HH, Mohanty SP, Rath HC, Tonkonogy S, Sartor RB. Interleukin-10 suppresses experimental chronic, granulomatous inflammation induced by bacterial cell wall polymers. Gut. 1996;39:836–845.
58. Kühn R, Löhler J, Rennick D, Rajewsky K, Müller W. Interleukin-10-deficient mice develop chronic enterocolitis. Cell. 1993;75:263–274.
59. Schreiber S, Heinig T, Panzer U et al. Impaired response of activated mononuclear phagocytes to interleukin-14 in inflammatory bowel disease. Gastroenterology. 1995;108:21–33.
60. West GA, Matsuura T, Levine AD, Klein JS, Fiocchi C. Interleukin-4 in inflammatory bowel disease and mucosal immune reactivity. Gastroenterology. 1996;110:1683–1695.
61. de Waal, Malefyt R, Figdor CG et al. Effects of IL-13 on phenotype, cytokine production, and cytotoxic function of human monocytes. Comparison with IL-4 and modulation with IFN-γ or IL-10. J Immunol. 1993;151:6370–6381.

62. Andrea A, Ma X, Aste-Amezaga M, Paganin C, Trinchieri G. Stimulatory and inhibitory effects of interleukin (IL)-4 and IL-13 on the production of cytokines by human peripheral blood mononuclear cells: priming for IL-12 and tumor necrosis factor-α production. J Exp Med. 1995;181:537–546.
63. Kornfeld S. Trafficking of lysosomal enzymes in normal and disease states. J Clin Invest. 1986;77:1–6.
64. Hasilik A, Neufeld EF. Biosynthesis of lysosomal enzymes in fibroblasts. Synthesis as precursors of higher molecular weight. J Biol Chem. 1980;255:4937–4945.
65. Lügering N, Kucharzik T, Lügering A, Winde G, Sorg C, Domschke W, Stoll R. Importance of combined treatment with IL-10 and IL-4, but not IL-13, for inhibiting monocyte release of the Ca^{2+}-binding protein MRP8/14. Immunology. 1997;91:130–134.
66. Kucharzik T, Lügering N, Adolf M, Domschke W, Stoll R. Synergistic effect of immuno-regulatory cytokines on peripheral blood monocytes from patients with inflammatory bowel disease. Dig Dis Sci. 1997;42:805–812.

32
Insensitivity towards inhibition by cyclosporin A, rapamycin, and tacrolimus in human intestinal lamina propria T lymphocytes

J. BRAUNSTEIN, F. AUTSCHBACH, B. SIDO, G. NEBL, A. SCHRÖDER, Y. SAMSTAG and S. C. MEUER

INTRODUCTION

The mucosal tissue of the intestine contains the vast majority (approximately 70%) of the body's lymphocyte population. Mucosal lymphocytes are constantly exposed to a multitude of exogenous antigens derived from food and microbial organisms. To avoid immunization against such beneficial foreign antigens, the functional behaviour of mucosal immunocompetent cells has to be different from that in other microenvironments, such as the lymph nodes, where exposure to foreign antigens leads to systemic immune responses. Otherwise, antigen encounter in the mucosal microenvironment would induce lymphocyte proliferation and cytokine production with the consequence of severe local inflammation. This may represent one important factor underlying inflammatory bowel diseases in man[1–6] and experimental animals[7,8].

T lymphocytes from the human intestinal lamina propria (LP-T) show a specialized state of differentiation, characterized by the predominant expression of CD45RO[9–11] and the α-E/β-7 integrin on approximately 40% of these cells[10–12]. In addition, when compared to T lymphocytes from peripheral blood (PB-T), LP-T exhibit a markedly reduced responsiveness to T cell receptor (TCR)/CD3 stimulation *in vitro*[13–16] while they are considerably more sensitive to triggering of the CD2 and the CD28 accessory receptors with regard to both proliferation and secretion of particular cytokines, including IL-2, IL-4 and IL-10[14,16–18].

Apart from a slightly reduced cell-surface density of TCR/CD3 complexes[14] the reasons for TCR/CD3 down-regulated signal transduction in LP-T are unclear at present. However, this state of transient local unresponsiveness may be an important factor underlying immune homeostasis at the body's interfaces with its exogenous environment.

LAMINA PROPRIA T LYMPHOCYTES ARE RATHER INSENSITIVE TO IMMUNOSUPPRESSIVE DRUGS

We have investigated the molecular basis of hyper-responsiveness of LP-T to activation through the CD2 receptor. In man, CD2 is restricted in its expression to T lymphocytes and the majority of natural killer-cells[19,20]. We reasoned that the enhanced sensitivity of LP-T to CD2 activation might be explained by the fact that particular steps of the intracellular activation cascades which lead to cellular proliferation and cytokine production could have already been induced *in vivo* in this population, thereby facilitating their responsiveness to subsequent stimulation *in vitro*.

One way to approach this question is to analyse the susceptibility of LP-T to inhibition by immunosuppressive agents capable of blocking intracellular enzymes which are involved in signal transduction from the cell surface towards the nucleus. In this regard, cyclosporin A (CSA) and tacrolimus (FK506), when complexed with their respective binding proteins cyclophilin and FKBP[21–28], inhibit the serine/threonine-phosphatase calcineurin[29,30] which dephosphorylates the transcription factor NFAT[31–37]. In contrast, rapamycin inhibits an as yet unknown Ser/Thr kinase which phosphorylates p70S6 kinase[38–42]. The latter is important for protein translation[41]. Moreover, rapamycin, which also binds to FKBP[32,42], inhibits the ubiquitin dependent proteolytic degradation of Kip1 following growth factor receptor engagement[43,44]. Kip1 negatively controls the G1-S transition step of the cell cycle[45,46].

These inhibitors, which are all derived from microbial antibiotic products[47–49], were used in *in vitro* experiments in which LP-T and PB-T from the same

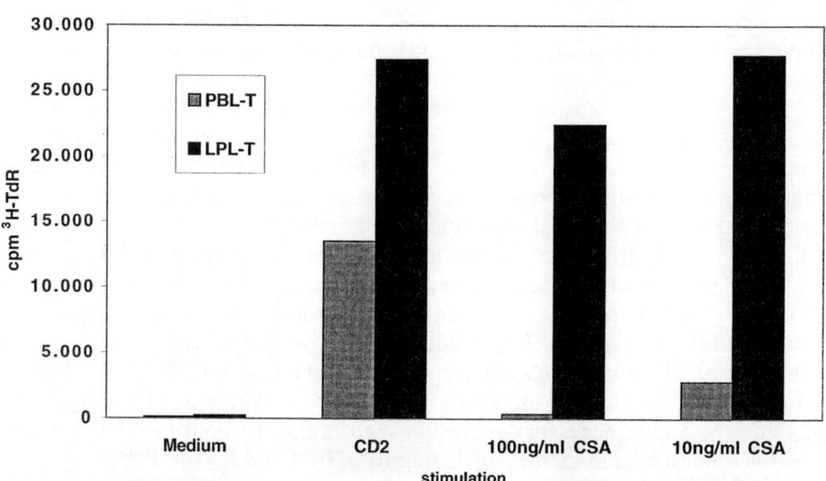

Figure 1   Effect of cyclosporin A (CSA) on LPL-T and PBL-T. PB-T and LP-T were activated by CD2 (monoclonal antibodies T11₂ (1/3000 v/v) and T11₃ (2.5 μg/ml) in the presence of SRBC) in the absence or presence of CSA (100 ng/ml and 10 ng/ml, respectively). Cell growth was measured by incorporation of [³H]thymidine after 4 days. Results are expressed as the mean cpm of triplicate cultures. SD < 20%

individual were tested for their proliferative responses and interleukin 2 (IL-2) production following activation to CD2 by mitogenic combinations of CD2 anti-monoclonal antibodies. As shown in Figure 1, LP-T mount a much stronger proliferative response than PB-T when exposed to a combination of mitogenic CD2 anti-antibodies, termed T11$_2$ and T11$_3$, respectively[19], in the presence of sheep red blood cells. Moreover, while the activation of PB-T is almost completely inhibited by therapeutic concentrations of CSA and FK506 (not shown), LP-T are much more resistant to this immunosuppressant. This is particularly obvious in the case of 10 ng/ml CSA and even visible at 10 times higher concentrations. An almost analogous result is obtained when rapamycin is introduced in such cultures. Thus, while LP-T are highly resistant to rapamycin, PB-T are completely blocked in their proliferative response under identical experimental conditions (Figure 2).

The differential susceptibility to inhibition by immunosuppressive drugs is even more obvious when IL-2 production is investigated following CD2 stimulation. IL-2 secretion by LP-T in response to CD2 activation exceeds the production of IL-2 by PB-T by more than 100-fold (Table 1). At low concentrations of CSA (10 ng/ml), LP-T were virtually resistant to inhibition, while IL-2 production by PB-T was completely abolished. Even at high concentrations of CSA (100 ng/ml) considerable quantities of IL-2 were produced by LP-T; this might explain their capacity to proliferate under such experimental circumstances. Despite its strong effect on lymphocyte proliferation, rapamycin did not, as expected, inhibit IL-2 production since, while it is known to block signal transduction through the IL-2 and other growth factor receptors, it does not affect those pathways which initiate transcription of the IL-2 gene[32,50–52].

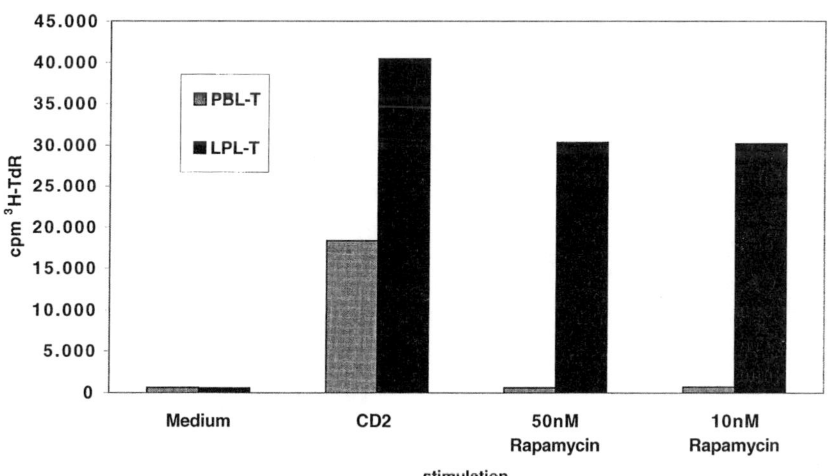

Figure 2 Effect of rapamycin on LPL-T and PBL-T. PB-T and LP-T were activated by CD2 (monoclonal antibodies T11$_2$ (1/3000 v/v) and T11$_3$ (2.5 μg/ml) in the presence of SRBC) in the absence or presence of rapamycin (50 nM and 10 nM, respectively). Cell growth was measured by incorporation of [³H]thymidine after 4 days. Results are expressed as the mean cpm of triplicate cultures. SD < 20%

Table 1 CSA blocks IL-2 production while rapamycin does not

	PBL-T	LPL-T
Stimulation		*IL-2 (pg/ml)[a]*
Medium	<min	<min
CD2	64	9450
CD2 + CSA (100 ng/ml)	<min	269
CD2 + CSA (10 ng/ml)	<min	8918
CD2	40	9831
CD2 + Rapa (50 nM)	26	7098
CD2 + Rapa (10 nM)	41	7247

PB-T and LP-T were activated by CD2 (monoclonal antibodies T11$_2$ (1/3000 v/v) and T11$_3$ (2.5 μg/ml) in the presence of SRBC) in the absence or presence of cyclosporin A (CSA; 100 ng/ml and 10 ng/ml, respectively) and rapamycin (Rapa; 50 nM and 10 nM, respectively). Supernatants were harvested after 60 h and the IL-2 content of each was determined by ELISA.
[a] Detection limit 16 pg/ml.

IL-2 REPRESENTS THE MAJOR GROWTH FACTOR FOR LP-T

The resistance of LP-T *in vitro* to inhibition by CSA might result from the action of a cytokine other than IL-2. This is, however, clearly not the case. As shown in Figure 3, addition of BT563, a monoclonal anti-CD25 antibody which blocks the human IL-2 receptor[53], results in a marked, but partial, inhibition of LP-T proliferation in response to CD2 simulation *in vitro*. Given the excessive production of IL-2 under these experimental conditions and the well known high

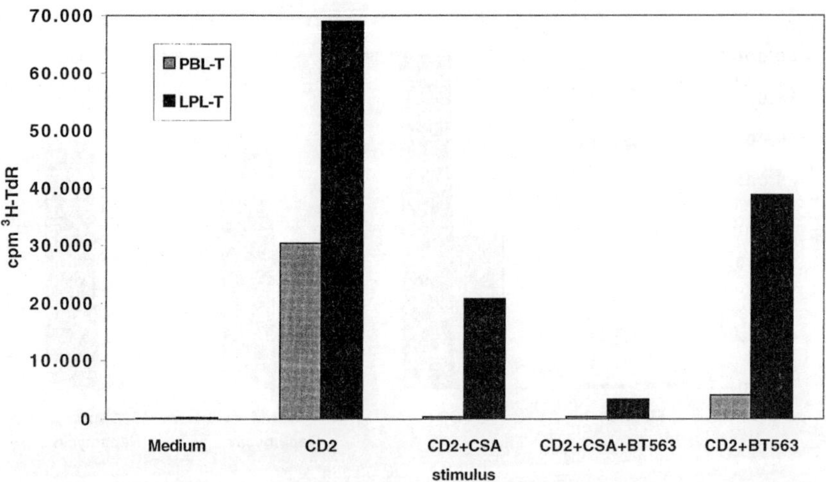

Figure 3 Cyclosporin (CSA) and IL-2R mAb synergize. PB-T and LP-T were activated by CD2 (monoclonal antibodies T11$_2$ (1/3000 v/v) and T11$_3$ (2.5 μg/ml) in the presence of SRBC) in the absence or presence of CSA (100 ng/ml) and IL-2RmAb BT563 (25 μg/ml). Cell growth was measured by incorporation of [^{3}H]thymidine after 4 days. Results are expressed as the mean cpm of triplicate cultures. SD < 20%

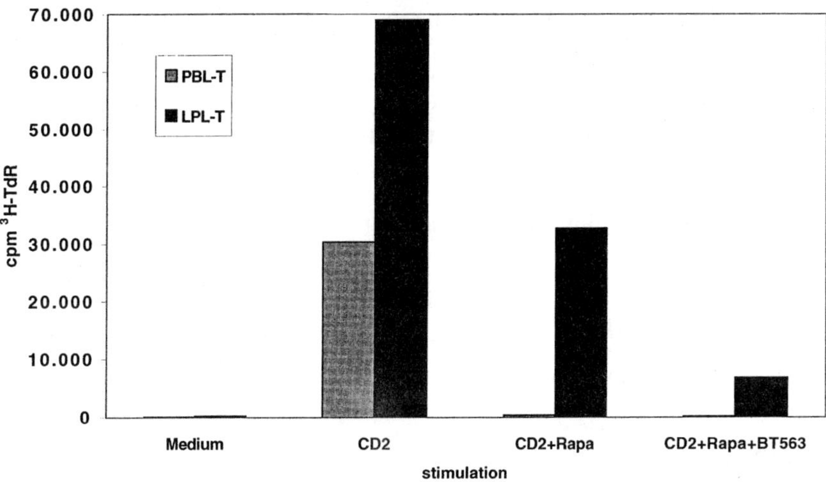

Figure 4 Rapamycin (Rapa) and IL-2R mAb synergize. PB-T and LP-T were activated by CD2 (monoclonal antibodies T11$_2$ (1/3000 v/v) and T11$_3$ (2.5 μg/ml) in the presence of SRBC) in the absence or presence of Rapa (50 nM) and IL-2RmAb BT563 (25 μg/ml). Cell growth was measured by incorporation of [^{3}H]thymidine after 4 days. Results are expressed as the mean cpm of triplicate cultures. SD < 20%

avidity of this cytokine for its receptor one could have not expected complete inhibition of IL-2-dependent proliferation by this antibody. However, when CSA was added at high concentrations (100 ng/ml), conditions under which considerable quantities of IL-2 are still produced (see Table 1), proliferation of LP-T is almost completely blocked. Moreover, BT563 is able to block CD2-induced proliferation of LP-T in the presence of rapamycin (Figure 4). These findings indicate that IL-2 represents the major growth factor promoting cellular proliferation of LP-T *in vitro*.

The relative resistance of LP-T to inhibition by CSA, FK506 and rapamycin is not without precedent. Earlier studies in non-human primates have already indicated such reactivity with CSA[54]. Moreover, CSA has only limited activity when administered to patients with inflammatory bowel disease[55,56]. The present findings may, thus, contribute to a better understanding of these clinical observations.

CONCLUSION

What could be a reason for the resistance of LP-T to inhibitory substances which block intracellular signal transducing processes and are derived from microbial production?

Given the tremendous number of bacterial and fungal organisms which are constitutively present in the gut flora and the potential food-related intake of additional microbial products, one might speculate that it is essential for the mucosal immune system to be resistant to inhibitory activities of antibiotic mediators that are capable of paralysing its reactivity by interfering with crucial intracellular signalling processes required for cellular activation. One would predict that the molecular basis of this resistance of the LP-T population exists in a functional state in which processes that are sensitive to such substances and essential for cell survival are constantly activated beyond a stage at which the local immune system can be negatively influenced. Investigations on the functional state of central transcription and survival factors such as NFAT[57], bcl-2, Bcl_{XL}[58], and cofilin[59] will be required to answer this question.

ACKNOWLEDGEMENTS

We are grateful to Gabriele Sturm for excellent technical assistance.

References

1. Autschbach F, Schürmann G, Qiao L, Merz H, Wallich R, Meuer SC. Cytokine messenger RNA expression and proliferation status of intestinal mononuclear cells in noninflamed gut and Crohn's disease. Virchows Arch. 1995;426:51–60.

2. Reinecker HC, Steffen M, Witthoeft T et al. Enhanced secretion of tumor necrosis factor-alpha, IL-6, and IL-1β by isolated lamina propria mononuclear cells from patients with ulcerative colitis and Crohn's disease. Clin Exp Immunol. 1993;94:174–181.

3. Fais S, Capobianchi MR, Pallone F et al. Spontaneous release of interferon γ by intestinal lamina propria lymphocytes in Crohn's disease. Kinetics of in vitro response to interferon γ inducers. Gut. 1991;32:403–407.

4. Breese E, Braegger CP, Corrigan CJ, Walker-Smith JA, MacDonald TT. Interleukin-2 and interferon-γ-secreting T cells in normal and diseased human intestinal mucosa. Immunology. 1993;78:127–131.

5. Fuss I, Neurath M, Boirivant M, Klein JS, de al Motte C, Strong SA, Fiocchi C, Strober W. Disparate CD4$^+$ lamina propria (LP) lymphokine secretion profiles in inflammatory bowel disease. Crohn's disease LP cells manifest increased secretion of IFN-γ, whereas ulcerative colitis LP cells manifest increased secretion of IL-5. J Immunol. 1996;157:1261–1270.

6. Monteleone G, Baincone L, Marasco R et al. Interleukin 12 is expressed and actively released by Crohn's disease intestinal lamina propria mononuclear cells. Gastroenterology. 1997;112: 1169–1178.

7. Neurath MF, Fuss I, Kelsall BL, Stuber E, Strober W. Antibodies to interleukin 12 abrogate established experimental colitis in mice. J Exp Med. 1995;182:1281–1290.

8. Neurath MF, Fuss I, Pasparakis M et al. Predominant pathogenic role of tumor necrosis factor in experimental colitis in mice. Eur J Immunol. 1997;27:1743–1750.

9. James SP, Fiocchi C, Graeff AS, Strober W. Phenotypic analysis of lamina propria lymphocytes: predominance of helper-inducer and cytolytic T cell phenotypes and deficiency of suppressor-inducer phenotypes in Crohn's disease and control patients. Gastroenterology. 1986;91: 1483–1489.

10. Schieferdecker HL, Ullrich R, Weiss-Breckwoldt AN et al. The HML-1 antigen of intestinal lymphocytes is an activation antigen. J Immunol. 1990;144:2541–2549.

11. Schieferdecker HL, Ullrich R, Hirseland H, Zeitz M. T cell differentiation antigens on lymphocytes in the human intestinal lamina propria. J Immunol. 1992;149:2816–2822.

12. Farstad IN, Halstensen TS, Lien B, Kilshaw PJ, Lazarovitz AI, Brandtzaeg P. Distribution of β7 integrins in human intestinal mucosa and organized gut-associated lymphoid tissue. Immunology. 1996;89:277–327.

13. Pirzer UC, Schürmann G, Post S, Betzler M, Meuer SC. Differential responsiveness to CD3-Ti vs CD2-dependent activation of human intestinal T lymphocytes. Eur J Immunol. 1990;20: 2339–2342.

14. Qiao L, Schürmann G, Betzler M, Meuer SC. Activation and signaling status of human lamina propria T lymphocytes. Gastroenterology. 1991;101:1529–1536.

15. De Maria R, Fais S, Silvestri M, Frati L et al. Continuous in vivo activation and transient hypo-responsiveness to TcR/CD3 triggering of human gut lamina propria lymphocytes. Eur J Immunol. 1993;23:3204–3208.

16. Boirivant M, Fuss I, Fiocchi C, Klein JS, Strong SA, Strober W. Hypoproliferative human lamina propria T cells retain the capacity to secrete lymphokines when stimulated via CD2/CD28 pathways. Proc Assoc Am Phys. 1996;108:55–67.

17. Targan ST, Deem RL, Liu M, Wang S, Nel A. Definition of a lamina propria T cell responsive state. Enhanced cytokine responsiveness of T cells stimulated through the CD2 pathway. J Immunol. 1995;154:664–675.

18. Braunstein J, Qiao L, Autschbach F, Schürmann G, Meuer SC. T cells of the human intestinal lamina propria are high producers of interleukin 10. Gut. 1997;41:215–220.

19. Meuer SC, Hussey R, Fabbi M et al. An alternative pathway of T-cell activation: a functional role for the 50 kd T11 sheep erythrocyte receptor protein. Cell. 1984;36:897–906.

20. Siciliano RF, Pratt JC, Schmidt RE, Ritz J, Reinherz EL. Activation of cytolytic T lymphocyte and natural killer cell function through the T11 sheep erythrocyte binding protein. Nature. 1985;317:428–430.

21. Handschumacher RE, Harding MW, Rice J, Drugge RJ, Speicher DW. Cyclophilin: A specific cytosolic binding protein for cyclosporin A. Science. 1984;226:544–547.

22. Harding MW, Handschumacher RE, Speicher DW. Isolation and amino acid sequence of cyclophilin. J Biol Chem. 1986;261:8547–8555.

23. Takahashi N, Hayano T, Suzuki M. Peptidyl-prolyl *cis-trans* isomerase is the cyclosporin A-binding protein cyclophilin. Nature. 1989;337:473–475.

24. Fischer G, Wittmann-Liebold B, Lang K, Kiefhaber T, Schmid FX. Cyclophilin and peptidyl-prolyl *cis-trans* isomerase are probably identical proteins. Nature. 1989;337:476–478.

25. Harding MW, Galat A, Uehling DE, Schreiber SL. A receptor for the immunosuppressant FK506 is a *cis-trans* peptidyl-prolyl isomerase. Nature. 1989;341:758–760.

26. Siekierka JJ, Hung SHY, Poe M, Lin CS, Sigal NH. A cytosolic binding protein for the immunosuppressant FK506 has peptidyl-prolyl isomerase activity but is distinct from cyclophilin. Nature. 1989;341:755–757.

27. Standaert RF, Galat A, Verdine GL, Schreiber SL. Molecular cloning and overexpression of the human FK506-binding protein FKBP. Nature. 1990;346:671–674.

28. Schreiber S. Chemistry and biology of the immunophilins and their immunosuppressive ligands. Science. 1991;251:283–287.

29. Liu J, Farmer JD, Lane WS, Friedman J, Weissman I, Schreiber SL. Calcineurin is a common target of cyclophilin-cyclosporin A and FKBP-FK506 complexes. Cell. 1991;66:807–815.

30. Fruman DA, Klee CB, Bierer B, Burakoff SJ. Calcineurin phosphatase activity in T lymphocytes is inhibited by FK506 and cyclosporin A. Proc Natl Acad Sci USA. 1992;89:3686–3690.

31. Emmel EA, Verweij CL, Durand DB, Higgins KM, Lacy E, Crabtree GR. Cyclosporin A specifically inhibits function of nuclear proteins involved in T cell activation. Science. 1989;246:1617–1620.

32. Bierer BE, Mattila PS, Standaert RF et al. Two distinct signal transmission pathways in T lymphocytes are inhibited by complexes formed between an immunophilin and either FK506 or rapamycin. Proc Natl Acad Sci USA. 1990;87:9231–9235.

33. Ho S, Clipstone N, Timmermann L et al. The mechanism of action of cyclosporin A and FK506. Clin Immunol Immunopathol. 1996;80:S40–S45.

34. Shaw KTY, Ho AM, Raghavan A et al. Immunosuppressive drugs prevent a rapid dephosphorylation of transcription factor NFAT1 in stimulated cells. Proc Natl Acad Sci USA. 1995;92:11205–11209.

35. Luo C, Shaw KTY, Raghavan A et al. Interaction of calcineurin with a domain of the transcription factor NFAT1 that controls nuclear import. Proc Natl Acad Sci USA. 1996;93:8907–8912.

36. Loh C, Shaw KTY, Carew J et al. Calcineurin binds the transcription factor NFAT1 and reversibly regulates its activity. J Biol Chem. 1996;271:10884–10891.

37. Wesselborg S, Fruman DA, Sagoo JK, Bierer BE, Burakoff SJ. Identification of a physical interaction between calcineurin and nuclear factor of activated T cells (NFATp). J Biol Chem. 1996;271:1274–1277.

38. Dumont FJ, Su Q. Mechanism of action of the immunosuppressant rapamycin. Life Sci. 1996;58:373–395.

39. Price DJ, Grove JR, Calvo V, Avruch J, Bierer BE. Rapamycin-induced inhibition of the 70-kilodalton S6 protein kinase. Science. 1992;257:973–976.

40. Kuo CJ, Chung J, Florentino DF, Flanagan WM, Blenis J, Crabtree GR. Rapamycin selectively inhibits interleukin-2 activation of p70 S6 kinase. Nature. 1992;358:70–73.
41. Jenö P, Ballou LM, Novak-Hofer I, Thomas G. Identification and characterization of a mitogen-activated S6 kinase. Proc Natl Acad Sci USA. 1988;85:406–410.
42. Dumont FJ, Melino MR, Staruch MJ, Koprak SL, Fischer PA, Sigal NH. The immuno-suppressive macrolides FK506 and rapamycin act as reciprocal antagonists in murine T cells. J Immunol. 1990;144:1418–1424.
43. Nourse J, Firpo E, Flanagan W et al. Interleukin-2 mediated elimination of the p27^{Kip1} cyclin-dependent kinase inhibitor prevented by rapamycin. Nature. 1994;372:570–573.
44. Pagano M, Tam SW, Theodoras AM et al. Role of the ubiquitin-proteasome pathway in regulating abundance of the cyclin-dependent kinase inhibitor p27. Science. 1995;269:682–685.
45. Polyak K, Kato JY, Solomon M, Sherr C, Massague J, Roberts JK, Koff A. p27^{Kip1}, a cyclin-cdk inhibitor, links transforming growth factor-β and contact inhibition to cell cycle arrest. Genes Dev. 1995;8:9–22.
46. Toyoshima H, Hunter T. p27, a novel inhibitor of G1 cyclin/cdk protein kinase activity, is related to p21. Cell. 1994;78:67–74.
47. Borel JF, Feurer C, Gubler H, Stahelin H. Biological effects of cyclosporin A: a new anti-lymphocytic agent. Agents Actions. 1976;6:468–475.
48. Kino T, Hatanaka H, Hashimoto M et al. FK506, a novel immunosuppressant isolated from a *Streptomyces*. I. Fermentation, isolation, and physico-chemical and biological characteristics. J Antibiotics. 1987;40:1249–1255.
49. Sehgal SN, Baker H, Vezina C. Rapamycin (AY-22.989), a new antifungal antibiotic. II. Fermentation, isolation and characterization. J Antibiotics. 1995;28:727–732.
50. Dumont FJ, Staruch MJ, Koprak SL, Melino MR, Sigal NH. Distinct mechanisms of suppression of murine T cell activation by the related macrolides FK506 and Rapamycin. J Immunol. 1990;144:251–258.
51. Henderson DJ, Naya I, Bundick RV, Smith GM, Schmidt JA. Comparison of the effects of FK506, cyclosporin A and rapamycin on IL-2 production. Immunology. 1991;73:316–321.
52. Bertagnolli MM, Yang L, Herrmann SH, Kirkman RL. Evidence that rapamycin inhibits interleukin-12-induced proliferation of activated T lymphocytes. Transplantation. 1994;58:1091–1096.
53. Otto G, Thies J, Kraus T et al. Monoclonal anti-CD25 for acute rejection after liver transplantation. Lancet. 1991;338:195.
54. Zeitz M, Quinn TC, Graeff AS, Schwarting R, James SP. Oral administration of Cyclosporin does not prevent expansion of antigen-specific, gut-associated, and spleen lymphocyte populations during *Chlamydia trachomatis* proctitis in nonhuman primates. Dig Dis Sci. 1989;34:585–595.
55. Feagan BG, McDonald JWD, Rochon J et al. Low-dose cyclosporin for the treatment of Crohn's disease. N Engl J Med. 1993;330:1846–1851.
56. Stange EF, Modigliani R, Pena AS, Wood AJ, Feutren G, Smith PR. The European Study Group. European trial of Cyclosporin in chronic active Crohn's disease: a 12-month study. Gastroenterology. 1995;109:774–782.
57. Rao A, Luo C, Hogan P. Transcription factors of the NFAT family: regulation and function. Annu Rev Immunol. 1997;15:707–747.
58. Cory S. Regulation of lymphocyte survival by the bcl-2 gene family. Annu Rev Immunol. 1995;13:513.
59. Samstag Y, Dreizler EM, Ambach A, Sczakiel G, Meuer SC. Inhibition of constitutive serin phosphatase activity in T lymphoma cells results in phosphorylation of pp19/cofilin and induces apoptosis. J Immunol. 1996;156:4167–4173.

33

Cyclosporin A resistant co-stimulatory signalling pathways in human T lymphocytes

Y. SAMSTAG, G. NEBL, A. AMBACH, J. SAUNUS and
S. C. MEUER

INTRODUCTION

Antigen encounter by T lymphocytes occurs in differential microenvironments within the body (lymph nodes, skin, mucosa of the gut or lung etc.). From a molecular viewpoint, the environment comprises a particular combination of ligands with which lymphocytes interact through their numerous specialized cell surface receptors. While the ligand (MHC + antigen-derived peptide) for an individual T cell receptor (TCR), which produces the initial activation signal in a T cell, is probably the same in any given microenvironment, it is the role of a second set of accessory receptor mediated signals to adjust an immune response to respective microenvironmental requirements. Thus, the functional outcome of antigen–MHC encounter by a given lymphocyte is determined by a multi-combinatorial event which is characteristic for the respective *in vivo* site (i.e. the ligand situation where it happens). Such a view suggests a dynamic concept of lymphocyte repertoires which is dictated by the respective microenvironment rather than the exclusive existence of genetically predetermined and fixed functional lymphocyte subsets.

To secure the antigen specificity of immunological reactions, the TCR–CD3 complex must exert control over accessory receptors. Therefore, a hierarchy has to exist for the multitude of receptor-mediated signals which a given lymphocyte can receive. Only following antigen recognition should the accessory receptors acquire functional competence for lymphocyte activation, because they are permanently exposed to endogenous ligands.

From an operational viewpoint one could perhaps distinguish the various receptor types of lymphocytes depending on the roles which their respective signals play for lymphocyte development and activation. These could be termed receptors for recognition (TCR/CD3); growth and survival (CD2, CD4, CD5, CD8, CD28 etc.); amplification (IL-1R, IL-2R, IL-6R, VLA, etc.);

down-regulation (CTLA 4, IL-10R, TGF-βR). Recognition of antigenic peptides bound to major histocompatibility complex molecules on antigen-presenting cells (APC) through the TCR–CD3 complex elicits the competence signal for activation. Full activation requires additional signals (co-stimulation). Such progression signals result from the interaction of accessory receptors (CD2, CD4, CD8 or CD28) with their natural ligands (CD58, MHC II, MHC I or CD80/CD86, respectively). Conversely, engagement of TCR–CD3 in the absence of co-stimulation leads to a state of unresponsiveness/anergy or even apoptosis (programmed cell death)[1–8]. Thus, accessory receptor signals have to differ from those elicited by the TCR–CD3. Accordingly, specialized intracellular costimulatory molecules must exist which transduce signals from accessory receptors to the nucleus.

INTRACELLULAR MEDIATORS OF CO-STIMULATORY SIGNALS

One approach to the identification of intracellular mediators of co-stimulatory second signals is the comparative analysis of *in vivo* phosphorylation events in reponse to TCR/CD3 triggering versus accessory receptor triggering, which can be performed employing monoclonal antibodies directed against the respective receptors. This approach yielded the recent identification of two intracellular phosphoproteins (pp19 and pp67) which are apparently regulated by an accessory signal either produced through triggering of the CD2 receptor complex or, alternatively, through co-crosslinking of CD4, CD8 or CD28 to the TCR–CD3 complex[9–12]. As shown in Figure 1, delivery of a second signal through CD2, CD4, and CD8 leads to *de novo* phosphorylation of a 67 kDa protein (pp67) and concomitant dephosphorylation of a 19 kDa protein (pp19) in human T cells. This is, however, clearly not the case when T cells are triggered through TCR/CD3 alone: despite the production of considerable quantities of interferon-γ (IFN-γ), p67 phosphorylation and pp19 dephosphorylation do not occur[10,11].

The mode of T cell triggering through CD2 *in vitro* can be interpreted as mimicking first and second signals simultaneously. Since analogous functional changes are produced when CD2, CD4, CD8 or CD28 are engaged during lymphocyte activation[10,11] one would propose that these cell surface receptors initiate a common intracellular pathway of T lymphocyte activation.

Based on its molecular weight, mobility upon isoelectric focusing and reactivity with specific antisera, p67 has been identified as the cytoplasmic protein L-plastin/fimbrin[11]. Interestingly, fimbrin represents an actin-binding protein which, in addition, expresses calmodulin binding motifs and calcium binding sites[13,14] suggesting functions influencing the conformation of cytoskeletal components as well as signal transducing properties. These activities are probably regulated through transient protein phosphorylation by accessory receptor-dependent second signals.

Slightly more information is available on pp19. Following its purification from preparative 2D-gels and microsequencing we found that this cytoplasmic molecule, which is constitutively phosphorylated on serine residues in human T cells, exhibits complete homology with a recently cloned small actin-binding protein from human placenta, named cofilin[15]. Pp19/cofilin dephosphorylation

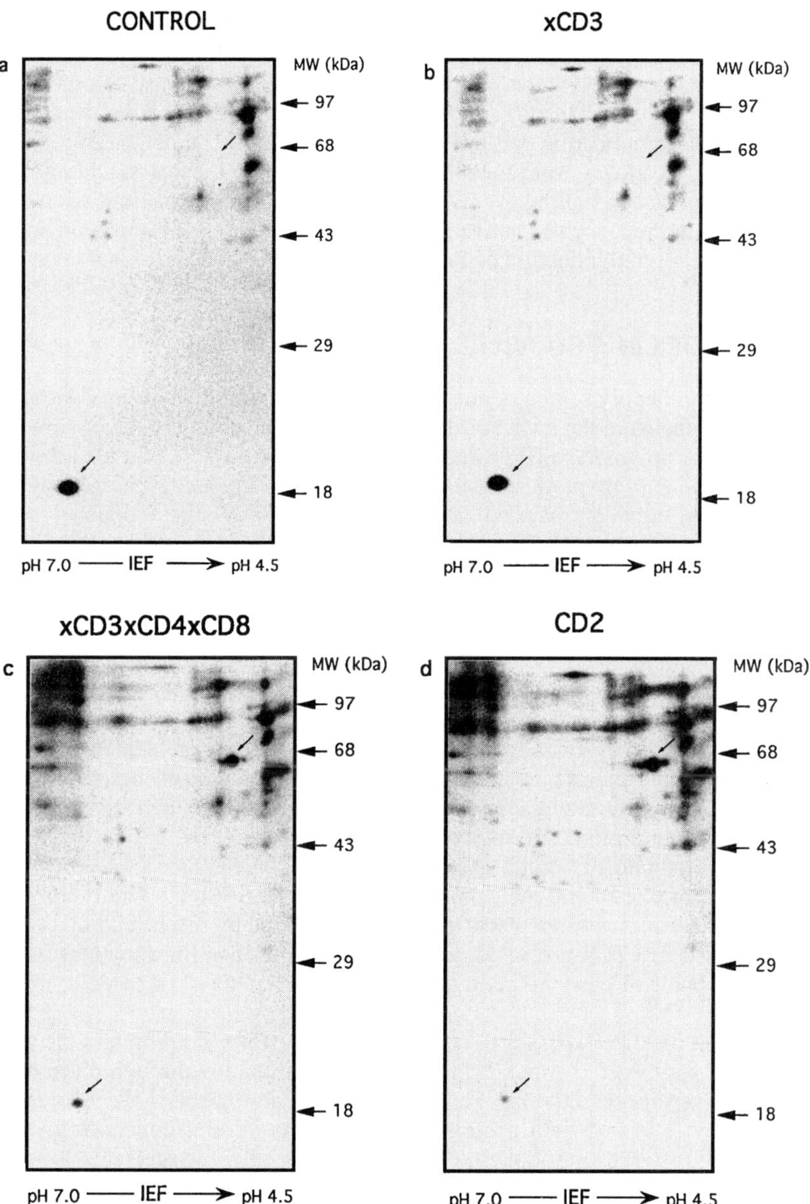

Figure 1 Peripheral human T lymphocytes were labelled with ^{32}P-orthophosphate. Subsequently, cells were exposed to monoclonal antibodies (b–d) or medium (a). Cells were lysed and postnuclear lysates subjected to isoelectric focusing followed by SDS-polyacrylamide gel electrophoresis. Stimulation through the accessory receptor CD2 (d) or co-stimulation through CD3/CD4/CD8 (c) led to phosphorylation of the 67 kDa protein L-plastin/fimbrin (small arrows) and dephosphorylation of the 19 kDa protein pp19/cofilin (large arrows). In contrast, triggering through TCR/CD3 alone did not induce these signalling events (b)

occurs on serine residues by a type 1 (PP1) or 2A (PP2A) serine phosphatase[9,16]. Importantly, this event is not susceptible to inhibition by the immunosuppressive drug cyclosporin A (CsA), an inhibitor of the serine phosphatase calcineurin[16]. Pp19/cofilin dephosphorylation is followed by its translocation from the cytosol into the nucleus, indicating that pp19/cofilin represents a component of a particular signalling pathway from the cytoplasm to the T cell nuclear machinery[15,17]. Other intracellular signalling events which are dependent on co-stimulation have also been identified, such as activation of JNK[18], PI3-kinase[19,20] and acid sphingomyelinase[21,22] and induction of Bcl-x$_L$ expression[7,8].

IS PP19/COFILIN A SURVIVAL FACTOR?

pp19/cofilin probably serves as an actin-transporter into the nucleus. Functional effects resulting from the nuclear import of cofilin/actin complexes may be activation of RNA polymerase II[23,24] and inhibition of DNase I[25], i.e. transcriptional activation and anti-apoptotic activity[26]. That pp19/cofilin dephosphorylation is a constitutively ongoing process in malignant T lymphoma cells[27] supports such a notion. Thus, an enhanced quantity of cofilin/actin complexes within nuclei could contribute to the autonomous proliferation and prolonged lifespan of transformed cells. In line with this view, blockade of pp19/cofilin dephosphorylation by okadaic acid, which results in a reduction of the nuclear cofilin/actin content, was found to be accompanied by apoptosis. Moreover, down-regulation of pp19/cofilin translation by expression of antisense-cofilin RNA *in vivo* leads to a markedly reduced tumour cell growth[27]. Importantly, recent data obtained in experimental yeast systems[28,29] as well as in *Xenopus laevis*[30] demonstrate that pp19/cofilin represents an essential protein for cell proliferation and survival.

Co-stimulation through CD28 has been demonstrated to enhance *in vitro* survival of peripheral blood T lymphocytes[7,8]. In this regard, inhibition of DNase I by nuclear actin/cofilin complexes, preventing DNA damage (see above)[25,26] may represent one of the mechanisms underlying this effect. The notion that nuclear actin exerts anti-apoptotic activity is supported by recent findings which demonstrated that ICE-proteases, which are key enzymes for apoptosis induction, are capable of cleaving actin into a form which is no longer able to inhibit DNase I[31,32].

Intriguing parallels exist between the regulation of pp19/cofilin and the well-established survival factor bcl-2: in both cases, inactivation through phosphorylation on serine residues is accompanied by apoptosis[27,33,34]. Moreover, dephosphorylation of both proteins is blocked by similar concentrations of okadaic acid, suggesting that they represent substrates for the same types of serine phosphatases. Finally, in transformed cells (e.g. Jurkat) both factors exist to a substantial degree in their unphosphorylated forms which may result from constitutive activation of PP1 and PP2A which are sensitive to inhibition by okadic acid.

Whether a functional relationship exists between dephosphorylation and nuclear translocation of pp19/cofilin and expression of Bcl-x$_L$, another potent anti-apoptotic protein which is regulated by co-stimulation[7,8], or whether these pp19/cofilin alterations by PP1 and/or PP2A belong to Bcl-x$_L$ independent anti-apoptotic pathways[35] remains to be determined. Note, however, that unlike dephosphorylation of pp19/cofilin, which is common for CD2 and CD28 signalling, induction of Bcl-x$_L$ expression is only observed in response to CD28 but not following CD2 co-stimulation[7]. Moreover, in untreated Jurkat lymphoma cells, which do not express Bcl-x$_L$[7], dephosphorylation and nuclear translocation of pp19/cofilin occur spontaneously[27]. Therefore, it seems more likely that dephosphorylation of pp19/cofilin by PP1 and/or PP2A represents a Bcl-x$_L$ independent survival mechanism.

PP1 AND/OR PP2A REGULATE BOTH COFILIN DEPHOSPHORYLATION AND IL-2 GENE TRANSCRIPTION

Dephosphorylation of pp19/cofilin as a consequence of co-stimulation correlates with the induction of IL-2 secretion and T cell proliferation[9–11]. Interestingly, we found that okadaic acid-sensitive serine/threonine phosphatases are not only responsible for pp19/cofilin dephosphorylation. Their activities are also required for the induction of transcription of the IL-2 gene: the serine/threonine phosphatase inhibitor okadaic acid specifically inhibited the expression of IL-2 mRNA following CD2 stimulation. Nuclear run-on experiments demonstrated that the prevention of IL-2 expression through okadaic acid occurred at the transcriptional level (Figure 2). However, okadaic acid treatment caused no general inhibition of transcription since other genes, such as β-actin, were still transcribed. Moreover, transcription of the c-*fos* and c-*jun* genes was enhanced under the same experimental conditions. Therefore, neither RNA polymerase II nor the basic transcriptional machinery is affected directly by inhibition of these serine/threonine phosphatases[36].

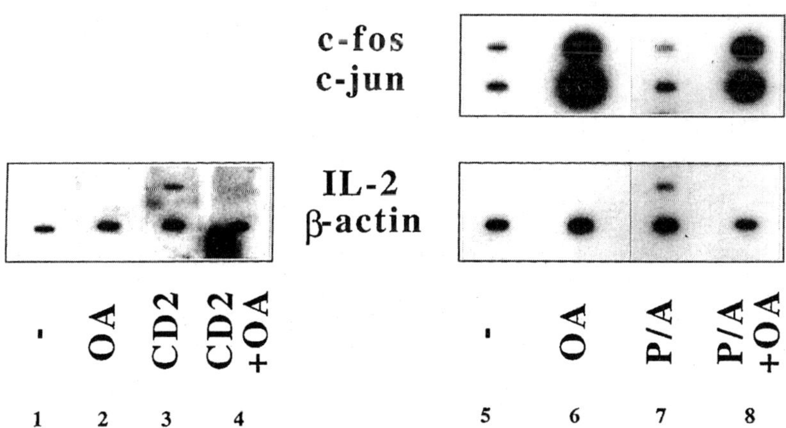

Figure 2 Transcription of the IL-2, c-*fos*, c-*jun* and β-actin genes in peripheral blood T lymphocytes was determined by nuclear run-on analysis. Cells were incubated with medium (lanes 1 and 5) or treated with okadaic acid (lanes 2 and 6). For activation, cells were stimulated for 6 h via CD2 triggering (lanes 3 and 4) or PMA/A23187 treatment (lanes 7 and 8) each in the absence (lanes 3 and 7) or presence (lanes 4 and 8) of okadaic acid

Interestingly, determination of the transactivating potencies of individual transcription factors regulating IL-2 transcription by transient transfections of AP1, NF-κB, Oct- and NFAT-reporter gene constructs demonstrated that okadaic acid differentially affects these transcription factors. Thus, while it inhibits NF-κB-, Oct- and NFAT-mediated transactivation processes during T cell activation, AP1 activity is markedly enhanced by okadaic acid. Therefore, okadaic acid-sensitive serine/threonine phosphatases are necessary for the transactivation of the IL-2 promoter by Oct, NF-κB and NFAT but not by AP1 proteins[36].

CONCLUSION

Taken together, activation of okadaic acid-sensitive serine/threonine phosphatases occurs through CD2, CD4, CD8 and CD28 receptors, and thus represents a common element in these co-activation pathways for human T cells (Figure 3). Perhaps more importantly, this co-stimulatory signalling pathway appears to be unaffected by the action of cyclosporin A, an inhibitor of the serine phosphatase PP2B/calcineurin. These findings provide explanations for the inability of cyclosporin A to induce tolerance because (1) important co-stimulatory signals are not inhibited and (2) cyclosporin A blocks signal transduction through the T cell antigen receptor, thus not allowing the induction of antigen-specific anergy.

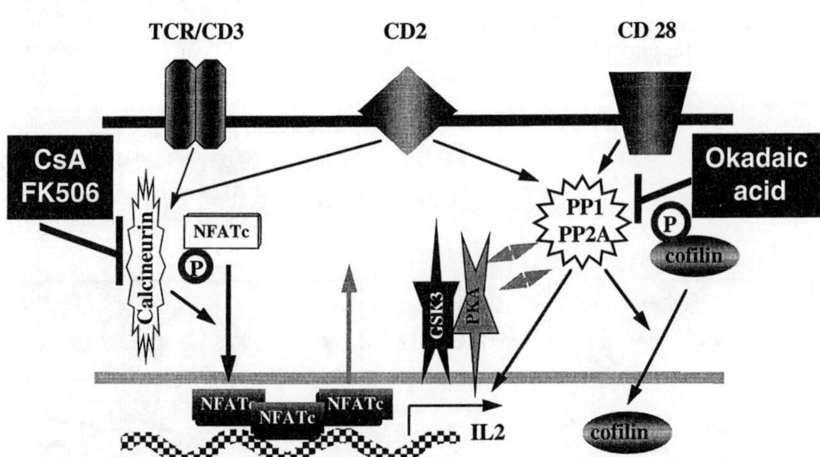

Figure 3 Calcineurin (PP2B) regulates activation and nuclear entry of the transcription factor NFATc in a cyclosporin A- and FK506-sensitive fashion. PP1 and PP2A catalyse dephosphorylation and nuclear translocation of cofilin. The latter process is resistant to inhibition by cyclosporin A but sensitive to okadaic acid. In addition, PP1 and PP2A influence serine kinases (GSK3 and PKA) which are involved in nuclear export of NFATc by means of phosphorylating its serine residues. Importantly, co-stimulation of T cells through e.g. CD2 or CD28 activates PP2B as well as PP1 and/or PP2A resulting in an altered balance between nuclear import and export of NFATc and cofilin with the consequence of their nuclear accumulation

It was demonstrated recently that stimulation through the CD2 receptor reverses tolerance induced by blockade of the CD80–CD28 interaction[37]. In a reciprocal fashion one would predict that immune tolerance induced through intervention at the CD2 level[38] can be broken by activating T cells through CD28. Therefore, it is rather unlikely to expect that 'complete' tolerance/anergy can be induced by inhibiting single receptors: this stresses the importance of targeting signal transducing elements (e.g. PP1, PP2A and pp19/cofilin) that are common for crucial pathways of co-stimulation. The identification of inhibitory components selectively affecting co-stimulatory signalling pathways and, unlike CsA[39], not blocking TCR–CD3 signalling, may provide novel tools for therapeutic immunosuppression with the perspective to inducing antigen specific tolerance. Since pp19/cofilin is a highly conserved and widely distributed protein it does itself not represent an ideal target for immune intervention. However, one might expect that proximal to this molecule components of this signalling pathway exist which are more tissue specific.

ACKNOWLEDGEMENTS

The authors thank Beate Funk, Jürgen Müller and Petra Quehl for excellent technical assistance. This work was supported by a grant from the Deutsche Forschungsgemeinschaft (SFB 405-A4) and the Forschungsschwerpunkt Transplantation Heidelberg.

References

1. Zanders ED, Lamb JR, Green N, Feldmann M, Beverley PC. Tolerance of T-cell clones is associated with membrane antigen changes. Nature. 1983;303:625–627.
2. Mueller DL, Jenkins MK, Schwartz RH. Clonal expansion versus functional clonal inactivation: a costimulatory signalling pathway determines the outcome of T cell antigen receptor occupancy. Annu Rev Immunol. 1989;7:445–480.
3. Murphy KM, Heimberger AB, Loh DY. Induction by antigen of intrathymic apoptosis of CD4+CD8+TCR[lo] thymocytes in vivo. Science. 1990,250:1720–1723.
4. Smith CA, Williams GT, Kingston R, Jenkinson EJ, Owen JJT. Antibodies to CD3/T-cell receptor complex induce death by apoptosis in immature T cells in thymic cultures. Nature. 1989;337:181–184.
5. Gimmi CD, Freeman GJ, Gribben JG, Gray G, Nadler LM. Human T-cell clonal anergy is induced by antigen presentation in the absence of B7 costimulation. Proc Natl Acad Sci USA. 1993;90:6586–6590.
6. Harding FA, McArthur JG, Gross JA, Raulet DH, Allison JP. CD28-mediated signalling co-stimulates murine T cells and prevents induction of anergy in T-cell clones. Nature. 1992;356:607–609.
7. Boise LH, Minn AJ, Noel PJ et al. CD28 costimulation can promote T cell survival by enhancing the expression of Bcl-x$_L$. Immunity. 1995;3:87–98.
8. Radvanyi LG, Shi Y, Vaziri H et al. CD28 costimulation inhibits TCR-induced apoptosis during a primary T cell response. J Immunol. 1996;156:1788–1798.
9. Samstag Y, Bader A, Meuer SC. A serine phosphatase is involved in CD2-mediated activation of human T lymphocytes and natural killer cells. J Immunol. 1991;147:788–794.
10. Samstag Y, Henning SW, Bader A, Meuer SC. Dephosphorylation of pp19: a common second signal for human T cell activation mediated through different accessory molecules. Int Immunol. 1992;4:1255–1262.
11. Henning SW, Meuer SC, Samstag Y. Serine phosphorylation of a 67kDa protein in human T lymphocytes represents an accessory receptor mediated signalling event. J Immunol. 1994;152:4808–4815.

12. Samstag Y, Henning S, Quehl P, Sturm G, Meuer SC. One costimulatory signal differentially regulates two actin-binding proteins in human T lymphocytes. In: Schlossman SF (ed). Leukocyte Typing V. Oxford: Oxford University Press, 1995:303–305.
13. de Arruda M, Watson S, Lin CS, Leavitt J, Matsudaira P. Fimbrin is a homologue of the cytoplasmic phosphoprotein plastin and has domains homologous with calmodulin and actin gelation proteins. J Cell Biol. 1990;111:1069–1079.
14. Zu Y, Shigesada K, Nishida E et al. 65-kilodalton protein phosphorylated by interleukin 2 stimulation bears two putative actin-binding sites and two calcium-binding sites. Biochemistry. 1990;29:8319–8324.
15. Samstag Y, Eckerskorn C, Wesselborg S, Henning S, Wallich R, Meuer SC. Costimulatory signals for human T cell activation induce nuclear translocation of pp19/cofilin. Proc Natl Acad Sci USA. 1994;91:4494–4498.
16. Ambach A, Saunus J, Wesselborg S, Meuer SC, Samstag Y. Delineation of serine phosphatases 1, 2A and cofilin as common cyclosporin A insensitive elements in the CD2 and CD28 pathways of T cell activation. submitted for publication.
17. Nebl G, Meuer SC, Samstag Y. Dephosphorylation of serine 3 regulates nuclear translocation of cofilin. J Biol Chem. 1996;271:26276–26280.
18. Su B, Jacinto E, Hibi M, Kallunki T, Karin M, Ben-Neriah Y. JNK is involved in signal integration during costimulation. Cell. 1994;77:727–736.
19. Ward SG, Wilson A, Turner L, Westwick J, Sansom DM. Inhibition of CD28-mediated T cell costimulation by the phosphoinositide 3-kinase inhibitor wortmannin. Eur J Immunol. 1995;25:526–532.
20. Ward SG, Westwick J, Hall ND, Sansom DM. Ligation of CD28 receptor by B7 induces formation of D-3 phosphoinositides in T lymphocytes independently of T cell receptor/CD3 activation. Eur J Immunol. 1993;23:2572–2577.
21. Boucher LM, Wiegmann K, Futterer A et al. CD28 signals through acidic sphingomyelinase [see comments]. J Exp Med. 1995;181:2059–2068.
22. Chan G, Ochi A. Sphingomyelin-ceramide turnover in CD28 costimulatory signaling. Eur J Immunol. 1995;25:1999–2004.
23. Scheer U, Hinssen H, Franke WW, Jockusch B. Microinjection of actin-binding proteins and actin antibodies demonstrates involvement of nuclear actin in transcription of lampbrush chromosomes. Cell. 1984;39:111–122.
24. Rungger D, Rungger-Brandle E, Chaponnier C, Gabbiani G. Intranuclear injection of anti-actin antibodies into *Xenopus* oocytes blocks chromosome condensation. Nature. 1979;282:320–321.
25. Blikstad I, Markey F, Carlsson L, Persson T, Lindberg U. Selective assay of monomeric and filamentous actin in cell extracts, using inhibition of desoxyribonuclease I. Cell. 1978;15:935–943.
26. Peitsch MC, Polzar B, Stephan H et al. Characterization of the endogenous deoxyribonuclease involved in nuclear DNA degradation during apoptosis (programmed cell death). EMBO J. 1993;12:371–377.
27. Samstag Y, Dreizler EM, Ambach A, Sczakiel G, Meuer SC. Inhibition of constitutive serine phosphatase activity in T lymphoma cells results in phosphorylation of pp19/cofilin and induces apoptosis. J Immunol. 1996;156:4167–4173.
28. Iida K, Moriyama K, Matsumoto S, Kawasaki H, Nishida E, Yahara I. Isolation of a yeast essential gene, COF1, that encodes a homologue of mammalian cofilin, a low-Mr actin-binding and depolymerizing protein. Gene. 1993;124:115–120.
29. Moon AL, Janmey PA, Louie KA, Drubin DG. Cofilin is an essential component of the yeast cortical cytoskeleton. J Cell Biol. 1993;120:421–435.
30. Abe H, Obinata T, Minamide LS, Bamburg JR. *Xenopus laevis* actin-depolymerizing factor/cofilin: a phosphorylation-regulated protein essential for development. J Cell Biol. 1996;132:871–885.
31. Kayalar C, Ord T, Testa MP, Zhong LT, Bredesen DE. Cleavage of actin by interleukin 1 beta-converting enzyme to reverse DNase inhibition. Proc Natl Acad Sci USA. 1996;93:2234–2238.
32. Ashkenas J, Werb Z. Proteolysis and the biochemistry of life-or-death decisions [comment]. J Exp Med. 1996;183:1947–1951.
33. Haldar S, Jena N, Croce CM. Inactivation of Bcl-2 by phosphorylation. Proc Natl Acad Sci USA. 1995;92:4507–4511.
34. Gajewski TF, Thompson CB. Apoptosis meets signal transduction: elimination of a BAD influence. Cell. 1996;87:589–592.

35. Miyawaki T, Uehara T, Nibu R et al. Differential expression of apoptosis-related Fas antigen on lymphocyte subpopulations in human peripheral blood. J Immunol. 1992;149:3753–3758.
36. Nebl G, Meuer SC, Samstag Y. CsA resistant transactivation of the IL-2 promoter requires activity of okadaic acid sensitive serine/threonine phosphatases. J Immunol. 1998;161: 1803–1810
37. Boussiotis VA, Freeman GJ, Griffin JD, Gray GS, Gribben JG, Nadler LM. CD2 is involved in maintenance and reversal of human alloantigen-specific clonal anergy. J Exp Med. 1994;180:1665–1673.
38. Gückel B, Berek C, Lutz M, Altevogt P, Schirrmacher V, Kyewsky BA. Anti-CD2 antibodies induce T cell unresponsiveness in vivo. J Exp Med. 1991;174:957–967.
39. Bloemens E, Vain Oers RHJ, Weinreich S, Stilma-Meinesz AP, Schellekens PThA, Van Lier RAW. The influence of cyclosporine A on the alternative pathways of human T cell activation in vitro. Eur J Immunol. 1989;19:943–946.

34
Immunomodulation in experimentally induced colitis using chimeric interleukin-2 fusion proteins

A. STALLMACH, B. WITTIG, K. PFISTER, J. C. HOFFMANN, C. PETERS, U. KUNZENDORF and M. ZEITZ

INTRODUCTION

The aetiology of the chronic human inflammatory bowel diseases (IBD), Crohn's disease (CD) and ulcerative colitis (UC) remains poorly understood. The development of the diseases may be a result of an uncontrolled or inadequately down-regulated cellular immune response in the intestinal mucosa towards a hitherto unknown pathogen, probably a constituent of the luminal content[1,2]. This leads to mucosal injury, breakdown of the epithelial barrier function and increased influx of luminal content to the lamina propria which might further exaggerate the uncontrolled immune response. Activated T lymphocytes with increased expression of the interleukin-2 (IL-2) receptor have been implicated in the pathogenesis of inflammatory bowel disease. Lymphocyte activation by antigen or mitogen results in expression of the high-affinity trimeric IL-2 receptor complex. This receptor in turn binds IL-2, resulting in activation, proliferation, and cytokine release by helper T cells[3]. In non-inflamed intestinal mucosa, few cells express this receptor, but in the inflamed intestinal mucosa of CD, UC and pouchitis, large numbers of T lymphocytes and macrophages expressing CD25 are found[4–6].

This enhanced understanding of the pathogenesis of IBD affords new opportunities to direct specific therapies at relevant molecules and cells. In particular, increasing evidence implicates both increased concentrations of proinflammatory cytokines such as interferon-γ (IFN-γ) or tumour necrosis factor-α (TNF-α) on one hand, and decreased local concentrations of contrainflammatory cytokines such as IL-10, as major mediators to the inflammatory and destructive reactions in IBD. Animal models increase the understanding of regulatory mechanisms behind the exaggerated immune response in diseases and offer the possibility to develop new more specific therapeutic strategies. One of the best described and most useful models to study the pathogenesis of IBD is the rectal administration of 2,4,6-trinitro-benzene sulphonic acid (TNBS). This agent haptenates autologous colonic proteins with trinitrophenyl (TNP), which then induce a massive transmural infiltration of T_H1 T cells producing IFN-γ (and TNF-α). These cytokines presumably cause mucosal inflammation by inducing macrophages to produce inflammatory cytokines and chemostatic factors. Successful experimental trials using antibodies to IL-12 or TNF-α or antisense oligonucleotides against NFκb indicate that the TNBS model is useful to prove new therapeutic strategies in colonic inflammation[7-9].

PROTECTION AGAINST TNBS-INDUCED COLITIS BY CHIMERIC PROTEINS

Current concepts for the medical treatment of severe IBD rely on the efficacy of drugs such corticosteroids, azathioprine and cyclosporine, that interfere with the immune response abrogating cytokine production and cell proliferation. Side effects and dose-limiting toxicity result from their limited specificity for the immune system. A more specific approach to inhibit selective immune functions became feasible with the application of genetically engineered immunoligands such as CTLA4–IgG or IL2–IgM in experimental models of organ transplantation and autoimmune diseases[10-13]. Previous data have demonstrated that the IL2–IgG2 fusion protein suppresses both cellular and humoral immune responses in a mouse model of DTH reaction after immunization with sheep erythrocytes[14]. Since a T_H1 pattern of cytokine responses in DTH reaction has been described and the presence of activated T cells with a predominant T_H1 reaction has been observed in TNBS-induced colitis, we determined whether IL2–IgG2 influences disease activity and analysed the immunomodulatory mechanisms of this fusion protein in experimental colitis.

TNBS colitis was induced as described by Neurath *et al.*[7]. Briefly, a 3.5 F catheter was carefully inserted into the colon such that the tip was 5 cm proximal to the anus. To induce colitis, 2.0 mg of the hapten reagent TNBS (depending on the weight of mice) in 50% ethanol was slowly administered into the lumen of the colon via the catheter fitted to a 1 ml syringe. Treatment consisted of intraperitoneal injections of 8 μg/200 μl PBS IL2–IgG2b or control mouse-anti-LFA3 IgG2b every 12 h.

As described by others, administration of TNBS resulted in a wasting disease with an increased mortality rate of approximately 60% after 5 days and a dramatic decrease in body weight (more than 15% after 3 days) (see also Table 1). Macroscopically, the wall of the colon was thickened and occasionally, small subserosal haemorrhagic spots were present. Microscopically, severe colitis was characterized by an inflammatory infiltrate in the colonic lamina propria and increased mitotic activity in the elongated epithelial crypts. When mice were treated with the fusion protein in a prevention trial (IL2–IgG2 was given twice daily starting 24 h before TNBS application (day −1)) mortality rate was reduced and loss of body weight was prevented. First, the mortality rate resulting from fulminant TNBS colitis decreased significantly. Second, mice that had received IL2–IgG2b usually obtained their initial body weight, whereas control IgG-treated mice continued to lose weight. Further, IL2–IgG2b treated mice became

Table 1 Effect of IL2-IgG2b on survival rate, body weight and cytokines

	TNBS	*TNBS + IL2-IgG2*
Survival rate	↓↓↓	↓ – =
Body weight	↓↓↓	↓ – =
Spleen weight	↑↑↑	↑ – =
Activation of T cells	↑	↑↑↑
TNF-α	↑↑↑	↑ – =
IL-10	=	↑↑↑

more active and lost their ruffled coat appearance when compared with untreated mice or mice given control mouse IgG. In order to analyse whether IL2–IgG2 treatment would be effective in established colitis, we started treatment 3 days after induction of TNBS colitis. A striking increase in the average weight of mice was found after IL2–IgG2b treatment but not after control IgG treatment. Interestingly, treatment with IL2–IgG2b resulted in a dramatic increase of spleen weight. When the spleen weights of TNBS mice receiving control and those treated with IL2–IgG2b were determined for comparison, the IL2–IgG2b-treated group showed a 110% weight increase (day 7).

Since these results showed that TNBS-induced colitis can be prevented by IL2–IgG2b, and to determine the mechanisms underlying the therapeutic effects, we next focused on the capacity of T cells to produce various cytokines (in cooperation with Thomas Giese, Department of Immunology, Heidelberg). Freshly isolated splenic cells were stimulated by PMA and ionomycin *in vitro* and stained for intracellular cytokines. A much larger fraction of the CD4-positive cells from IL2–IgG-treated mice stained positive for IL-10 than from untreated TNBS-mice. In parallel to flow cytometry analysis, preliminary data from semiquantitative RT-PCR studies demonstrated an increased IL-10 mRNA concentration in IL2–IgG2b-treated mice after induction of TNBS colitis. Levels of mucosal mRNA coding for TNF-α and IFN-γ seem to be decreased in IL2–IgG-treated mice when compared with diseased mice.

DISCUSSION

Various Ig fusion proteins using cytokines or extracellular domains of integral membrane proteins to replace the variable regions of immunoglobulins have been developed recently to interfere with inflammatory immune responses. In this study, we investigated the *in vivo* effects of a murine IL2–IgG2b fusion protein in TNBS-induced colitis. IL-2 was fused to IgG2b, a mouse isotype with little *in vivo* complement fixationability. Binding of this chimeric protein to IL-2 receptors or cellular Fc receptors was previously demonstrated *in vitro*. Soluble but also cell-bound IL2–IgG2b supported IL-2-dependent cell proliferation. Thus, both parts of the fusion protein remain functional[14]. Despite the absence of immunosuppressive properties *in vitro*, the IL2–IgG2b fusion protein effectively abrogated wasting disease in TNBS induced colitis. This inhibition occurred despite a profound proliferation and accumulation of splenic T cells. The IL2–IgG2b fusion protein bound to high-affinity IL-2 receptors and supported proliferation of T cells *in vitro*. While IL-2 can trigger T cells to undergo apoptosis after T cell receptor stimulation[15], expansion of splenic T cells consistent with a vigorous proliferative response was observed after application of IL2–IgG2b; this finding strongly argues against T cell apoptosis as the underlying mechanism by which IL2–IgG2b suppresses inflammatory activity in TNBS colitis. Similar findings have been reported after application of the CTLA4–IgG fusion protein. This fusion protein very effectively suppresses cell-mediated and humoral immune responses in mice[10,16] but causes no deletion of T cells[17]. It has been suggested that CTLA4–IgG exerts its immunosuppressive action by interfering with the CD28–B7 signalling pathway; *in vivo* evidence to support this mode of action is sparse, and targeting of B cells to the reticuloendothelial system may alter B and T cell responses. This mechanism has also been discussed for nondepleting anti-CD25 mAb. Since IL-2 displays high receptor affinity compared with blocking anti-CD25 antibodies, enormous amounts of antibodies would be required to inhibit IL-2-dependent cell proliferation *in vivo* but *in vivo* effects have been achieved using amounts of anti-CD25 mAb that would not inhibit proliferation *in vitro*[18]. It appears that the immunosuppressive mechanism of nondepleting antibodies and potentially chimeric proteins, such as the IL2–IgG2b fusion, may depend on opsonization of target cells. These, in turn, are retained in the reticuloendothelial system of the spleen and liver[19] and, despite vigorous proliferation, are unable to take part in the cellular immune response. The observed increase of both T cell numbers

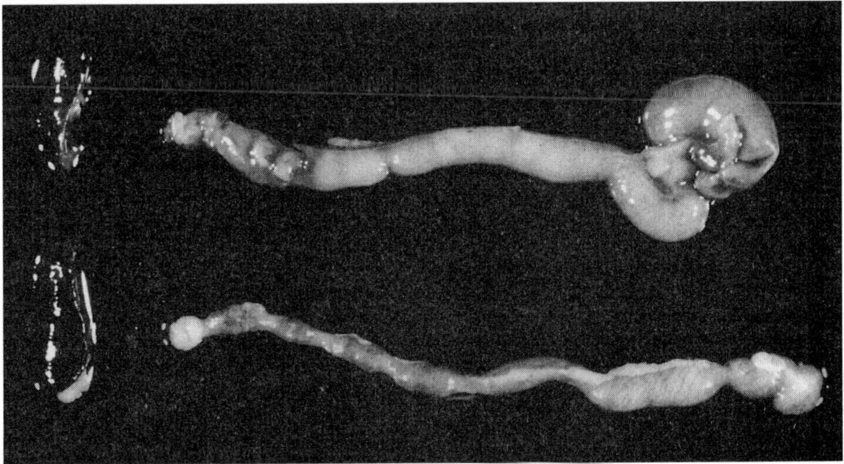

Figure 1 Macroscopic changes of colon and spleen in TNBS-treated mice. Photographs of dissected large intestine and spleen of a mouse 7 days after application of TNBS in 50% ethanol (top) and a mouse treated with IL2–IgG2b after induction of TNBS colitis (bottom). The colon of the TNBS-treated mouse was severely inflamed and hyperaemic. The dramatic increase of spleen size after IL2-IgG2b treatment is also clearly visible

in the spleen in IL2–IgG2b-treated animals support this hypothesis. Another hypothesis which explained the therapeutic effects of IL2–IgG2b based on the observed increase of IL-10 production. It is tempting to speculate that the IL2-IgG2b fusion protein binds on one side to CD25[+] T cells and on the other side to monocytes/macrophages. This antigen-independent cell–cell interaction could result in the induction of IL-10 translation in T cells. IL-10 is important for the prevention of T cell-mediated inflammation in the gut, as IL-10-deficient mice develop inflammatory bowel disease, which is thought to be mediated by physiological enteric antigens. In addition, administration of IL-10 to young IL-10-deficient mice prevents inflammatory bowel disease[20]. IL-10 also significantly inhibits the development of inflammatory bowel disease induced by transfer of CD4/CD45RB[hi]-positive T cells into SCID mice or by intrarectal administration of TNBS[21]. Clinical trials in patients with Crohn's disease using recombinant IL-10 have provided first evidence that contrainflammatory cytokines might be useful therapeutic agents. First in three patients with ulcerative colitis[22] and later in a double-blind, placebo-controlled trial, clinical disease activity decreased in patients with Crohn's disease[23]. The mechanism of action of IL-10 is still unknown, but the observed anti-inflammatory effects may be partly attributable to down-regulation of the production of TNF-α, IL-1, IL-12, and IL-6, inhibition of synthesis of matrix metalloproteinases and/or nitric oxide, and/or increased secretion of natural contrainflammatory cytokines, such as IL-1 receptor antagonist and soluble TNF receptor.

Another group of chimeric proteins induce cytotoxicity as mode of action. Diphtheria toxin-related ligand fusion proteins are one such group of agents, in which the cytotoxic portion of diphtheria toxin catalytic domain and transmembrane domain is fused to the receptor-binding portion of a known ligand. Wiliams *et al.* described the genetic construction and functional properties of the prototypic fusion toxin DAB_{486}–IL-2, consisting of a truncated form of diphtheria toxin fused to human IL-2[24]. This fusion protein is internalized and catalyses ADP-ribosylation of elongation factor 2, resulting in inhibition of translation, decrease in protein synthesis and cell death. Since activated lymphocytes produce higher levels of proinflammatory cytokines than resting cells, selectively depleting activated lymphocytes can potentially reduce inflammation while leaving resting and memory lymphocyte function unimpaired. Bousvaros and coworkers demonstrated that the IL-2 diphtheria toxin fusion protein specifically targets activated (CD25-positive) lamina propria lymphocytes[25]. This fusion protein inhibited in these cells protein synthesis and IFN-γ levels by 80% in 24 h cultures[25]. In this context it is important to note that specific deletion of antigen-activated T cell clones has been demonstrated *in vivo* for IL-2–diphtheria toxin fusion protein[26]. Further the IL-2 toxins have been administered with encouraging results to patients with haematological malignancies and refractory rheumatoid arthritis[27–29]. These and our results justify further investigations of the IL-2–diphtheria toxin fusion proteins in IBD.

In summary, genetically engineered fusion proteins can profoundly alter the immune response in murine T_H1 models of chronic intestinal inflammation. This inflammation is abrogated in the absence of detectable side effects may prove useful in the treatment of inflammatory bowel disease.

References

1. Duchmann R, Schmitt E, Knolle P, Meyer zum Büschenfelde KH, Neurath M. Tolerance towards resident intestinal flora in mice is abrogated in experimental colitis and restored by treatment with interleukin-10 or antibodies to interleukin-12. Eur J Immunol. 1996;26:934–938.

2. Duchmann R, Neurath M, Merker-Hermann E, Meyer zum Büschenfelde KH. Immune responses towards intestinal bacteria – current concepts and future perspectives. Z Gastroenterol. 1997;35:337–346.

3. Zeitz M, Greene WC, Pfeffer NJ, James SP. Lymphocytes isolated from the intestinal lamina propria of normal nonhuman primates have increased expression of genes associated with T-cell activation. Gastroenterology. 1988;94:647–655.

4. Pallone F, Fais S, Squarcia O, Biancone L, Pozzilli P, Boirivant M. Activation of peripheral blood and intestinal lamina propria lymphocytes in Crohn's disease. In vivo state of activation and in vitro response to stimulation as defined by the expression of early activation antigens. Gut. 1987;28:745–753.

5. Choy MY, Walker SJ, Williams CB, MacDonald TT. Differential expression of CD25 (interleukin-2 receptor) on lamina propria T cells and macrophages in the intestinal lesions in Crohn's disease and ulcerative colitis. Gut. 1990;31:1365–1370.

6. Stallmach A, Schäfer F, Weber S et al. Increased state of activation of CD4-positive T cells and elevated interferon-g production in pouchitis. Gut. 1998; in press.

7. Neurath MF, Fuss I, Kelsall BL, Stuber F, Strober W. Antibodies to interleukin 12 abrogate established experimental colitis in mice. J Exp Med. 1995;182:1281–1290.

8. Neurath MF, Fuss I, Kelsall B, Meyer zum Büschenfelde KH, Strober W. Effect of IL-12 and antibodies to IL-12 on established granulomatous colitis in mice. Ann NY Acad Sci. 1996;795:368–370.

9. Neurath MF, Pettersson S, Meyer zum Büschenfelde KH, Strober W. Local administration of antisense phosphorothioate oligonucleotides to the p65 subunit of NF-kappa B abrogates established experimental colitis in mice. Nature Med. 1996;2:998–1004.

10. Lenschow DJ, Zeng Y, Thistlethwaite JR et al. Long-term survival of xenogeneic pancreatic islet grafts induced by CTLA4Ig. Science. 1992;257:789–792.

11. Turka LA, Linsley PS, Lin H et al. T-cell activation by the CD28 ligand B7 is required for cardiac allograft rejection in vivo. Proc Natl Acad Sci USA. 1992;89:11102–11105.

12. Bogers WM, Lang F, Parker KE et al. Rat interleukin-2 immunoglobulin M fusion proteins are cytotoxic in vitro for cells expressing the IL-2 receptor and can abolish cell-mediated immunity in vivo. Transplantation. 1994;58:932–939.

13. Finck BK, Linsley PS, Wofsy D. Treatment of murine lupus with CTLA4Ig. Science. 1994;265:1225–1227.

14. Kunzendorf U, Pohl T, Bulfone Paus S et al. Suppression of cell-mediated and humoral immune responses by an interleukin-2-immunoglobulin fusion protein in mice. J Clin Invest. 1996;97:1204–1210.

15. Lenardo MJ. Interleukin-2 programs mouse alpha beta T lymphocytes for apoptosis. Nature. 1991;353:858–861.

16. Linsley PS, Wallace PM, Johnson J et al. Immunosuppression in vivo by a soluble form of the CTLA-4 T cell activation molecule. Science. 1992;257:792–795.

17. Baliga P, Chavin KD, Qin L et al. CTLA4Ig prolongs allograft survival while suppressing cell-mediated immunity. Transplantation. 1994;58:1082–1090.

18. Diamantstein T, Osawa H. The interleukin-2 receptor, its physiology and a new approach to a selective immunosuppressive therapy by anti-interleukin-2 receptor monoclonal antibodies. Immunol Rev. 1986;92:5–27.

19. Jonker M, Goldstein G, Balner H. Effects of in vivo administration of monoclonal antibodies specific for human T cell subpopulations on the immune system in a rhesus monkey model. Transplantation. 1983;35:521–526.

20. Kühn R, Lohler I, Rennick D, Rajewsky K, Müller W. Interleukin-10-deficient mice develop chronic enterocolitis. Cell. 1993;75:263–274.

21. Powrie F, Leach MW, Mauze S, Menon S, Caddle LB, Coffman RL. Inhibition of Th1 responses prevents inflammatory bowel disease in scid mice reconstituted with CD4SRBhi CD4+ T cells. Immunity. 1994;1:553–562.

22. Schreiber S, Heinig T, Thiele HG, Raedler A. Immunoregulatory role of interleukin 10 in patients with inflammatory bowel disease. Gastroenterology. 1995;108:1434–1444.

23. van Deventer SJ, Elson CO, Fedorak RN. Multiple doses of intravenous interleukin 10 in steroid-refractory Crohn's disease. Crohn's Disease Study Group. Gastroenterology. 1997;113:383–389.
24. Williams DP, Parker K, Bacha P et al. Diphtheria toxin receptor binding domain substitution with interleukin-2: genetic construction and properties of a diphtheria toxin-related interleukin-2 fusion protein. Protein Eng. 1987;1:493–498.
25. Bousvaros A, Stevens AC, Strom TB, Murphy J, Lamont JT. Interleukin-2 fusion protein (DAB389IL-2) selectively targets activated human peripheral blood and lamina propria lymphocytes. Dig Dis Sci. 1997;42:1542–1548.
26. Bastos MG, Pankewycz O, Rubin KV, Murphy JR, Strom TB. Concomitant administration of hapten and IL-2-toxin (DAB486-IL-2) results in specific deletion of antigen-activated T cell clones. J Immunol. 1990;145:3535–3539.
27. LeMaistre CF, Rosenblum MG et al. Therapeutic effects of genetically engineered toxin (DAB486IL-2) in patient with chronic lymphocytic leukaemia. Lancet. 1991;337:1124–1125.
28. Sewell KL, Parker KC, Woodworth TG, Reuben J, Swartz W, Trentham DE. DAB486IL-2 fusion toxin in refractory rheumatoid arthritis. Arthritis Rheum. 1993;356:1223–1233.
29. Tepler I, Schwartz G, Parker K et al. Phase I trial of an interleukin-2 fusion toxin (DAB486IL-2) in hematologic malignancies: complete response in a patient with Hodgkin's disease refractory to chemotherapy. Cancer. 1994;73:1276–1285.

35
Anti-T cell strategies

J. EMMRICH

INTRODUCTION

A number of observations suggest that T cells and their associated cytokines play a central role in the pathogenesis of inflammatory bowel diseases (IBD). Evidence for activation of mucosal T cells is provided by several findings: expanded mucosal T cell population, increased expression of activation markers on surface of mucosal T cells, increased cytotoxic T cell function, and increased production of cytokines[1-3]. Recently developed mouse models of IBD have shown that a dysregulated T cell response in the gut can result in chronic colitis[4]. In one of these models T cells induce extensive mucosal inflammation after transfer to SCID mice that lack T cells[5]. Therefore, T cells are main targets for therapeutic activity in Crohn's disease (CD) as well as in ulcerative colitis (UC).

There are different strategies to treat patients with IBD using T cell-directed therapies. T cell apheresis, blocking of T cell activation, blocking of co-stimulatory signals, inhibition of CD4, and immunomodulatory cytokines are principal

Table 1 Anti-T cell strategies

---

1. *T cell apheresis*

2. *Blocking of T cell activation*
   Anti-IL-2 receptor antibodies
   IL-2 fusion toxin
   Anti-CD2 antibodies

3. *Blocking of co-stimulatory signals*
   Soluble class II MHC–peptide complexes
   CTLA4Ig
   Specific blockade of B7-1
   Interruption of the CD40–CD40L interaction

4. *Inhibition of CD4*
   Anti-CD4 antibodies
   CD4 V1 CDR3 analogue peptide

5. *Immunomodulatory cytokines*
   IL-4, IL-10, TGF-ß
   Neutralization of T_H1 cytokines (anti-IFN-γ, anti-IL-12)

---

approaches to decrease inflammatory activity by influencing T cells (Table 1). Strategies using immunomodulatory cytokines as well as antibodies against immunomodulatory cytokines to inhibit the development of T cells are the subject of another chapter in this book.

T CELL APHERESIS

T cell apheresis is used to reduce the number of T cells. Uncontrolled trials have suggested that T cell apheresis may be efficacious in a high proportion of patients with CD[6]. A controlled trial reported a steroid sparing effect with T cell apheresis in patients with CD but with a high incidence of early relapse in the responder group[7]. Because of the expense and inconvenience of apheresis, in addition to the lack of studies demonstrating long-term efficacy, alternative strategies directed at removing selected subsets of T cells are more attractive.

BLOCKING OF T CELL ACTIVATION

The initiating events of IBD are likely to centre on a specific immune response triggered by an antigen. Because this antigen, or class of antigens, has not been defined, effective strategies directed at antigen are lacking, and therapeutic approaches directed against activation of the T cells have, therefore, been developed. After activation T cells produce interleukin-2 (IL-2) as a critical co-factor for the initiation and perpetuation of a specific immune response. Activated T cells elaborate IL-2 receptor, completing an autocrine and paracrine loop promoting clonal expansion. Anti-IL-2 receptor antibodies have been used with some success in autoimmune diseases to block T cell activation[8,9]. Another strategy has been the creation of a chimeric IL-2 receptor-targeted toxin. In this hybrid molecule the receptor binding domain of diphtheria toxin is replaced by IL-2 (DAB 486 IL-2) to kill cell populations expressing the high-affinity IL-2 receptor on the cell surface[10]. No studies in IBD have yet been reported.

Proliferation of intestinal T lymphocytes *in vitro* can be achieved via the CD2 molecule[11]. Anti-CD2 monoclonal antibodies were reported to induce donor-specific tolerance in murine heart transplantation[12]. Using these antibodies Hoffmann *et al.*[13] could show reduction of arthritis score in an adjuvant arthritis model in mice compared with control antibody. Therefore, anti-CD2 antibodies could be helpful also in IBD. Studies in animal models are ongoing.

BLOCKING OF CO-STIMULATORY SIGNALS

Activation of T cells occurs when the T cell receptor binds the specific antigen presented by MHC. T cell activation can be prevented by the application of a pathogenetically relevant antigen linked to a modified MHC molecule lacking co-stimulation via MHC. This could be shown using soluble complexes of MHC class II–encephalitogenic peptide to treat experimental allergic encephalomyelitis[14]. It was suggested that the soluble class II MHC–peptide complexes induced clonal deletion, long-term tolerance being due to the delivery of the antigen signal without the co-stimulation which is essential for T cell activation[15]. However, this approach needs the identification of relevant antigens, and these are not known in IBD.

Antigen recognition by T cell receptor and MHC is not sufficient to activate naive T cells. Simultaneous binding of a second, antigen-nonspecific binding ligand is necessary. This co-stimulatory signal may be provided by the interaction of B7-1 or B7-2 molecules on the cell surface of antigen-presenting cells with CD28 on the T cell surface[16]. Cytotoxic T cell antigen 4 (CTLA-4) presented by T cells binds to B7 with greater affinity than CD28, and inhibits T cell proliferation as well as the production of IL-2[17,18]. Therefore, a fusion protein of immunoglobulin and CTLA-4 (CTLA4Ig) was created to block co-stimulatory signals provided by B7. CTLA4Ig was an effective treatment in animal models of autoimmune disease[19,20], but no studies in IBD are available.

An interesting new field of therapeutic approaches is to block co-stimulatory signals to modify the ratio of T_H1/T_H2 reactions: binding of the co-stimulatory molecule B7-1 stimulates a T_H1 response, whereas B7-2 favours T_H2[21]. This observation might be of therapeutic relevance since there is evidence that especially CD is mediated by dominance of T_H1-type reaction[22,23].

Interactions between the accessory molecule CD40 on antigen-presenting cells and CD40 ligand on activated T cells promote the development of T_H1 by inducing secretion of IL-12 by macrophages[24]. This suggests that the interruption of the CD40–CD40 ligand interaction may be an effective treatment in IBD[25]. The administration of anti-gp39 (CD40L) antibodies during the induction phase of TNBS-induced experimental colitis in mice prevented interferon-γ (IFN-γ) production by lamina propria CD4+ T cells and also prevented clinical and histological evidence of this disease[26].

INHIBITION OF CD4

The CD4 molecule is intimately involved in antigen recognition by T cells. It interacts with MHC class II molecules on the antigen-presenting cells, thus stabilizing antigen recognition by the T cell receptor. Moreover, when cross-linked to the T cell receptor it provides a co-stimulatory signal[27].

Beneficial prophylactic and therapeutic effects of monoclonal antibodies directed against CD4 surface molecules have been demonstrated in animal models and clinical trials of autoimmune diseases. These trials have demonstrated immunomodulatory effects and clinical improvements[28–30]. However, the choice of a suitable anti-CD4 monoclonal antibody is obviously of critical importance. Some antibodies led only to a coating of the CD4+ cells, while others induced strong modulation. Many of the immunomodulatory effects appear to depend on the proximity of the recognized epitope to the HLA-binding region[30].

In human pilot studies anti-CD4 antibodies have been administered to patients with therapy-refractory IBD, with controversial results. Different antibodies have been used in these studies, including the monoclonal mouse antibodies MAX.16H5 and B5 as well as the chimeric antibody cM-T412 (Table 2).

The monoclonal antibody cM-T412 (Centocor, Malvern, PA, USA) is a chimeric molecule that contains the V domains of the mouse anti-CD4 antibody,

Table 2 Anti-CD4 antibodies in IBD

Monoclonal antibodies	Characterization	References
MAX.16H5	Murine monoclonal antibody IgG1	35,36
cM-T412	Chimeric monoclonal antibody (mouse–human)	31,32
B-F5	Murine monoclonal antibody IgG1	34

grafted onto the human IgG1κ constant domains. It recognizes epitopes located in V1–2 domains of the CD4 molecule. Six patients with CD and four patients with UC were treated in an open-label fashion with cM-T412[31]. Treatment was given intravenously at 20 mg/day for 7 days, with retreatment at 40 mg/day for 4 days between 2 and 16 weeks later. All patients achieved clinical and endoscopic remission with a mean duration of 11 months in CD and 12 months in UC. Administration of the antibody cM-T412 resulted in a striking depletion of CD4[+] T cells. One year after the first antibody cycle all patients had CD4 cell counts < 550 cells/μl. The same monoclonal antibody was used in a second study as a daily infusion of 10, 30, or 100 mg for a week to treat three groups of four patients with active, intractable CD[32]. The mean reduction in Crohn's disease activity index (CDAI[33]) was 25%, 24%, and 36%, respectively, at 4 weeks, and 24% and 52% at 10 weeks in the 30 mg and 100 mg groups. CD4[+] cell counts were decreased to nearly 25% of the baseline. The authors concluded that treatment of patients with CD using monoclonal antibody cM-T412 has moderate potential efficacy[32].

The antibody B-F5, a murine monoclonal of IgG1 isotype, was also used for therapy of patients with CD[34]. Twelve patients with severe refractory CD were treated in an open clinical trial with intravenous B-F5 (0.5 mg/day/kg for 7 consecutive days in eight patients). Four patients received the antibody at a dose of 0.5 mg/kg on the first day and 1 mg/kg/day for the next 6 days. No depletion of CD4[+] cells was observed. Among the 11 patients who received the complete course of treatment, two had prolonged clinical improvement and two had partial clinical improvement. In this trial, monoclonal anti-CD4 B-F5 antibody was not successful in treating severe CD[34].

We performed a clinical trial using the monoclonal mouse IgG1 antibody MAX.16H5[35,36] to treat 12 individuals with chronic active UC or CD. In an open clinical trial monoclonal antibody 16H5 was infused daily in a concentration of 0.3 mg/kg body weight for 7 days. Four of these patients received a second therapy cycle 4 weeks later in the same manner. For evaluation of the clinical response, we used the CDAI[33] and the clinical activity index according to Rachmilewitz *et al.*[37] for UC.

One cycle of antibody therapy was used to treat five patients suffering from UC and three patients with CD. In one patient with CU a longer lasting remission of 3 years was observed, but the other four patients had no or short remissions only. In the three patients with Crohn's disease remission lasted 4–16 weeks. All four patients treated with a second therapy cycle achieved

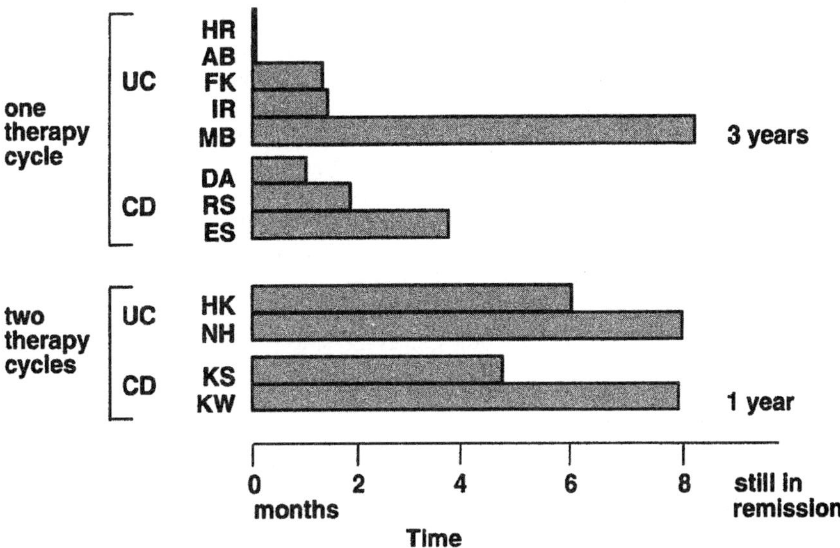

Figure 1   Anti-CD4 Antibody Therapy

remission which lasted for longer than that in patients treated with a single cycle. Figure 1 shows the remission time of all treated patients. In patients with remission a reduced CRP was a good serological indicator of inflammation.

There are reports about a long-lasting CD4 cell depletion after application of a chimeric anti-CD4 antibody. In our study CD4+ cell counts were slightly decreased immediately after therapy; this was followed by nearly normal values with a wide variation. The other lymphocyte subpopulations like suppressor cells, B cells or NK cells were not affected by the therapy.

Our findings demonstrate that anti-CD4 antibody therapy can be successful in IBD. The population of patients treated in this open, nonrandomized trial consisted of individuals with high levels of inflammatory activity. These patients had been refractory to several conventional treatment regimens and had been hospitalized many times without significant improvement in the disease activity. It was therefore surprising that changes in laboratory and clinical parameters occurred in parallel within the 1 week of treatment. However, a single cycle of anti-CD4 at the doses we used is not sufficient to persistently suppress disease activity in all patients.

Taken together, anti-CD4 treatment appeared to produce significant changes in laboratory and clinical parameters of disease activity. Additional carefully controlled studies are required to investigate the clinical use of anti-CD4 antibodies. Prolonged or repeated courses of antibody therapy or in combination with immunosuppressive drugs should be considered.

The immunological mechanisms upon which anti-CD4 therapy is based are still not fully understood[30,38]. Immediate effects are probably due to blocking of antigen recognition and influence of cellular interaction. However, the mechanism underlying the long-term effects of this therapy remains unknown. Three hypotheses should be discussed. It is known that T cell activation against luminal antigens in the gut of patients plays an important role in pathogenesis. One effect of anti-CD4 antibodies could be their capability to induce tolerance[39,40]. Conversely, it has been suggested that anti-CD4 transmits a negative signal to T cells if ligation occurs without simultaneous triggering of the T cell receptor[41]. The third way in which CD4 antibodies may have a therapeutic effect may depend on the T_H1/T_H2 imbalance, in which they induce T_H2 type reactions more than T_H1 type reactions[39,42]. Preliminary data indicate that the anti-CD4 antibody MAX.16H5 induces a switch from the T_H1 to the T_H2 reaction *in vitro*. IL-4 secretion was increased after incubation of isolated and activated lymphocytes with anti-CD4 antibodies, in contrast to IFN-γ.

CONCLUSION

Anti-T cell strategies hold great potential for the improved therapy of CD and UC. However, the long-term role of these immunomodulatory agents as part of standard therapy is not clear. The efficacy as well as the side effects of antibodies and other immunomodulatory mediators have to be evaluated. Furthermore, studies on immunomodulatory agents will provide new insights into the pathogenesis and improved treatment of IBD.

References

1. Zeitz M. Immunoregulatory abnormalities in inflammatory bowel disease. Eur J Gastroenterol Hepatol. 1990;2:246–250.
2. Podolsky DK. Inflammatory bowel disease. N Engl J Med. 1991;325:928–937.
3. Sartor RB. Cytokines in intestinal inflammation: pathophysiological and clinical considerations. Gastroenterology. 1994;106:533–539.
4. Strober W, Ehrhardt RO. Chronic intestinal inflammation: an unexpected outcome in cytokine or T cell receptor mutant-mice. Cell. 1993;75:203–205.
5. Morissey PJ, Charrier K, Braddy S, Liggitt D, Watson JD. CD4+ T cells that express high levels of CD45RB induce wasting disease when transferred into congenic severe combined immunodeficient mice. Disease development is prevented by cotransfer of purified CD4+ T cells. J Exp Med. 1993;178:237–244.
6. Bicks RO, Groshart KD. Editorial: the current status of T-lymphocyte apheresis (TLA) treatment of Crohn's disease. J Clin Gastroenterol. 1989;11:136–138.
7. Lerebours E, Bussel A, Modigliani R et al. Treatment of Crohn's disease by lymphocyte apheresis: a randomized controlled trial. Gastroenterology. 1994;107:357–361.
8. Kelley VE, Gaulton GN, Hattori M et al. Anti-interleukin-2 receptor antibody suppresses murine diabetic insulinitis and lupus nephritis. J Immunol. 1988;140:59–61.
9. Kroemer G, Wick G. The role of interleukin 2 in autoimmunity. Immunol Today. 1989;10:246–251.
10. Strom TB, Kelley VR, Murphy JR, Nichols JM, Woodworth TG. Interleukin-2 receptor-directed therapies: antibody- or cytokine-based targeting molecules. Annu Rev Med. 1993;44:343–353.
11. Zeitz M, Quinn TC, Graeff AS, James JP. Mucosal T cells provide helper function but do not proliferate when stimulated by specific antigen in lymphogranuloma venerum proctitis. Gastroenterology. 1988;94:353–366.
12. Kriger NR, Most D, Bromberg B et al. Coexistence of Th1- and Th2-type cytokine profiles in anti-CD2 monoclonal antibody-induced tolerance. Transplantation. 1996;62:1285–1292.
13. Hoffmann JC, Herklotz C, Zeidler H, Bayer B, Westermann J. Anti-CD2 (OX 34) mAB treatment of adjuvant arthritic rats: attenuation of established arthritis, selective depletion of CD4+ T cells, and CD2 downmodulation. Clin Exp Immunol. 1997;110:63–70.

14. Sharma SD, Nag B, Su XM et al. Antigen-specific therapy of experimental allergic encephalomyelitis by soluble class II major histocompatibility complex–peptide complexes. Proc Natl Acad Sci USA. 1991;88:11465–11469.

15. Nicolle MW, Nag B, Sharma SD et al. Specific tolerance to an acetylcholine receptor epitope induced in vitro in myasthenia gravis CD4+ lymphocytes by soluble major histocompatibility complex class II-peptide complexes. J Clin Invest. 1994;93:1361–1369.

16. Janeway CA, Bottomly K. Signals and signs for lymphocyte responses. Cell. 1994;76:275–285.

17. Allison JP, Krummel MF. The yin and yang of T cell costimulation. Science. 1995;270:932–933.

18. Krummel MF, Allison JP. CTLA-4 engagement inhibits IL-2 accumulaiton and cell cycle progression upon activation of resting T cells. J Exp Med. 1996;183:2533–2540.

19. Finck BK, Linsley PS, Wofsy D. Treatment of murine lupus with CTLA4Ig. Science. 1994;265:1225–1227.

20. Judge TA, Tang A, Turka LA. Immunosuppression through blockade of CD28: B7-mediated co-stimulatory signals. Immunol Res. 1996;15:38–49.

21. Kuchroo VK, Das MP, Brown JA et al. B7-1 and B7-2 co-stimulatory molecules activate differentially the Th1/Th2 developmental pathways: application to autoimmune disease therapy. Cell. 1995;80:707–718.

22. Mullin GE, Lazenby AJ, Harris ML et al. Increased interleukin-2 messenger RNA in the intestinal mucosal lesions of Crohn's disease but not ulcerative colitis. Gastroenterology. 1992;102:1620–1627.

23. Niessner M, Volk BA. Altered Th1/Th2 cytokine profiles in the intestinal mucosa of patients with inflammatory bowel disease as assessed by quantitative reversed transcribed polymerase chain reaction (RT-PCR). Clin Exp Immunol. 1995;101:428–435.

24. Shu U, Kiniwa M, Wu CY et al. Activated T cells induce interleukin-12 production by monocytes via CD40–CD40 ligand interaction. Eur J Immunol. 1995;25:1125–1128.

25. Buhlmann JE, Noelle RJ. Therapeutic potential for blockade of the CD40 ligand, gp39. J Clin Immunol. 1996;16:83–89.

26. Stüber E, Strober W, Neurath M. Blocking the CD40L-CD40 interaction in vivo specifically prevents the priming of T helper 1 cells through the inhibition of interleukin 12 secretion. J Exp Med. 1996;183:693–698.

27. Emmrich F, Rieber P, Kurrle R, Eichmann K. Selective stimulation of human T lymphocyte subsets by heteroconjugates of antibodies to the T cell receptor and to subset-specific differentiation antigens. Eur J Immunol. 1988;18:645–648.

28. Horneff G, Burmester GR, Emmrich F, Kalden JR. Treatment of rheumatoid arthritis with an anti-CD4 monoclonal antibody. Arth Rheum. 1991;34:129–140.

29. Olive D, Mawas C. Therapeutic applications of anti-CD4 antibodies. Crit Rev Ther Drug Carrier Sys. 1993;10:29–63.

30. Emmrich F, Schulze-Koops H, Burmester G. Anti-CD4 and other antibodies to cell surface antigens for therapy. In: Davies ME, Dingle JT (eds) Immunopharmacology of Joints and Connective Tissue. London: Academic Press, 1994:87–117.

31. Deusch K, Mauthe B, Reiter C, Riethmüller G, Classen M. CD4-Antibody treatment of inflammatory bowel disease: One-year follow up. Gastroenterology. 1993;104:A691

32. Stronkhorst A, Radema S, Yong S-L, Bijl H, ten Berge IJM, Tytgat GNJ, van Deventer SJH. CD4 antibody treatment in patients with active Crohn's disease: a phase 1 dose finding study. Gut. 1997;40:320–327.

33. Best WR, Becktel JM, Singleton JW, Kern F Jr. Development of a Crohn's disease activity index. Gastroenterology. 1976;70:439–444.

34. Canva-Delcambre V, Jacquot S, Robinet E et al. Treatment of severe Crohn's disease with anti-CD4 monoclonal antibody Aliment Pharmacol Ther. 1996;10:721–727.

35. Emmrich J, Seyfarth M, Fleig WE, Emmrich F. Treatment of inflammatory bowel disease with anti-CD4 monoclonal antibody. Lancet. 1991;338:570–571.

36. Emmrich J, Seyfarth M, Liebe S, Emmrich F. Anti-CD4 antibody treatment in inflammatory bowel disease without a long CD4+-cell depletion. Gastroenterology. 1995;108:A815.

37. Rachmilewitz D. Coated mesalazine (5-aminosalicylic acid) versus sulphasalazine in the treatment of active ulcerative colitis: A randomized trial. Br Med J. 1989;298:82–86.

38. Alters SE, Sakai K, Steinman L, Oi VT. Mechanisms of anti-CD4-mediated depletion and immunotherapy. A study using a set of chimeric anti-CD4 antibodies. J Immunol. 1990;144:4587–4592.

39. Siegling A, Lehmann M, Riedel H et al. A non-depleting anti-rat CD4 monoclonal antibody that suppresses T helper 1-like but not T helper 2-like intragraft lymphokine secretion induces long-term survival of renal allografts. Transplantation. 1994;57:464–466.
40. Lehmann M, Sternkopf F, Metz F et al. Induction of long-term survival of rat skin allografts by a novel, highly efficient anti-CD4 monoclonal antibody. Transplantation. 1992;54:959–962.
41. Bröker BM, Tsygankov AY, Fickenscher H et al. Engagement of the CD4 receptor inhibits the interleukin-2-dependent proliferation of human T cells transformed by herpes virus saimiri. Eur J Immunol. 1994;24:843–850.
42. Stumbles P, Mason D. Activation of CD4+ T cells in the presence of a nondepleting monoclonal antibody to CD4 induces a Th2-type response in vitro. J Exp Med. 1995;182:5–13.

Index

Falk Symposium Series

43. Reutter W, Popper H, Arias IM, Heinrich PC, Keppler D, Landmann L, eds.: *Modulation of Liver Cell Expression*. Falk Symposium No. 43. 1987   ISBN: 0-85200-677-2*

44. Boyer JL, Bianchi L, eds.: *Liver Cirrhosis*. Falk Symposium No. 44. 1987   ISBN: 0-85200-993-3*

45. Paumgartner G, Stiehl A, Gerok W, eds.: *Bile Acids and the Liver*. Falk Symposium No. 45. 1987   ISBN: 0-85200-675-6*

46. Goebell H, Peskar BM, Malchow H, eds.: *Inflammatory Bowel Diseases – Basic Research & Clinical Implications*. Falk Symposium No. 46. 1988   ISBN: 0-7462-0067-6*

47. Bianchi L, Holt P, James OFW, Butler RN, eds.: *Aging in Liver and Gastrointestinal Tract*. Falk Symposium No. 47. 1988   ISBN: 0-7462-0066-8*

48. Heilmann C, ed.: *Calcium-Dependent Processes in the Liver*. Falk Symposium No. 48. 1988   ISBN: 0-7462-0075-7*

50. Singer MV, Goebell H, eds.: *Nerves and the Gastrointestinal Tract*. Falk Symposium No. 50. 1989   ISBN: 0-7462-0114-1

51. Bannasch P, Keppler D, Weber G, eds.: *Liver Cell Carcinoma*. Falk Symposium No. 51. 1989   ISBN: 0-7462-0111-7

52. Paumgartner G, Stiehl A, Gerok W, eds.: *Trends in Bile Acid Research*. Falk Symposium No. 52. 1989   ISBN: 0-7462-0112-5

53. Paumgartner G, Stiehl A, Barbara L, Roda E, eds.: *Strategies for the Treatment of Hepatobiliary Diseases*. Falk Symposium No. 53. 1990   ISBN: 0-7923-8903-4

54. Bianchi L, Gerok W, Maier K-P, Deinhardt F, eds.: *Infectious Diseases of the Liver*. Falk Symposium No. 54. 1990   ISBN: 0-7923-8902-6

55. Falk Symposium No. 55 not published

55B. Hadziselimovic F, Herzog B, Bürgin-Wolff A, eds.: *Inflammatory Bowel Disease and Coeliac Disease in Children*. International Falk Symposium. 1990 ISBN 0-7462-0125-7

56. Williams CN, eds.: *Trends in Inflammatory Bowel Disease Therapy*. Falk Symposium No. 56. 1990   ISBN: 0-7923-8952-2

57. Bock KW, Gerok W, Matern S, Schmid R, eds.: *Hepatic Metabolism and Disposition of Endo- and Xenobiotics*. Falk Symposium No. 57. 1991   ISBN: 0-7923-8953-0

58. Paumgartner G, Stiehl A, Gerok W, eds.: *Bile Acids as Therapeutic Agents: From Basic Science to Clinical Practice*. Falk Symposium No. 58. 1991   ISBN: 0-7923-8954-9

59. Halter F, Garner A, Tytgat GNJ, eds.: *Mechanisms of Peptic Ulcer Healing*. Falk Symposium No. 59. 1991   ISBN: 0-7923-8955-7

60. Goebell H, Ewe K, Malchow H, Koelbel Ch, eds.: *Inflammatory Bowel Diseases – Progress in Basic Research and Clinical Implications*. Falk Symposium No. 60. 1991   ISBN: 0-7923-8956-5

61. Falk Symposium No. 61 not published

62. Dowling RH, Folsch UR, Löser Ch, eds.: *Polyamines in the Gastrointestinal Tract*. Falk Symposium No. 62. 1992   ISBN: 0-7923-8976-X

63. Lentze MJ, Reichen J, eds.: *Paediatric Cholestasis: Novel Approaches to Treatment*. Falk Symposium No. 63. 1992   ISBN: 0-7923-8977-8

64. Demling L, Frühmorgen P, eds.: *Non-Neoplastic Diseases of the Anorectum*. Falk Symposium No. 64. 1992   ISBN: 0-7923-8979-4

64B. Gressner AM, Ramadori G, eds.: *Molecular and Cell Biology of Liver Fibrogenesis*. International Falk Symposium. 1992   ISBN: 0-7923-8980-8

*These titles were published under the MTP Press imprint.

Falk Symposium Series

65. Hadziselimovic F, Herzog B, eds.: *Inflammatory Bowel Diseases and Morbus Hirschprung*. Falk Symposium No. 65. 1992   ISBN: 0-7923-8995-6

66. Martin F, McLeod RS, Sutherland LR, Williams CN, eds.: *Trends in Inflammatory Bowel Disease Therapy*. Falk Symposium No. 66. 1993   ISBN: 0-7923-8827-5

67. Schölmerich J, Kruis W, Goebell H, Hohenberger W, Gross V, eds.: *Inflammatory Bowel Diseases – Pathophysiology as Basis of Treatment*. Falk Symposium No. 67. 1993   ISBN: 0-7923-8996-4

68. Paumgartner G, Stiehl A, Gerok W, eds.: *Bile Acids and The Hepatobiliary System: From Basic Science to Clinical Practice*. Falk Symposium No. 68. 1993   ISBN: 0-7923-8829-1

69. Schmid R, Bianchi L, Gerok W, Maier K-P, eds.: *Extrahepatic Manifestations in Liver Diseases*. Falk Symposium No. 69. 1993   ISBN: 0-7923-8821-6

70. Meyer zum Büschenfelde K-H, Hoofnagle J, Manns M, eds.: *Immunology and Liver*. Falk Symposium No. 70. 1993   ISBN: 0-7923-8830-5

71. Surrenti C, Casini A, Milani S, Pinzani M , eds.: *Fat-Storing Cells and Liver Fibrosis*. Falk Symposium No. 71. 1994   ISBN: 0-7923-8842-9

72. Rachmilewitz D, ed.: *Inflammatory Bowel Diseases – 1994*. Falk Symposium No. 72. 1994   ISBN: 0-7923-8845-3

73. Binder HJ, Cummings J, Soergel KH, eds.: *Short Chain Fatty Acids*. Falk Symposium No. 73. 1994   ISBN: 0-7923-8849-6

73B. Möllmann HW, May B, eds.: *Glucocorticoid Therapy in Chronic Inflammatory Bowel Disease: from basic principles to rational therapy*. International Falk Workshop. 1996   ISBN 0-7923-8708-2

74. Keppler D, Jungermann K, eds.: *Transport in the Liver*. Falk Symposium No. 74. 1994   ISBN: 0-7923-8858-5

74B. Stange EF, ed.: *Chronic Inflammatory Bowel Disease*. Falk Symposium. 1995   ISBN: 0-7923-8876-3

75. van Berge Henegouwen GP, van Hoek B, De Groote J, Matern S, Stockbrügger RW, eds.: *Cholestatic Liver Diseases: New Strategies for Prevention and Treatment of Hepatobiliary and Cholestatic Liver Diseases*. Falk Symposium 75. 1994.   ISBN: 0-7923-8867-4

76. Monteiro E, Tavarela Veloso F, eds.: *Inflammatory Bowel Diseases: New Insights into Mechanisms of Inflammation and Challenges in Diagnosis and Treatment*. Falk Symposium 76. 1995.   ISBN 0-7923-8884-4

77. Singer MV, Ziegler R, Rohr G, eds.: *Gastrointestinal Tract and Endocrine System*. Falk Symposium 77. 1995.   ISBN 0-7923-8877-1

78. Decker K, Gerok W, Andus T, Gross V, eds.: *Cytokines and the Liver*. Falk Symposium 78. 1995.   ISBN 0-7923-8878-X

79. Holstege A, Schölmerich J, Hahn EG, eds.: *Portal Hypertension*. Falk Symposium 79. 1995.   ISBN 0-7923-8879-8

80. Hofmann AF, Paumgartner G, Stiehl A, eds.: *Bile Acids in Gastroenterology: Basic and Clinical Aspects*. Falk Symposium 80. 1995   ISBN 0-7923-8880-1

81. Riecken EO, Stallmach A, Zeitz M, Heise W, eds.: *Malignancy and Chronic Inflammation in the Gastrointestinal Tract – New Concepts*. Falk Symposium 81. 1995   ISBN 0-7923-8889-5

82. Fleig WE, ed.: *Inflammatory Bowel Diseases: New Developments and Standards*. Falk Symposium 82. 1995   ISBN 0-7923-8890-6

Falk Symposium Series

99. Goebell H, Holtmann G, Talley NJ, eds. *Functional Dyspepsia and Irritable Bowel Syndrome: Concepts and Controversies.* Falk Symposium 99. 1998
ISBN 0-7923-8735-X

100. Blum HE, Bode Ch, Bode JCh, Sartor RB, eds. *Gut and the Liver.* Falk Symposium 100. 1998
ISBN 0-7923-8736-8

101. Rachmilewitz D, ed. *V International Symposium on Inflammatory Bowel Diseases.* Falk Symposium 101. 1998
ISBN 0-7923-8743-0

102. Manns MP, Boyer JL, Jansen PLM, Reichen J, eds. *Cholestatic Liver Diseases.* Falk Symposium 102. 1998
ISBN 0-7923-8746-5

102B. Manns MP, Chapman RW, Stiehl A, Wiesner R, eds. *Primary Sclerosing Cholangitis.* International Falk Workshop. 1998.
ISBN 0-7923-8745-7

103. Häussinger D, Jungermann K, eds. *Liver and Nervous System.* Falk Symposium 102. 1998
ISBN 0-7924-8742-2

103B. Häussinger D, Heinrich PC, eds. *Signalling in the Liver.* International Falk Workshop. 1998
ISBN 0-7923-8744-9

103C. Fleig W, ed. *Normal and Malignant Liver Cell Growth.* International Falk Workshop. 1998
ISBN 0-7923-8748-1

104. Stallmach A, Zeitz M, Strober W, MacDonald TT, Lochs H, eds. *Induction and Modulation of Gastrointestinal Inflammation.* Falk Symposium 104. 1998
ISBN 0-7923-8747-3